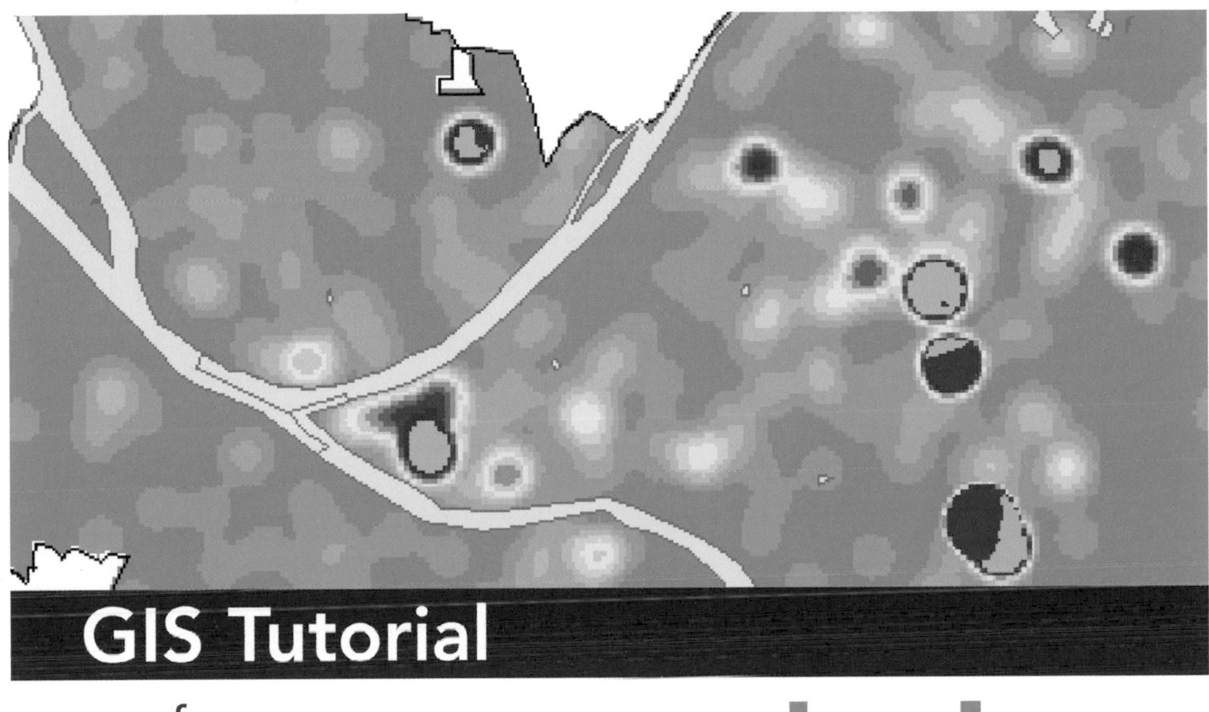

GIS Tutorial for Health

Fifth Edition

Kristen S. Kurland
Wilpen L. Gorr

Esri Press
REDLANDS | CALIFORNIA

Cover map designed by Kristen Kurland; cover photograph courtesy of Nattika/Shutterstock.

Esri Press, 380 New York Street, Redlands, California 92373-8100

Printed in the United States of America

19 18 17 16 15   2 3 4 5 6 7 8 9 10

Ask for Esri Press titles at your local bookstore or order by calling 800-447-9778, or shop online at esri.com/esripress. Outside the United States, contact your local Esri distributor or shop online at eurospanbookstore.com/esri.

Esri Press titles are distributed to the trade by the following:

In North America:
Ingram Publisher Services
Toll-free telephone: 800-648-3104
Toll-free fax: 800-838-1149
E-mail: customerservice@ingrampublisherservices.com

In the United Kingdom, Europe, Middle East and Africa, Asia, and Australia:
Eurospan Group
3 Henrietta Street
London WC2E 8LU
United Kingdom
Telephone: 44(0) 1767 604972
Fax: 44(0) 1767 601640
E-mail: eurospan@turpin-distribution.com

Contents

Part 2: Preparation of map data

Part 4: GIS case studies

Preface

GIS Tutorial for Health is a unique textbook for teaching geographic information systems (GIS) to health professionals, medical residents, nursing students, and students interested in health IT and informatics, health-care administration, and health policy. It embeds lessons on GIS software in health-care scenarios to solve real-world problems. The book provides students many opportunities to visualize and analyze health-related data. Its health-care scenarios address substantive issues of health care, decision support requirements for policy and planning, and technical requirements of spatial data sources and processing.

This fifth edition of *GIS Tutorial for Health* includes improvements and updates to tutorials and assignments using ArcGIS 10.2 for Desktop, as well as an introduction to ArcGIS Online. It also features downloading international health data as well as downloading raster maps from the US Geological Survey.

The book has four parts. Part 1, "GIS benefits and map basics," is essential for all beginning students. Part 2, "Preparation of map data," and part 3, "Spatial analysis," are largely independent of each other, and you can use these chapters in the order that best fits your needs. The fourth part, "GIS case studies," contains two chapters that each present a relevant case study for you to work through on your own. Each case study has a series of requirements, input datasets, instructions on the structure required for GIS analysis, and maps and reports for you to produce.

Chapters 1–9 use tutorials and assignments to explore health-care issues, while chapters 10 and 11 involve independent case studies. Chapters 1–9 use the following structure:

- Each chapter begins with a health issue or problem in a health-care scenario that has a spatial component. Learning a new tool or software package works best in the context of work that is interesting to you. So, we begin by stating a health issue or problem that can be better understood or solved by using GIS and, by extension, ArcGIS software.
- Each chapter follows with a conceptual section that details the solution approach. General knowledge is often needed to understand specific steps and workflows using GIS. This section provides knowledge and principles on underlying GIS methods. Whenever possible, we have separated this material into brief descriptions preceding chapter tutorials. As a result, you can read this material before sitting down at a computer to work with ArcGIS.
- Each chapter includes a series of tutorials to carry out the solution using ArcGIS. Each tutorial contains step-by-step exercises and corresponding screen captures as well as user dialog boxes and resulting outputs. The steps follow workflows that you can use in a variety of projects. "Your Turn"

exercises interspersed throughout the tutorials are designed to reinforce the lessons you learn. These exercises can help you internalize ArcGIS steps and workflows.

- Each chapter ends with hands-on assignments that require independent thinking to apply the knowledge and skills gained from the tutorials. By working through these assignments, you will make ArcGIS part of your routine and a reliable tool for analysis of health care and other issues.

The target audience for the book includes health management students and practitioners, computer specialists who want to work in the health field, and health-care managers and researchers who want to gain proficiency in GIS. This book serves primarily as a computer-lab textbook, but it can also be used for self-study. The beginning chapters of *GIS Tutorial for Health* can be used for short, two- to three-day courses.

If you are new to ArcGIS for Desktop and are using the book as a self-study guide, we recommend you work through the chapters in sequence. However, because the chapters are largely independent of each other, you can use them in the order that best fits your needs.

Data for the book is available to download on the Esri Press "Book Resources" webpage, esripress.esri.com/bookresources. Click the appropriate book title, and then click the data link under "Resources" to download the exercise data. A 60-day trial of ArcGIS for Desktop software and extensions is available for readers at esri.com/trydesktop. You will need the exercise data and access to ArcGIS 10.2 for Desktop to perform the exercises in this book. Access to Microsoft Word, Excel, and PowerPoint, and an Internet connection are also necessary for some tutorials.

For more information about this book, including how to obtain instructor resources, please go to esri.com/esripress.

After teaching GIS for over 20 years, we know that you—like our own students—will enjoy this subject and software. Go to it!

Acknowledgments

We would like to thank all who made this book possible.

GIS Tutorial for Health was used by students at Carnegie Mellon University before it went to Esri Press for publication. The students and teaching assistants who used the book provided us with significant feedback. Their thoughtful comments guided our revisions and helped improve the content and overall quality of this book.

We are very grateful to the many individuals, organizations, and vendors who have generously supplied us with interesting GIS cases and data. These include Dr. Bruce Dixon, Gerald Barron, Jo Ann Glad, Dr. LuAnn Brink, Glenda Christy, Dan Cinpinski, Mike Diskin, Bruce Good, Dave Namey, and Thom Stulginski of the Allegheny County Health Department; Ross Capaccio of röös design + consulting, and Thom D. Freyer, CAE of the American College of Healthcare Executives, for the datasets used in the Partners for Success chapter deployment project; Carl Kinkade of the Centers for Disease Control and Prevention (CDC); Noel S. Zuckerbraun, MD, MPH, assistant professor of pediatrics, Department of Pediatrics, Division of Pediatric Emergency Medicine, Children's Hospital of Pittsburgh, University of Pittsburgh School of Medicine; Barbara A. Gaines, MD, director, Benedum Trauma Program, assistant professor of surgery, Children's Hospital of Pittsburgh, University of Pittsburgh School of Medicine; Noor Ismail, Mike Homa, and Lena Andrews of the City of Pittsburgh, Department of City Planning; the Trustees of Dartmouth College, the Dartmouth Atlas of Health Care; Linda Williams Pickle, PhD, and David Stinchcomb of the National Cancer Institute, Cancer Mortality Maps website; Chris Chalmers, GIS coordinator, Nebraska Health and Human Services, Bioterrorism Response Section director for GIS Public Health Research, University of Nebraska-Lincoln, CALMIT; Maurie Kelly of Pennsylvania Spatial Data Access (PASDA); Clara Burgert and Blake Zachary, IFC Marco, funding provided by US President's Emergency Plan for AIDS Relief (PEPFAR) through the MEASURE DHS project; Nathan Heard, US Department of State; US Geological Survey and US Census Bureau; and Tele Atlas for use of its USA datasets contained within the Esri Data & Maps 2004 Media Kit.

Finally, thanks to the entire team at Esri and Esri Press.

Part 1

GIS benefits and map basics

Chapter 1

Introducing GIS and health applications

Objectives

- Define GIS
- Define spatial data for graphic and image map layers
- Review the national infrastructure for spatial data
- Review the unique capabilities of GIS
- Demonstrate how GIS can be used for health applications
- Introduce ArcGIS and its user interface
- Introduce online GIS tools

Geographic information systems (GIS) is a technology that has unique and valuable applications for policy makers, planners, and managers in many fields, including public health and health care. GIS health applications include an academic organization's use of GIS for medical research, a hospital or managed-care organization's improved delivery of health-care services, and a public health department's use of mapping and spatial statistics for disease surveillance and analysis. GIS software and applications allow visualization and processing of data in ways that were not possible in the past. The purpose of this book is to provide hands-on experience with the use of ArcGIS for Desktop software in the context of health applications. You need no previous experience using GIS.

This chapter describes GIS and its inputs and special capabilities and follows with a discussion of health issues and GIS applications. We also preview the upcoming tutorials in this book, and then use short tutorials in this chapter to introduce you to the use of ArcGIS software.

What is GIS?

GIS is computer technology that engages geographers, computer scientists, social scientists, planners, engineers, and others in spatially analyzing issues. Consequently, it has been defined from several different perspectives (see Clarke 2003). We prefer a definition that emphasizes GIS as an information system:

GIS is a system for input, storage, processing, and retrieval of spatial data. Except for the additional word "spatial," this is a standard definition of an information system. Spatial components include a digital map infrastructure, GIS software with unique functionality that focuses on location, and new mapping applications for organizations of all kinds. Definitions of these distinctive aspects of GIS follow.

Spatial data

Spatial data includes the locations and shapes of geographic features, in the form of either vector or raster data. Vector maps have features drawn using points, lines, and polygons to represent discrete geographic objects such as automobile accident locations, streets, and counties. (A polygon is a closed area that has a boundary consisting of connected straight lines.) Raster maps are generally aerial photographs, satellite images, or representations of surfaces such as elevation, which are used to represent continuous geographies.

For example, figure 1.1 is a vector map that has three polygon map layers (state and county boundaries and lakes), a line layer of rivers, and a point layer of cities that have populations of 250,000 or more. The state and county boundaries are coterminous—that is, they share boundaries and do not overlap each other. Color fill is used within the county polygons to show the mortality of lung cancer for white males. This map has some striking geographic patterns that are discussed later in this chapter.

Associated with individual point, line, or polygon features are data records that provide identifying and descriptive data attributes. For example, in figure 1.1, the

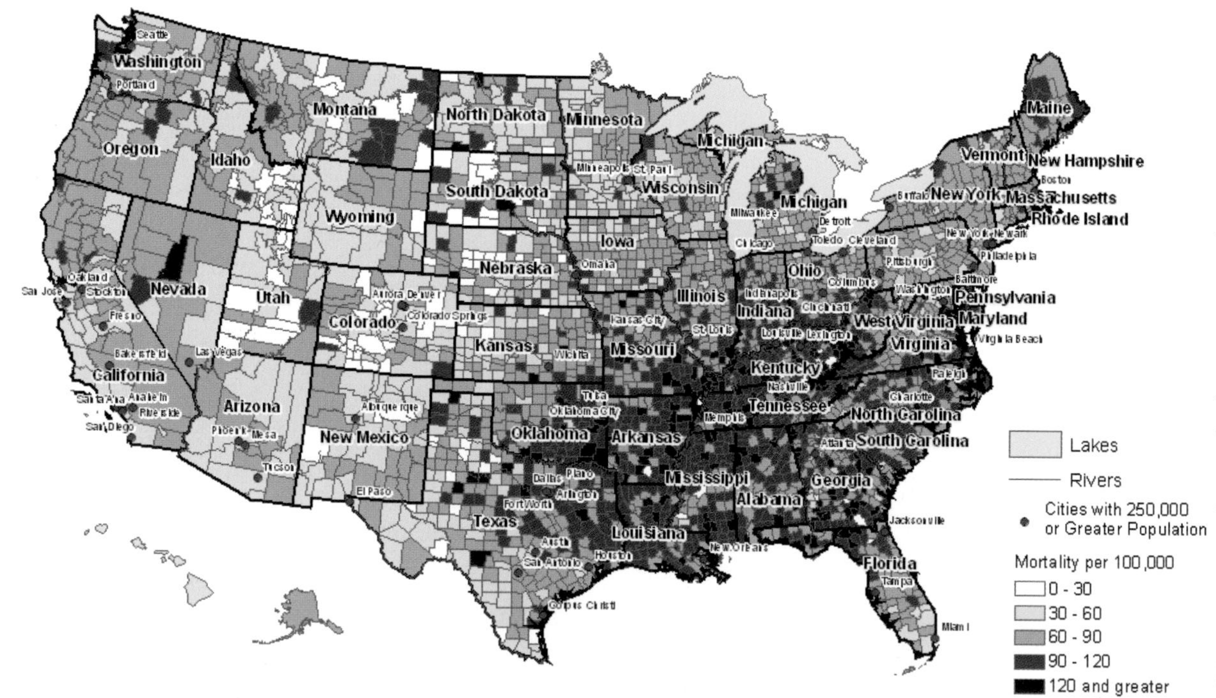

Figure 1.1 Lung cancer mortality per 100,000 white males, 2000–2004.

Sources: (a) Esri Data & Maps; (b) Cancer Mortality Maps website, National Cancer Institute.

labels for the names of states and cities come from tables of attribute records associated with each map layer. You will revisit this map in tutorials 1-3 and 1-4 in this chapter where you will use ArcGIS to explore map layers and spatial patterns of cancer mortality.

Raster maps are stored in standard digital image formats, such as tagged image file format (TIFF) and Joint Photographic Experts Group (JPEG) files. An image file is a rectangular array, or raster, of very small, square pixels. Each pixel, or cell, has a single value and solid color and corresponds to a small, square area on the ground, from 6 in. to 3 ft on a side for high-resolution images. Accompanying the image files are world files that provide georeferencing data, including the upper-left pixel's location coordinates and the width of each pixel in ground units. Using world file information, GIS software can assemble individual raster datasets into larger areas and overlay them with aligned vector datasets.

Viewed on a computer screen or on a paper map, a raster map can provide a detailed backdrop of physical features. In figure 1.2, an aerial photograph overlaid with vector map layers shows locations where serious injuries of child pedestrians occurred in relation to public parks that have playgrounds. The two boundaries surrounding the parks are 600 ft and 1,200 ft buffers used to study injury rates near parks. You will explore the GIS data behind this map in depth in

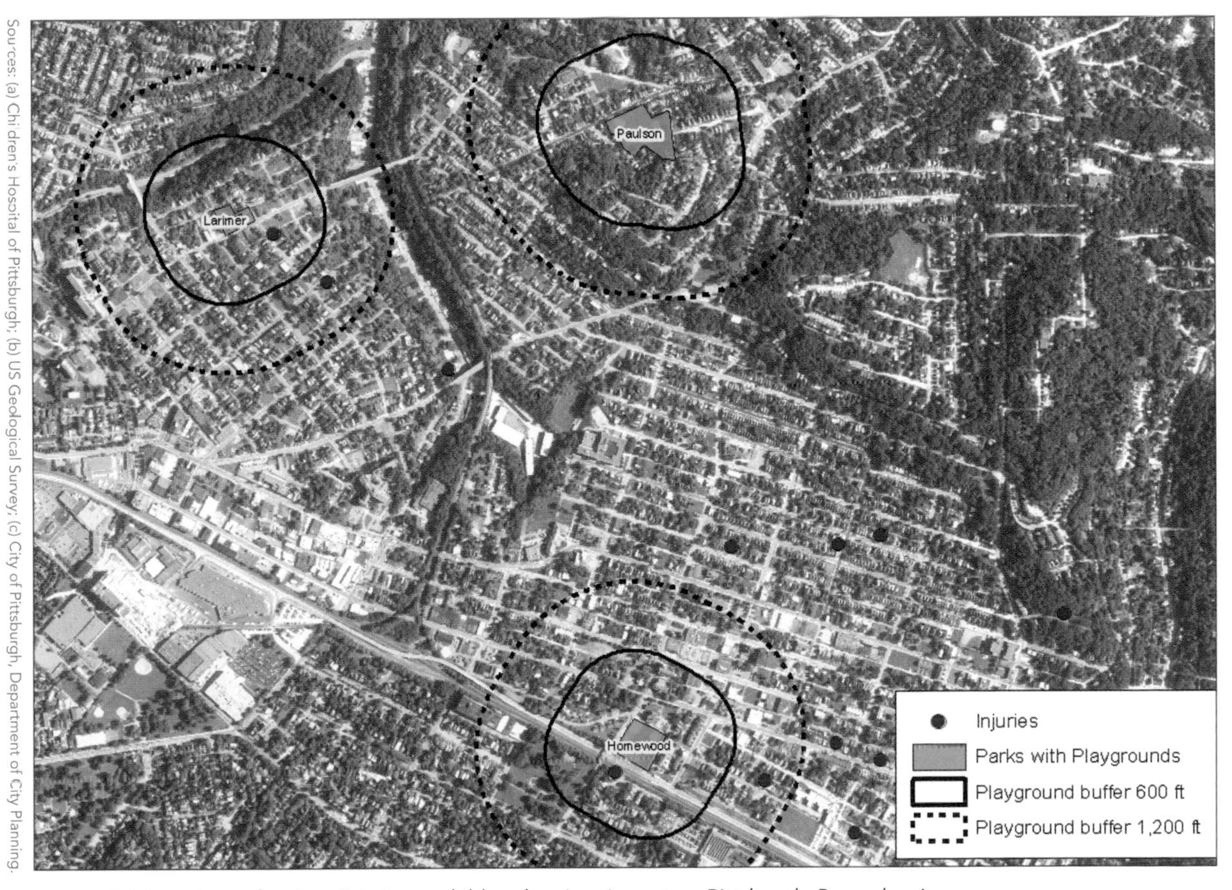

Sources: (a) Children's Hosital of Pittsburgh; (b) US Geological Survey; (c) City of Pittsburgh, Department of City Planning.

Figure 1.2 Locations of serious injuries to child pedestrians in eastern Pittsburgh, Pennsylvania.

chapters 4 and 7, where you will download similar orthoimagery and create and use buffers similar to those in figure 1.2.

Map layers have geographic coordinates, projections, and scale. Geographic coordinates for the nearly spherical world are measured in polar coordinates, and the angles of rotation are measured in degrees, minutes, and seconds, or decimal degrees. The (0,0) origin of the coordinate system is generally taken as the intersection of the equator and the prime meridian (great circle), which passes through the poles and an observatory in Greenwich, England. Latitude is measured north and south for up to 90 degrees in each direction. Longitude is measured to the east and west of the origin for up to 180 degrees in each direction.

The world is not quite a sphere because the poles are slightly flattened and the equator is slightly bulged out. The world's surface is better modeled by a spheroid, which has elliptical cross sections and two radii, instead of the one radius of a sphere. The mathematical representation of the world as a spheroid is called a datum; for example, a datum commonly used for North America is North American Datum of 1983 (NAD 1983). If you use the same projection but two different datums for your maps, each corresponding map will have small but noticeable differences in location.

A point, line, or polygon feature on the surface of the world is on a three-dimensional spheroid, whereas features on a paper map or computer screen are on a flat surface. The mathematical transformation of a world feature into a flat map is called a projection. There are many projections, some of which you will use in chapter 4. Each projection has its own rectangular coordinate system and a (0,0) origin conveniently located so that coordinates are positive and have distance units, usually in feet or meters.

All projections necessarily cause distortion of direction, shape, area, or length in some combination. So-called conformal projections preserve shape at the expense of distorting area. Some examples are the Mercator cylindrical and Lambert conic projections. Equal-area projections are the opposite of conformal projections: They preserve area while distorting shape. An example is the Albers equal-area projection (Clarke 2003, 42–44).

Map scale is often stated as a unitless, representative fraction; for example, 1:24,000 is a map scale where 1 in. on the map represents 24,000 in. on the ground, and any distance units can be substituted for inches. Small-scale maps have a vantage point far above the earth and large-scale maps are zoomed in on relatively small areas. Distortions are considerable for small-scale maps but negligible for large-scale maps relative to policy, planning, and research applications.

GIS maps are composites of overlying map layers. For large-scale maps such as figure 1.2, the bottom layer can be a raster map that has one or more vector layers on top, placed in order so that smaller or more important features are on top and not covered up by larger contextual features. Small-scale maps, such as figure 1.1, often consist solely of vector-map layers. Each vector layer consists of a homogeneous type of feature—points, lines, or polygons.

Digital map infrastructure

GIS is perhaps the only information technology that requires a major digital infrastructure. The map layers of the infrastructure are referred to as basemaps—namely, a collection of standards, codes, and data designed, built, and maintained by government. Vendors provide valuable enhancements to the digital map infrastructure, but for the most part, it is a public good financed by tax dollars. Without this infrastructure, GIS would not be a viable technology.

The National Spatial Data Infrastructure (NSDI), developed by the Federal Geographic Data Committee (FGDC at http://www.fgdc.gov), incorporates policies, standards, and procedures that allow organizations to produce and share geographic data. The Geospatial One-Stop website (http://geo.data.gov/geoportal), which is part of the NSDI, provides access to spatial data. Websites change often. The websites noted in this book could be named differently or redirected to different sites, but the information will still be available if you search for it. GIS provides a way to use this wealth of publicly available data in your own studies.

Perhaps the most useful spatial data for health applications comes from the US Census Bureau in the form of TIGER/Line maps. These maps are available by state and county for many classes of layers. These classes, and examples of each, include the following:

- *Political:* states, counties, county subdivisions (towns and cities), and voting districts
- *Statistical:* census tracts, block groups, and blocks
- *Administrative:* ZIP Codes and school districts
- *Physical:* highways, streets, rivers, streams, lakes, and railroads

You can download TIGER/Line map layers in GIS-ready formats at no cost from the US Census Bureau website (http://www.census.gov). Steps for doing so are included in chapter 5.

Census data that corresponds to TIGER/Line maps of statistical boundaries is tabulated by census-area codes and American National Standards Institute (ANSI) codes (http://www.census.gov/georeference/ansi.html). ANSI codes are "a standardized set of numeric or alphabetic codes issued by the American National Standards Institute (ANSI) to ensure uniform identification of geographic entities through all federal government agencies," according to the ANSI website. Data from the decennial census is available at no cost from the Census Bureau. Steps for downloading census data and preparing it for GIS use with TIGER/Line maps are included in chapter 5.

The US Geological Survey (http://www.usgs.gov/aboutusgs/) is the "nation's largest water, earth, and biological science and civilian mapping agency . . . [and it] collects, monitors, analyzes, and provides scientific understanding about natural resource conditions, issues, and problems," according to the USGS website. Among its products that are useful for health applications are national map orthoimagery aerial photographs (such as the one used in figure 1.2). Full national coverage of the most recent national map orthoimagery is available from USGS via The National Map at http://viewer.nationalmap.gov/viewer/. Steps for downloading USGS maps are included in chapter 4.

Local governments provide many of the large-scale map layers in the United States, and most features in this data are smaller than a city block. This data includes deeded land parcels and corresponding real property data files on land parcels, structures, owners, building roof footprints, and pavement digitized from aerial photographs. You can often obtain such map layers and data for nominal prices from local governments. Some local health departments provide limited health data.

Unique capabilities of GIS

Maps were historically made for reference purposes. Street maps, atlases, and USGS topographic maps are all reference maps. It wasn't until the advent of GIS, however, that analytic mapping became widely possible. For analytic mapping, an analyst collects and compiles related map layers, builds a database, and then uses GIS functionality to provide information for understanding or solving a problem. Before GIS, analytic mapping was limited to organizations such as city planning departments. Analysts did not have digital map layers, so they made hard-copy drawings on acetate sheets that could be overlaid and switched in and out to show before-and-after maps for a new facility such as a baseball stadium or a hospital. Using GIS, however, anyone can easily add, subtract, turn on and off, and modify map layers in an analytic map composition. This capacity has led to a revolution in geography and an entirely new tool for organizations of all kinds.

As figures 1.1 and 1.2 show, maps use symbols, which are defined in map legends. Graphical elements of symbols include fill color, pattern, and boundaries for polygons; width, color, and type (solid, dashed, curved) for lines; and shape, color, and outline for points. A GIS analyst does not individually apply symbols to features, but applies and renders a layer at a time based on attribute values associated with geographic features.

For example, given a code attribute for schools that has the values "public," "private," and "parochial," a GIS analyst can choose a green, circular, 10-point marker for public schools; a blue, square, 8-point marker for private schools; and an orange, triangular, 8-point marker for parochial schools. These three steps render all schools in a map layer by the desired point markers.

Similarly, we created the color-shaded county map layer in figure 1.1 based on an attribute that provides the lung cancer mortality rate of white males by county. A map that uses fill color in polygons for coding is called a choropleth map. In this case, it shows an equal-interval numeric scale, rendered using a gray monochromatic color scale. The darker the shade of gray, the higher the interval of the numeric scale. By making selections and setting parameters, the GIS analyst accomplishes all this coding and rendering using a simple graphic user interface (GUI).

Most organizations generate or collect data that includes street addresses, ZIP Codes, or other georeferences. GIS is able to spatially enable this data—that is, add geographic coordinates or make data records joinable to boundary maps.

Geocoding, also known as address matching, uses street addresses as input and assigns point coordinates to address records on or adjacent to street centerlines, such as in the TIGER/Line street maps. Geocoding uses a sophisticated program that has built-in intelligence—similar to that of a postal delivery person delivering your mail—that can interpret misspellings, variations in abbreviations, and rearrangement of certain address components.

Policy, planning, and research activities often require data aggregated over space and time, rather than individual points. For example, in a study of demand patterns for locating a satellite medical clinic, it may be desirable to aggregate patient residence data to counts per census tract or ZIP Code boundaries for a recent year. GIS has the unique capacity to determine the areas in which points lie, using a spatial join or overlay function that allows the analyst to count points or summarize their attributes by area, using sums or averages.

This leads to the last GIS capability to be described in this section, proximity analysis. As an example, we conducted a study to determine whether the decline in the use of senior centers was affected by the distance from the seniors' residences (Johnson et al. 2005). We geocoded the senior centers that provided human services and where the senior citizens lived, placing them as points on a map, and included the total target population using census data by city block. Then we used ArcGIS to create buffers around the facilities using a radius of 0.5 mi, 1 mi, 1.5 mi, 2 mi, and so on. We used spatial joins to assign buffer identifiers to residence points and blocks, count clients by buffer area, and sum up the population by block group.

Next, through careful subtraction of counts and sums, we were able to get the total number of clients and the target population in each ring around facilities (such as 0.5 mi, 1 mi, 1.5 mi), calculate use rates for each ring by dividing the count of clients by the sum of the target population, and plot the relationship of use rate versus mean distance of each ring from facilities. We found that the use rate by clients, who were elderly users of the senior center facilities in our county, declined rapidly with distance, presumably because of the seniors' mobility limitations. The policy implication is that senior centers need to be located in areas that have high densities of elderly populations so that more of the elderly will be able to use them. You will conduct similar buffer analyses in chapters 7, 9, and 10 in a variety of health contexts.

Summary of chapters

Following is a brief summary of chapters. Chapters 1–9 include tutorials for learning GIS and chapters 10 and 11 are optional case studies that reinforce the skills learned in the previous chapters.

Chapter 1: Introducing GIS and health applications

Health care is a large, growing, and complex sector of economies around the world. The United States, like other countries, faces many challenges in providing the best health care for its citizens and at the lowest possible cost. Currently, many health informatics systems are manual and/or nonintegrated (*The Economist* 2005) in that interacting organizations have in-house information systems that are not connected to each other in ways that would allow beneficial sharing of data. This has led to top-heavy administrations, high costs of transactions (Hagland 2004), medical errors, and duplication of efforts, such as unnecessary medical tests (Protti 2005). Additional health policy issues can arise from too much emphasis on the treatment of sickness and not enough on the prevention of illness (Kennedy 2004), enormous numbers of uninsured persons, the overuse of emergency rooms, nursing shortages, and the lack of preparedness for bioterrorism (Featherly 2004).

One clear trend in health policy, research, planning, and management is the increasingly important role of health informatics. More systems will become automated and integrated, at a large cost but with even larger benefits. What does this mean for GIS applications? One consequence is that there will be even more data available for possible input to GIS—additional data on patients, facilities, programs, and events that include disease incidence, medical diagnostics, and treatments. Much of the additional data will have street addresses, ZIP Codes, or other location elements that will make it applicable to GIS processing.

In addition to ArcGIS for Desktop, there are online and mobile applications that allow you to view, download, and share basemaps. ArcGIS.com map viewer is a free web application that allows sharing and searching of geographic information, as well as content published by Esri, ArcGIS users, and other authoritative data providers. ArcGIS.com map viewer allows users to create and join groups and to control access to items shared publicly or within groups. For those wanting to explore using GIS on mobile devices, ArcGIS for iOS is a free application that runs on an iOS device such as iPad or iPhone. You can download this free application to your iOS device to view web maps created in ArcGIS Online and perform simple GIS functions such as measuring distances and areas.

In this chapter, you begin to explore the online sites by creating layer packages in ArcMap, one of the primary components of ArcGIS for Desktop, to upload to ArcGIS.com as well as explore health content already available on this website.

The book overall contains a sampling of health GIS applications that cut a wide path across the landscape we have just described.

Chapter 2: Visualizing health data

Chapter 2 uses a simple public health application for visualizing breast cancer mortality rates at the state and county levels across the United States. In the tutorials, you work with breast cancer data. While valuable for providing a snapshot of cancer mortality, the primary purpose of the application is to get you comfortable with map navigation in ArcGIS. ArcGIS provides many ways to change scales and views of a map in search of information, as well as ways to work with the data records behind the map features. You will get experience with some of them in this chapter.

Chapter 3: Designing maps for a health study

In chapter 3, you learn about uninsured populations in a state and their health-care financial needs. In the tutorials, you analyze where to locate programs that provide health-related financial support for uninsured populations in Texas counties. You use an advanced map with a bivariate analysis to contrast the magnitude of uninsured populations with measures of poverty by county.

GIS can provide many kinds of outputs. In this chapter, you build stand-alone map layouts that contain components such as multiple map frames, legends, and scale bars for use in presentations and reports.

Chapter 4: Projecting, downloading, and using spatial data

What are the most appropriate ways to map disease incidence (numbers of cases) versus prevalence (numbers of cases per population of 10,000)? In the first health application in chapter 4, you visualize a communicable disease—HIV infection and AIDS. You build two kinds of map layers to encode data: one for disease incidence based on polygon centroids (points) using size-graduated point markers and the other for disease prevalence represented by the fill color for polygons.

A second application teaches you how to download international HIV/AIDS data from a website for a selected country.

A third application uses local data to pursue the problem of child obesity. Your objective in these tutorials is to identify green spaces in the vicinity of schools that could possibly be used in physical education programs. You will also learn how to download aerial images from USGS.

GIS issues pursued in these applications involve downloading and importing spatial data into ArcGIS and projecting map layers based on the application and geographic scale at hand.

Chapter 5: Downloading and preparing spatial and tabular data

Where are the concentrations of a city's older houses that are likely to have lead-based paint? Do children who have elevated levels of lead in their blood live in those areas? The purpose of the study in chapter 5 is to identify clusters of children who have elevated blood lead levels for the targeting of lead-screening programs. You work with elevated blood lead level samples that have been aggregated to census tracts and census tract data on housing built before 1970, when lead-based paints were still used.

In chapter 5, you download and prepare US Census data. You must clean up the data by renaming variables and deleting rows that do not conform to data table formats and by modifying census tract identifiers in the table so that they match comparable identifiers in the census tract map layer. Then you join them to a downloaded census tract boundary map. Ultimately, you will produce a very nice bivariate map using choropleth and dot-density displays. In that map, you will place randomly located points within polygons in proportion to an attribute of interest. The tutorials in chapter 5 seek additional explanation of observed clusters by using additional census variables to spatially explore a public health problem.

Chapter 6: Geocoding tabular data

General spatial information is available from basemaps, but how do you format the data your organization has so it can be converted to points on a map? Data of interest often includes point locations of patients' or clients' residences and health care or other service delivery locations, such as the scenes of traffic accidents. If data includes street addresses, ZIP Codes, or other spatial identifiers, GIS has the tools to plot points of interest for use in analysis.

For the example in chapter 6, you need to spatially enable data that is in tabular form. You'll geocode existing facilities within a county so they can be placed as points on a map. You also place patients on a ZIP Code map over a wide area. Having this data mapped, you can readily see potential service gaps. Then you map suitability measures for a health clinic location to aid in identifying locations in gap areas that would be an attractive site for a new facility.

Chapter 7: Processing and analyzing spatial data

What are some neighborhood factors that lead to child pedestrian injuries in a city? Is poverty a factor? What about the lack of safe public areas for play? In chapter 7, you explore the determinants of serious juvenile-pedestrian injuries for the purpose of designing prevention programs. The basis of your study is a sample of serious-injury data that has been geocoded and can be compared to census data on poverty and to map layers for streets, neighborhoods, and parks that have playgrounds and playing fields.

The GIS work in chapter 7 includes preparatory steps for extracting study region maps from county maps, and then focuses on detailed proximity analyses using park buffers, like those seen in figure 1.2.

Chapter 8: Transforming data using approximate methods

How can health-care analysts combine data from different, incompatible polygon boundary sets? Chapter 8 explores how to transform this data so it can be used for comparative analysis. Often the spatial unit of analysis for a health study is a custom set of polygon boundaries designed for the phenomenon at hand. An example is the hospital service areas and hospital referral regions used in the Dartmouth Atlas of Health Care Project (http://www.dartmouthatlas.org) at the Center for the Evaluative Clinical Sciences at Dartmouth Medical School in Hanover, New Hampshire. Although appropriate for studying patterns in the quality of health care across the country, these custom areas have the limitation of not sharing boundaries with census statistical areas (that is, they are noncoterminous sets of boundaries). Thus, census data cannot be used directly for supportive analysis of these custom areas and must be spatially apportioned to the noncoterminous boundaries.

Another common case of noncoterminous data involves regional analysis of spatial areas such as emergency management service zones for a city where such zones become the de facto unit of spatial analysis. Detailed census variables on income, poverty, educational attainment, and so on are not easily attainable at these levels. Advanced GIS functionality such as using spatial joins, however, can produce some very accurate approximations (or apportionments) for transforming data from one set of polygons to another incompatible set.

Chapter 9: Using ArcGIS Spatial Analyst for demand estimation

Chapter 9 is an introduction to the ArcGIS Spatial Analyst extension. Spatial Analyst uses or creates raster datasets composed of grid cells to display data that is distributed continuously over space as one continuous surface. In this chapter, you prepare and analyze a demand surface map for the location of heart defibrillators in Pittsburgh, where demand is based on the number of out-of-hospital cardiac arrests in which potential bystander help is available. You also learn how to use ArcGIS Spatial Analyst to create a poverty index surface combined with several census data measures from block and block group polygon layers.

Chapter 10: Studying food-borne-disease outbreaks

Chapters 10 and 11 provide a change of pace—opportunities for you to apply and extend the GIS skills and health applications you have learned in the previous nine chapters to new case studies that you develop. We provide the source data and guidelines for analysis, as well as a broad outline of steps; however, it is up to you to carry out the GIS work on your own in an independent case study. In chapter 10, you prepare map layers, including geocoding incidence addresses as the basis for analyzing outbreaks of food-borne illness. Then you use data to simulate the impact of an outbreak. You also do a proximity analysis based on patterns in reported disease cases.

Chapter 11: Forming local chapters of ACHE

Chapter 11 concludes this workbook with a second independent case study, following a setup similar to that in chapter 10. Staff members of the American College of Healthcare Executives (ACHE) want you to use GIS to help them set up ACHE chapters across the country that provide educational and other services to health-care professionals.

In chapter 11, you perform a buffer analysis of existing affiliates that propose becoming ACHE chapters. The buffers will help determine the territories that are served as well as the gaps that suggest where new chapters should be established. You do some work interactively using ArcGIS, but for steps that must be done repeatedly over time, you build an ArcGIS model that generates a macro to automate these steps.

Introduction to ArcGIS and map documents

This book is designed for use with ArcGIS 10.2 for Desktop software. ArcGIS is a full-featured GIS software application for visualizing, managing, creating, and analyzing geographic data. The more advanced levels of ArcGIS offer advanced data conversion and geoprocessing capabilities. ArcGIS has numerous extensions that include ArcGIS 3D Analyst for three-dimensional rendering of surfaces, ArcGIS Network Analyst for routing and other street network applications, and ArcGIS Spatial Analyst for generating and working with raster maps.

ArcGIS includes four application programs: ArcCatalog, ArcGlobe, ArcMap, and ArcScene. ArcCatalog is a utility program for file browsing, data importing and converting, and file maintenance functions (such as create, copy, and delete)—all with special features for GIS source data. You will use ArcCatalog instead of the Microsoft Windows utilities My Computer or Windows Explorer to manage GIS source data. ArcGlobe provides 3D capabilities to work seamlessly on a 3D globe. ArcMap is the primary interface for building, viewing, and analyzing conventional two-dimensional (2D) maps. ArcScene is comparable to ArcMap but for 3D maps.

GIS analysts use ArcMap to compose a map from basemap layers, and then carry out many kinds of analysis and produce several types of GIS outputs. A map composition is saved to a map document file and has a name, chosen by the user, and the .mxd file extension. For example, you will soon open the first map document in the chapter, Tutorial1-3.mxd.

A map document stores pointers (paths) to map layers, data tables, and other data sources for use in a map composition, but it does not store a copy of any data source. Consequently, map layers can be stored anywhere on your computer, local area network, or even on an Internet server, and be part of your map document. In this book, you will use data sources available from the data you will download from the Esri Press "Book Resources" webpage (see the following section).

Exercise data and software

Data for the book is available to download on the Esri Press "Book Resources" webpage, esripress.esri.com/bookresources. Click the appropriate book title, and then click the data link under "Resources" to download the exercise data. A 60-day trial of ArcGIS for Desktop software and extensions is available for readers at esri.com/trydesktop. You must download the data and have access to ArcGIS 10.2 for Desktop software to complete the tutorials in this book.

Learning about ArcGIS

The following tutorials will acquaint you with the functionality and user interface of ArcMap and ArcCatalog. You will start by using ArcCatalog to browse through the data sources used in figure 1.1, and then examine the completed project itself. In the remaining chapters, you will learn how to build, modify, and query data.

In the tutorials that follow, you need to be at your computer to carry out the numbered steps. Screen captures accompanying the steps illustrate important dialog boxes and output. Occasionally, we have added "Your turn" exercises after a series of steps. It is critical that you do these brief exercises to internalize the processes covered. Note that the appearance of the user interface is contantly changing, depending on your operating system and customization choices, so the windows in this book may not appear exactly like the windows on your screen.

Tutorial 1-1

Exploring the ArcCatalog user interface

1 **Start Windows, and then click Start to start your programs. Click All Programs > ArcGIS > ArcCatalog 10.2.** Depending on how ArcGIS has been installed, you may have a different navigation menu or a name other than ArcGIS. The left panel of ArcCatalog is called the Catalog tree. It is used to navigate to the data on your computer or network server, much like Windows Explorer.

2 **Use the Connect to Folder tool on the ArcCatalog toolbar to make a connection to the \EsriPress\GISTHealth folder. In the Connect to Folder dialog, browse to GISTHealth and click OK. This will create a connection you will use to navigate to the tutorial data for the rest of this book.**

3 **In the Catalog tree, browse to \EsriPress\GISTHealth\Data\ by clicking the small plus signs (+) to expand the folders in which the GISTHealth data is installed.** The default location for this folder is C:\EsriPress\GISTHealth\Data, but it may be in a different location depending on where you or your instructor installed it. If you cannot find this folder, make sure it was installed properly.

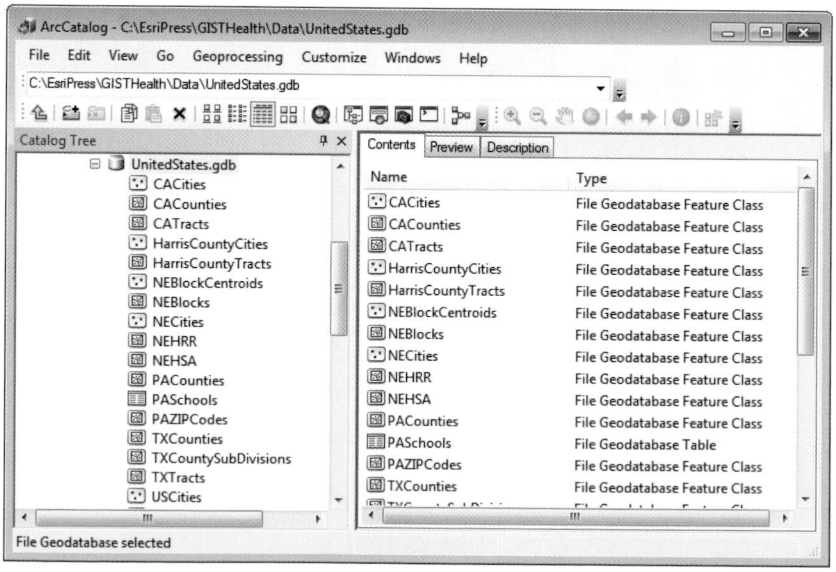

4 **After navigating to the Data folder, expand the United States geodatabase, UnitedStates.gdb.** The right panel, called the Catalog display, contains three tabs: Contents, Preview, and Description. When you click the Contents tab, the datasets in the current folder are listed. The datasets currently listed represent spatial data, and the icon next to each file name indicates what type of geometry the data is built in: point, line, or polygon. (See facing page.)

5 **In the Catalog tree, click USStates and click the Preview tab.** Previewing data this way allows you to get a quick glimpse of the data without actually loading it into a map. You can also use this tab to preview the contents of a table.

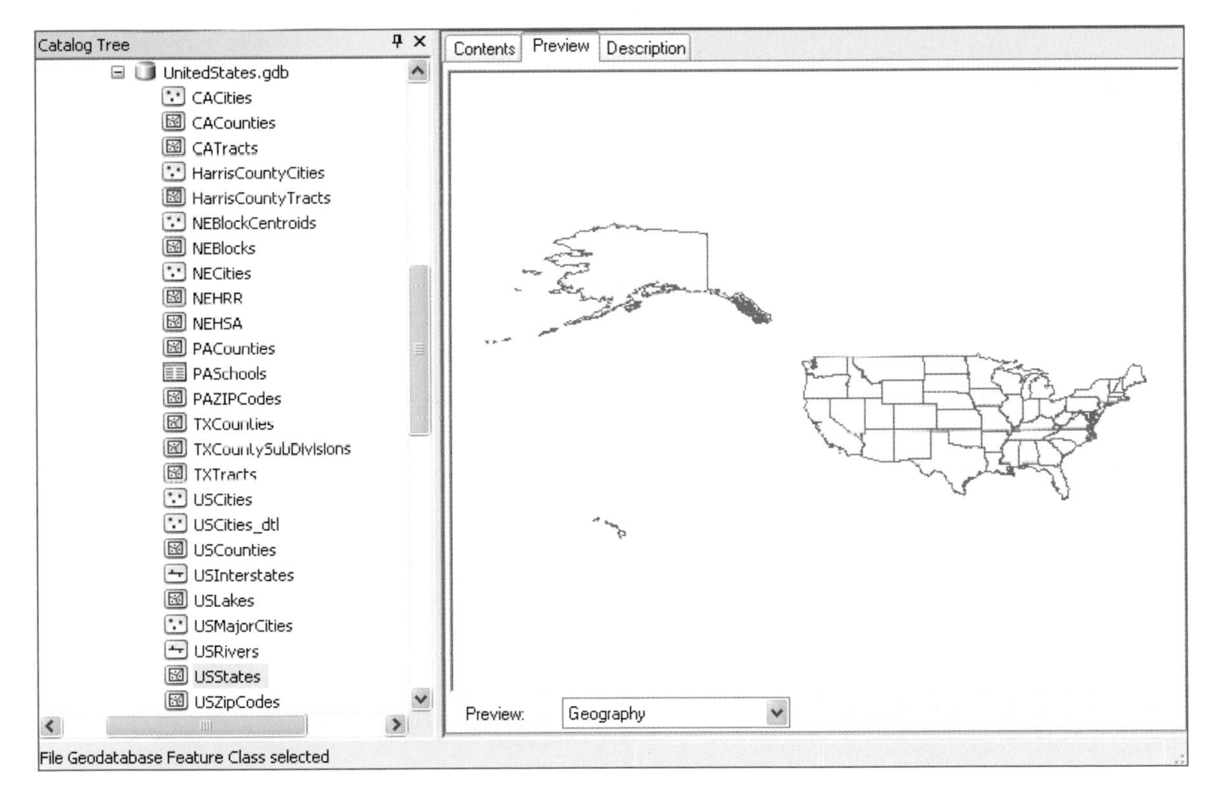

6 **At the bottom of the Catalog display, click the Preview arrow, click Table, and then use the horizontal scroll bar to view the attribute fields in the table.** Each record in the table corresponds to one of the state polygons you previewed in the preceding step, and as you can see, there are quite a few attributes stored for each state, most of which are demographic. For example, by reading across the table, you could identify that the state of Washington is in the Pacific subregion and had a population of 5,894,121 in 2000 and 6,756,150 in 2010. We used the STATE_NAME attribute to label states in figure 1.1.

Contents | Preview | Description

OBJECTID *	Shape *	STATE_NAME	STATE_FIPS	SUB_REGION	STATE_ABBR	POP2000	POP2010
1	Polygon	Hawaii	15	Pacific	HI	1211537	1309580
2	Polygon	Washington	53	Pacific	WA	5894121	6756150
3	Polygon	Montana	30	Mountain	MT	902195	983932
4	Polygon	Maine	23	New England	ME	1274923	1338645
5	Polygon	North Dakota	38	West North Central	ND	642200	662194
6	Polygon	South Dakota	46	West North Central	SD	754844	827263
7	Polygon	Wyoming	56	Mountain	WY	493782	548154
8	Polygon	Wisconsin	55	East North Central	WI	5363675	5741617
9	Polygon	Idaho	16	Mountain	ID	1293953	1581697
10	Polygon	Vermont	50	New England	VT	608827	626078
11	Polygon	Minnesota	27	West North Central	MN	4919479	5334772
12	Polygon	Oregon	41	Pacific	OR	3421399	3865839
13	Polygon	New Hampshire	33	New England	NH	1235786	1329915
14	Polygon	Iowa	19	West North Central	IA	2926324	3057995
15	Polygon	Massachusetts	25	New England	MA	6349097	6555736
16	Polygon	Nebraska	31	West North Central	NE	1711263	1822473
17	Polygon	New York	36	Middle Atlantic	NY	18976457	19543731
18	Polygon	Pennsylvania	42	Middle Atlantic	PA	12281054	12574407
19	Polygon	Connecticut	09	New England	CT	3405565	3535787
20	Polygon	Rhode Island	44	New England	RI	1048319	1058412
21	Polygon	New Jersey	34	Middle Atlantic	NJ	8414350	8822373
22	Polygon	Indiana	18	East North Central	IN	6080485	6479832

0 (of 51)

Preview: Table

7 **Click the Description tab at the top of the Catalog display.** This tab describes metadata, which is data about data.

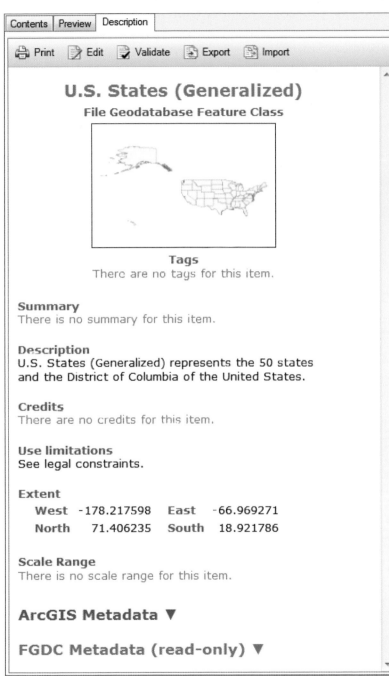

8 In the Catalog display, click the Contents tab.

Other folders in the \EsriPress\GISTHealth\ Catalog tree include Maps, where original map document files are located; MyAssignments, where you will save files to chapter folders if you are working in a classroom and are required to complete the assignments at the end of each chapter; and MyExercises, where you will save files as you complete tutorial exercises in each chapter. MyExercises contains a subfolder called FinishedExercises, which includes tutorial exercises completed by the book's authors that you can use as needed.

YOUR TURN

Explore additional layers in UnitedStates.gdb. When you are finished, click the toggle key that has the minus sign (-) to the left of the UnitedStates.gdb folder icon in the Catalog tree to collapse that folder. Then close ArcCatalog.

Tutorial 1-2
Reviewing data source types

You will do most GIS file maintenance work in ArcCatalog, although it is instructive to view GIS files in a conventional file utility program. In this tutorial, you will examine two common Esri file formats used in GIS: a shapefile and a file geodatabase. A shapefile map layer has three or more files that have the same name but different file extensions, all stored in the same folder. A file geodatabase is a folder that has one or more map layers (and possibly other kinds of data) stored as feature classes. Both of these data types are common in the GIS industry, where the file geodatabase is a more modern format. Other less common GIS and spatial data formats that can be stored in this folder include an ArcInfo coverage and a CAD DXF (drawing exchange format). You will learn more about these formats in chapter 4.

1 **On the taskbar, click Start, and then click Computer.** The path to Computer may differ depending on which operating system you are using.

2 **Browse to where your GISTHealth folder is installed (for example, C:\EsriPress\GISTHeath\).**

3 **Double-click Data > DataFiles to view the available data files.**

Name	Size	Type
Clinics	3 KB	Microsoft Excel Comma Separated Values File
cs42_d00.e00	6,700 KB	E00 File
Rivers	489 KB	AutoCAD Drawing Interchange
Rivers.dxf	61 KB	XML Document
Rivers.prj	1 KB	PRJ File
Tracts.dbf	82 KB	DBF File
Tracts.prj	1 KB	PRJ File
Tracts.sbn	5 KB	SBN File
Tracts	1 KB	Adobe Illustrator Tsume File
Tracts	236 KB	AutoCAD Shape Source
Tracts.shp	10 KB	XML Document
Tracts	4 KB	AutoCAD Compiled Shape

Now you can review the Tracts shapefile, which actually consists of seven files that all have the same name, Tracts. These are US Census tracts for Allegheny County, Pennsylvania.

- The Tracts file that has the .shp extension has the features geometry and coordinates. For points, each record has a point and an x,y location. For line and polygon layers, each shape record has coordinates of a line segment or a polygon. Tracts, of course, consist of polygons.
- The Tracts file that has the .dbf extension has the feature attribute table in dBASE format. You can open and edit this file as a Microsoft Excel spreadsheet and as a Microsoft Access database, but such work must be done carefully and without deleting or adding records or changing the order of rows, which could result in corrupted data. The relationship between the .shp and .dbf files of a shapefile depends on the one-to-one physical arrangement of records in both files.
- The .sbx and .shx files contain indexes for speeding up searches and queries. The .prj file is a simple text file that has the map projection parameters of the layer.
- Finally, the .shp.xml file has the layer metadata, and you can open this file in a Web browser to read it.

4 In Computer, navigate up one level to GISTHealth\Data. The remaining folders in the Data folder are file geodatabases. Each file geodatabase includes a .gdb extension. A single file geodatabase can have one or more vector-map layers and data tables.

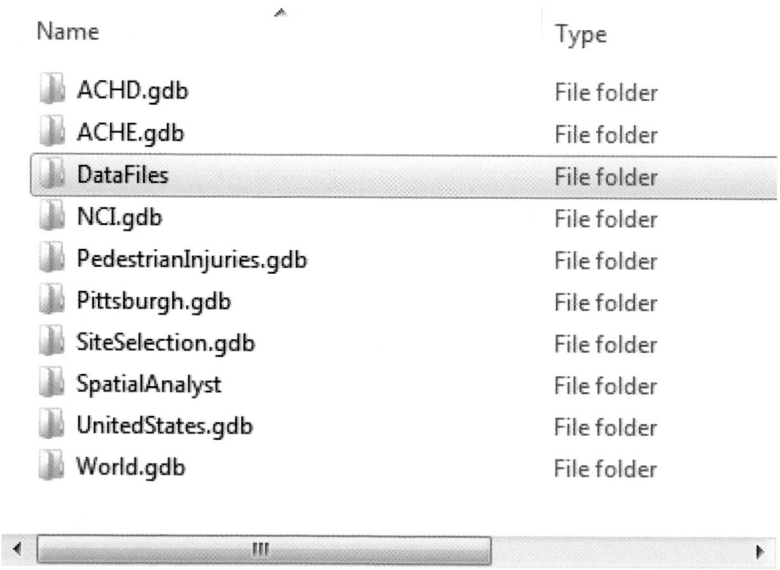

Name	Type
ACHD.gdb	File folder
ACHE.gdb	File folder
DataFiles	File folder
NCI.gdb	File folder
PedestrianInjuries.gdb	File folder
Pittsburgh.gdb	File folder
SiteSelection.gdb	File folder
SpatialAnalyst	File folder
UnitedStates.gdb	File folder
World.gdb	File folder

5 **Double-click the UnitedStates.gdb folder icon.** You cannot identify the files contained in a file geodatabase in My Computer. Always use ArcCatalog to maintain map layers and data tables stored in a personal geodatabase; otherwise, you will likely corrupt the layers.

6 **Close My Computer.**

YOUR TURN

Start ArcCatalog and explore the file geodatabases in the Data folder. Preview the feature classes in each geodatabase. Then close ArcCatalog.

Tutorial 1-3
Exploring the ArcMap user interface

To get started, you will open a completed map document that has health and other data to get the feel for ArcMap and health layers.

Open a map document

1. **On the taskbar, click Start, and then click All Programs > ArcGIS > ArcMap10.2.** Depending on how ArcGIS and ArcMap have been installed, you may have a different navigation menu or a name other than ArcGIS.

2. **In the ArcMap - Getting Started dialog box, click Existing Maps > Browse for more.**

3. **In the Open ArcMap Document dialog box, browse to the drive where you installed the \EsriPress\GISTHealth\Maps folder (for example, C:\EsriPress\GISTHealth\Maps), select Tutorial1-3.mxd, and click Open.**

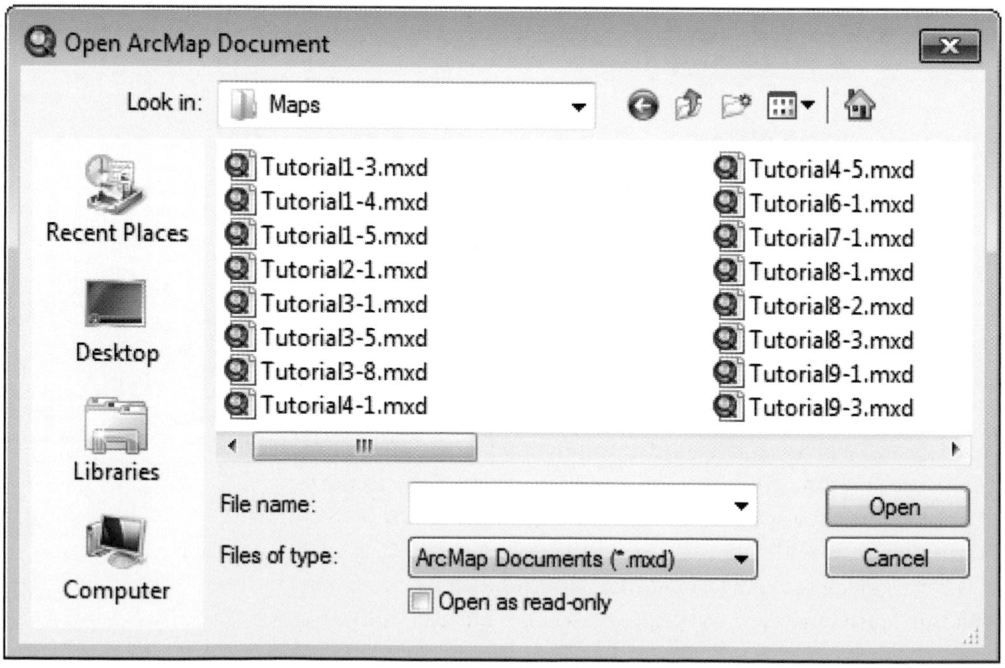

Tutorial1-3.mxd is displayed in the ArcMap application window. The map currently contains the contiguous United States showing demographics related to female-headed households as both point and polygon features and male lung cancer mortality rates. The major components of the ArcMap interface are also identified.

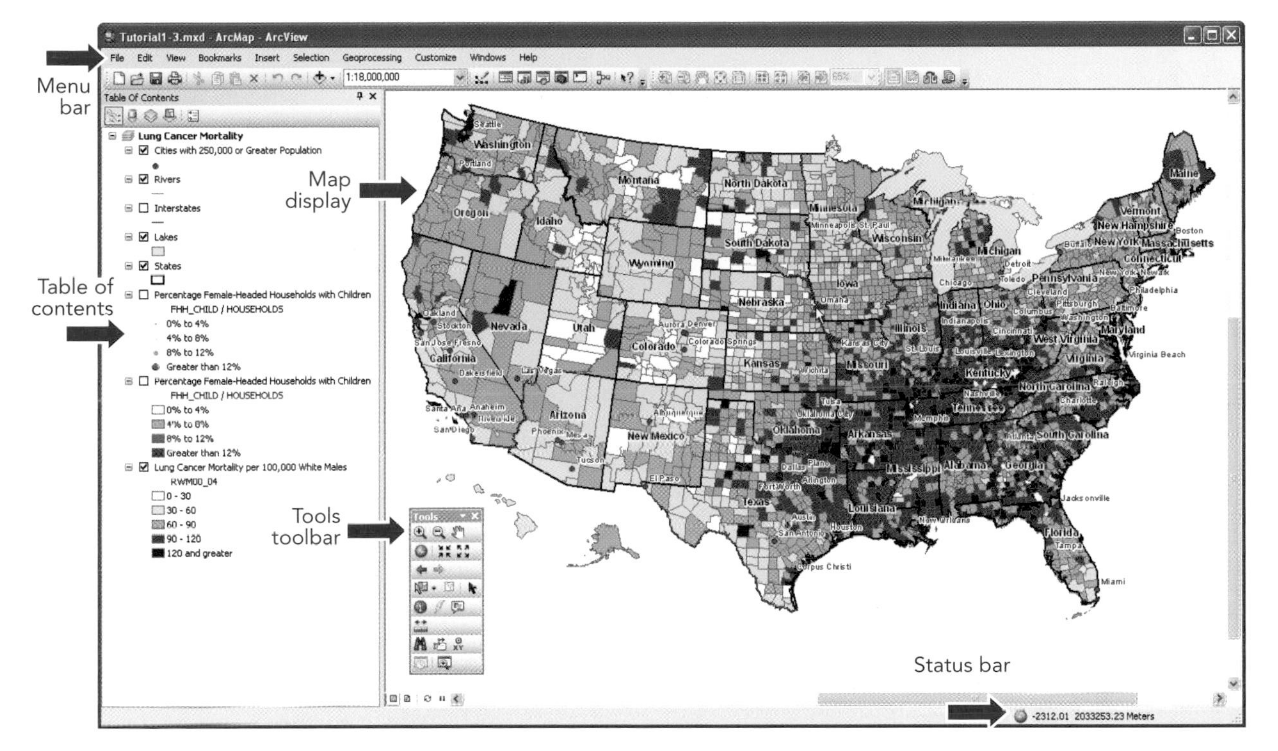

The major components of the ArcMap application window include the following:

- The *Menu bar* has some items common to most Windows application packages, plus some that are unique to GIS.

- The *map display* is where the feature classes loaded into the map are drawn.

- The *table of contents* lists all the data in the map document by layer and allows you to change layer visibility and access layer properties. Currently, the List By Drawing Order button is selected at the top of the table of contents showing the order of map layers and their legends. By clicking the List By Source button at the top of the table of contents, you can also see the folder and file path to the source data of map layers and tables. ArcMap draws maps from the bottom up in the table of contents, so polygon feature layers, such as Lung Cancer Mortality, that would cover line or point feature layers, such as Rivers, must go on the bottom. You can see that only some of the layers are turned on—those that have selected check boxes in the Table of Contents.

- The *Tools toolbar* has frequently used tools and can be docked, if desired, by dragging it by its title bar to any boundary in the ArcMap interface. Similarly, you can undock it by dragging it to the desired location.

- The *Status bar* displays the map coordinates of the pointer location in the map display. In the preceding graphic, the pointer is over Omaha, Nebraska, and the coordinates for Omaha are displayed on the Status bar.

YOUR TURN

Experiment with turning map layers on and off by selecting and then clearing the check boxes to the left of each map layer in the table of contents. Start with layers currently turned off, from the top down, and turn each one on and then off. Then try various combinations. Keep in mind that the Female-Headed Households with Children layer is a strong indicator of poverty. Of course, not every such household is in poverty, but the tendency is strong. When you are finished, return the map document to its original condition, with layers turned on or off as shown in the preceding figure.

View map-layer attribute tables

1 **In the table of contents, right-click Cities with 250,000 or Greater Population and click Open Attribute Table.** The attribute table for Cities with 250,000 or Greater Population is displayed. This is the same sort of table you previewed in ArcCatalog.

2 **Visually scan the map for a few cities listed in the table. Verify that there is a point plotted for each corresponding record in the table.**

Table

Cities with 250,000 or Greater Population

OBJECTID *	Shape *	NAME	CLASS	ST	STFIPS	PLACEFIP	CAPITAL	AREALAND	AREAWATER	POP_CLASS	POP2000	POP2007
4	Point	Seattle	City	WA	53	63000		83.872	58.671	9	563374	593350
5	Point	Portland	City	OR	41	59000		134.32	11.048	9	529121	551302
7	Point	Oakland	City	CA	06	53000		56.055	22.098	8	399484	411240
8	Point	San Francisco	City	CA	06	67000		46.694	185.221	9	776733	796417
10	Point	San Jose	City	CA	06	68000		174.863	3.315	9	894943	946979
14	Point	Stockton	City	CA	06	75000		54.71	1.239	8	243771	293097
15	Point	Sacramento	City	CA	06	64000	State	97.157	2.083	8	407018	462910
16	Point	Fresno	City	CA	06	27000		104.363	0.441	8	427652	475005
17	Point	San Diego	City	CA	06	66000		324.341	47.69	10	1223400	1301514
21	Point	Los Angeles	City	CA	06	44000		469.072	29.216	10	3694820	3908521
22	Point	Long Beach	City	CA	06	43000		50.44	15.426	8	461522	486861

68 (0 out of 68 Selected)

Cities with 250,000 or Greater Population

3 Close the table.

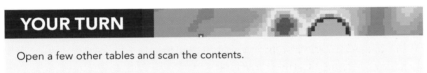

Open a few other tables and scan the contents.

View map layer properties

1 In the table of contents, right-click Cities with 250,000 or Greater

Layer Properties

General | Source | Selection | Display | Symbology | Fields | Definition Query | Labels | Joins & Relates | Time | HTML Popup

Layer Name: Ciities with 250,000 or Greater Population ☑ Visible

Description: Represents locations for cities within United States with populations of 250,000 or greater (based on Census 2007 figures).

Credits:

Scale Range

You can specify the range of scales at which this layer will be shown:

◉ Show layer at all scales

○ Don't show layer when zoomed:

Out beyond: <None> (minimum scale)

In beyond: <None> (maximum scale)

OK | Cancel | Apply

Population and click Properties. In the Layer Properties dialog box, click the General tab. Layer Properties is an important dialog box for managing how layers behave and appear in ArcMap. Although there are many properties that can be set, it is good to review a few useful ones for now. For example, in the General window of Layer Properties, you can change the layer name by typing the name of your choice into the Layer Name text box.

2 **In the Layer Properties dialog box, click the Source tab.** The Source window provides bounding coordinates of the map layer (that is, its extent), the data type, location on the server or computer, geometry type, and projection.

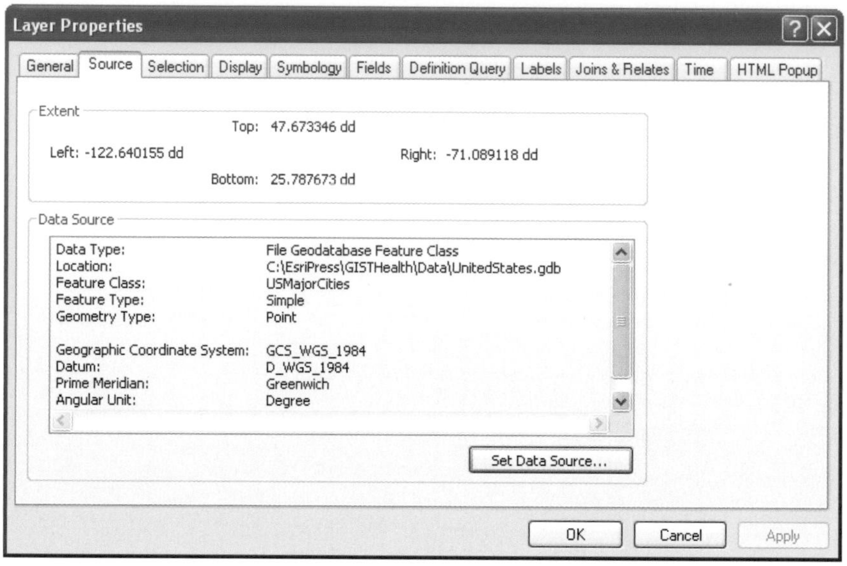

3 **Click the Symbology tab.** The Symbology window provides many options for symbolizing vector-map layers. The cities layer uses a single symbol chosen by the authors, a purple circular point marker that has a black outline.

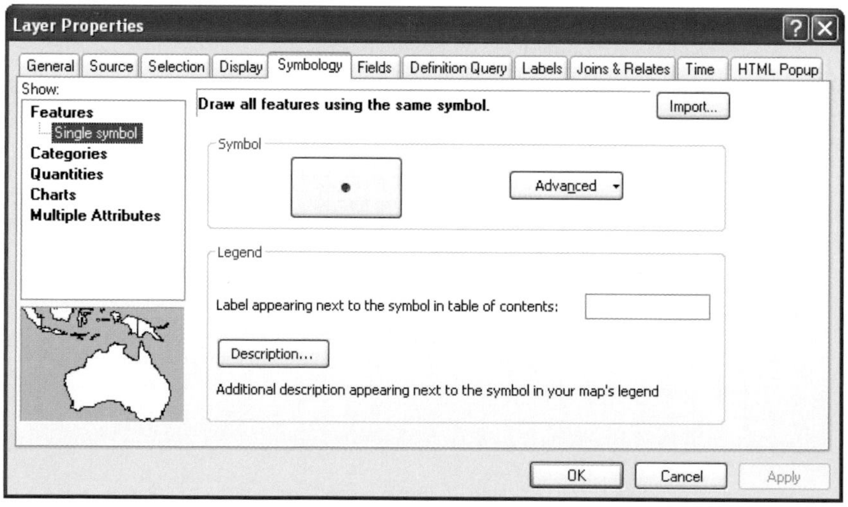

4 **Click the Fields tab.** The Fields window lists the layer's attribute fields and their properties.

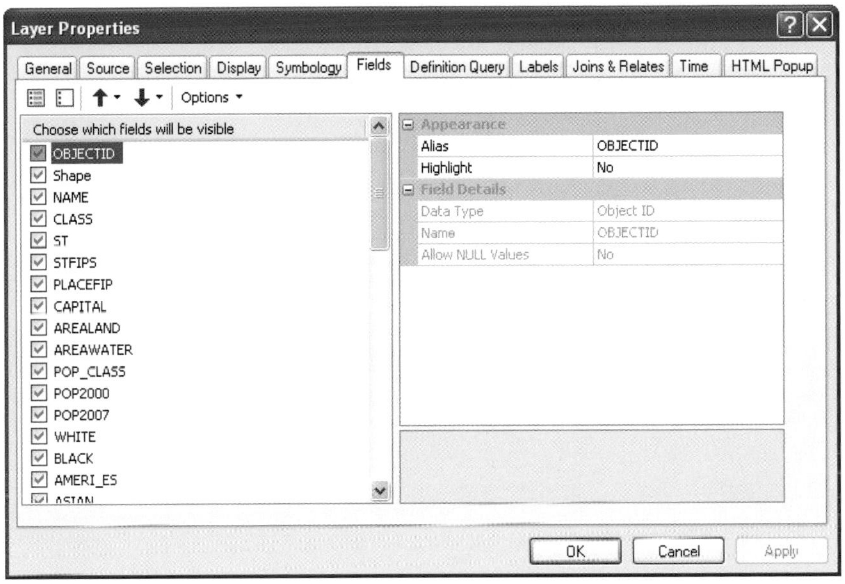

5 **Click the Definition Query tab.** The Definition Query window allows you to restrict what is displayed in a map layer. In this case, we used the POP2007 attribute to limit the cities displayed to those that had a population of 250,000 or more in the year 2007. This window changes only the display and does not remove the records from the source data.

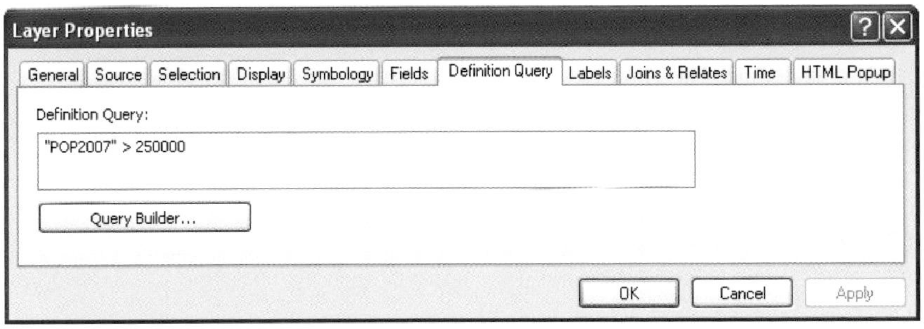

6 **Click the Labels tab.** The Labels window allows you to label features using an attribute from the feature attribute table. We used NAME, which is the name of cities, in a purple font and a white halo mask. We also turned labeling on by selecting the check box at the top of the form.

Layer Properties
General | Source | Selection | Display | Symbology | Fields | Definition Query | Labels | Joins & Relates | Time | HTML Popup
Label features in this layer
Method: Label all the features the same way.
All features will be labeled using the options specified.
Text String
Label Field: NAME
Expression...
Text Symbol
AaBbYyZz
Arial 8
B I U Symbol...
Other Options
Placement Properties... Scale Range...
Pre-defined Label Style
Label Styles...
OK Cancel Apply

T 1-3

7 **Close Layer Properties.**

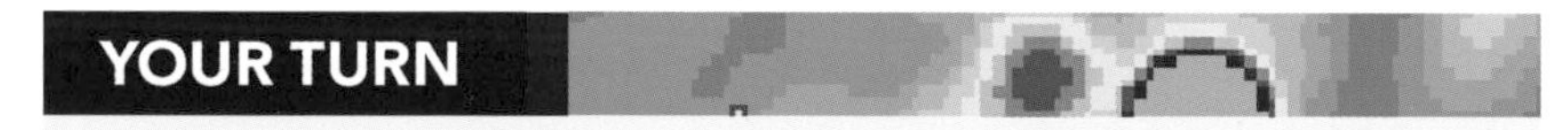

Examine the properties of a few more layers, but do not make any changes. When you are finished, close ArcMap but do not save any changes.

Tutorial 1-4
Using and exporting a map

Fundamentally, when you use GIS for analysis, you are observing spatial patterns related to a problem, phenomenon, or issue of interest. In this case, the phenomenon is mortality of white males from lung cancer.

In this tutorial, you will clearly see strong spatial patterns and concentrations of mortality along the southeastern coast of the United States and other locations. You can recognize some correlations on the map, based on spatial arrangement alone. For example, the band of high mortality along the eastern border of Kentucky is in that state's coal mining belt. Perhaps the white males succumbing to lung cancer in that area tend to be coal miners.

Some of the southeastern peak areas for mortality correspond to tobacco-growing areas of Virginia, the Carolinas, and Georgia, but high-mortality areas run beyond the tobacco fields. Perhaps being near tobacco-growing areas increases the likelihood of smoking and, therefore, lung cancer. The question then becomes, how far beyond the immediate tobacco-growing areas could such an influence exist? Regardless, it cannot account for the high mortality observed along the Mississippi River.

An additional correlation is poverty, which contributes to many health problems and perhaps increases exposure to factors leading to lung cancer. A strong indicator of poverty, and the only poverty indicator available in the working US counties data, is the percentage of female-headed households with children. As an example of the effectiveness of this indicator, in Pittsburgh at the tract level, the simple correlation between percentage of female-headed households with children and the percentage of total population below the poverty line is 0.67. Now you can see if there is any visual evidence of a positive correlation between this poverty indicator and white male lung cancer incidence.

For this poverty indicator, we used a size-graduated point marker and a dichromatic color scale. We used an equal-interval numeric scale of 4 percent width, where the darker shade of green signifies the lowest-value interval and the darker shade of orange signifies the highest-value interval. Also, the larger the diameter of circular point marker used, the higher the interval of the indicator variable.

Find and export a map

1 **Start ArcMap and open Tutorial1-4.mxd. Select the check box to the left of the Percentage Female-Headed Households with Children map layer in the table of contents to turn that layer on.** Immediately, you can see that this variable is promising as a correlation to the male lung cancer deaths because it is high in many of the same areas where lung cancer mortality is high. The current map, however, is zoomed out too far. You need a closer look at the southeastern United States. We have built a spatial bookmark for this purpose, which you will use next, to get an uncluttered, zoomed-in view of the map. Notice that the map scale in the figure is 1:20,000,000 for the entire United States. It will be different on your screen, because your screen is likely a different physical size from ours. Make a note of your scale.

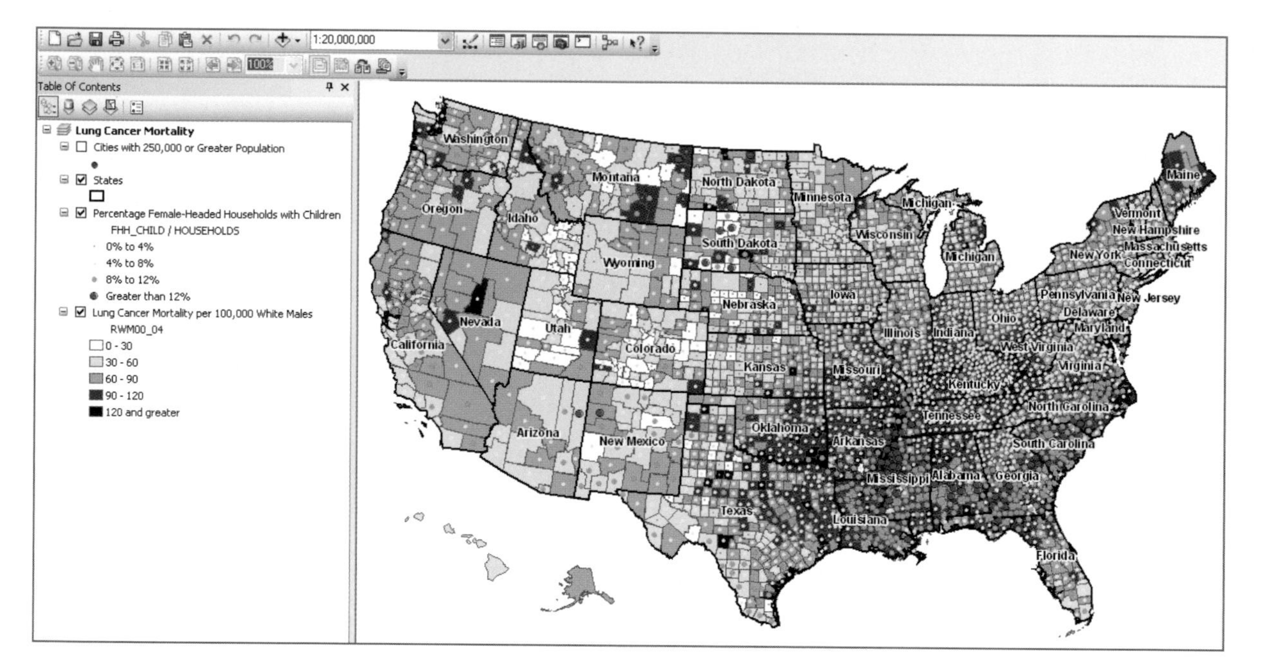

2 On the Menu bar, click Bookmarks > Southeast. Using this bookmark helps considerably. There is a visual correlation between the variables, with both tending to be high in the same areas. Clearly, further examination would require a multivariate model. We have identified some promising variables: coal production, tobacco crops, adjacency to tobacco-growing areas, and poverty. For the present, however, you need a professional-quality map that could be used in a Microsoft Word document or a Microsoft PowerPoint presentation. We have built a map layout for this purpose, which you will view next. Note that the map scale is much larger when zoomed in to 1:9,000,000, as shown in the figure.

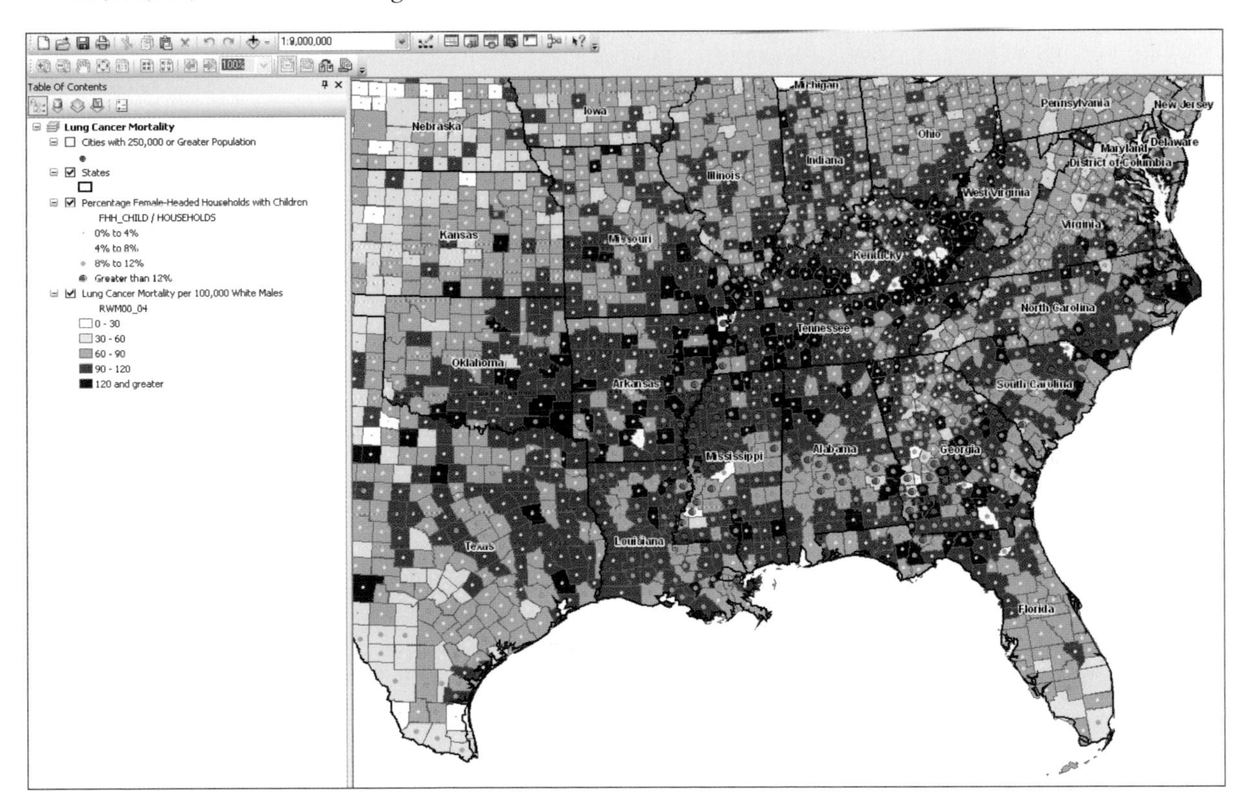

3 On the Menu bar, click View > Layout View. The resulting map, which you will learn how to export for use in a document in chapter 3, is in layout view. ArcMap provides two general views: data view and layout view. Typically, you use data view to interact with your map data by browsing, symbolizing, and editing. You can also interact with your data in layout view, but its primary purpose is to finalize a map composition. In layout view, you can add a north arrow, a scale bar, a legend, and other map elements.

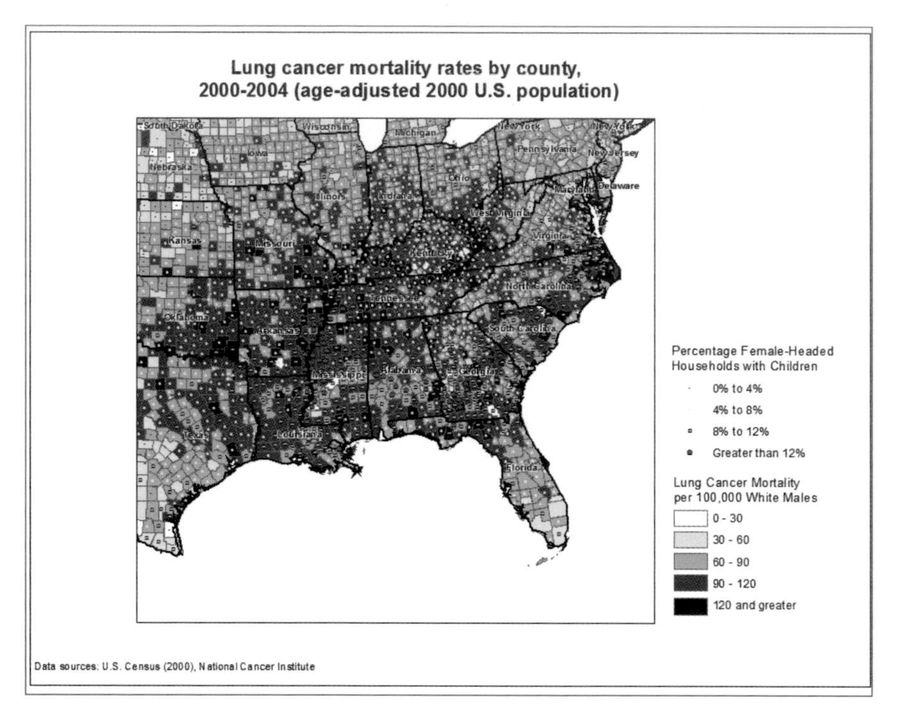

4 On the Menu bar, click File > Export Map.

5 Browse to \EsriPress\GISTHealth\MyExercises\Chapter1\ and save the map as a JPEG file, resolution 150 dpi, called Tutorial1-4YourName.jpg.

6 On the Menu bar, click Bookmarks > U.S.

7 Close ArcMap. Do not save your changes.

Learning about GIS websites

Esri offers a website for sharing maps and map layers: ArcGIS Online (http://www.arcgis.com).

ArcGIS Online is a cloud-based system for sharing your data with others and accessing shared data that others have posted. One thing you can do with ArcGIS Online is share your symbolized data with others. If you create a map in ArcMap showing the results of an analysis, you can make a layer of that data in ArcMap, then post it to the Internet on ArcGIS Online, and share it with the public or selected colleagues.

A second thing you can do with ArcGIS Online is make a web-based map, using data available on ArcGIS Online that others have posted or Esri has made available. You can share that map with the public or selected colleagues.

In the following tutorials, you will be trying out these capabilities of ArcGIS Online. First you will be posting a layer file from ArcMap. Then you will be creating and saving a webmap.

Tutorial 1-5
Creating and sharing map layers

You can use ArcGIS Online to publish maps you create in ArcGIS for Desktop on the Internet. To do so, you'll need to create layer packages for your map layers. Here are the major steps:

1. Create a map document in ArcMap.
2. After the map is symbolized and labeled, and each layer is documented in Layer Properties using the General tab, right-click the layer and click Create Layer Package. Then choose a storage location and file name on your computer.

A layer package is an .lpk file you save locally that encapsulates both data and symbolization. Layer packages can be used in ArcMap, ArcGIS Online and ArcGIS Explorer Desktop.

Note: If you have a group layer in ArcMap, you can save the entire group layer (and all its map layers and layer symbolization) in a single layer package. So one "trick" is to put your entire map document's map layers into a group layer. Then you can publish the entire map document easily, although using a group layer does not allow reuse of individual map layers by others. In this tutorial, a group layer has already been created for you. You will learn how to create group layers in chapter 3.

Create a layer package in ArcMap

1 **Start ArcMap and open Tutorial1-5.mxd.** The map document includes three layers: the percentage of female-headed households (single moms) by census tract in California, and major cities and counties for the state. All three layers are contained in one group layer called California Female-Headed Household Population Study.

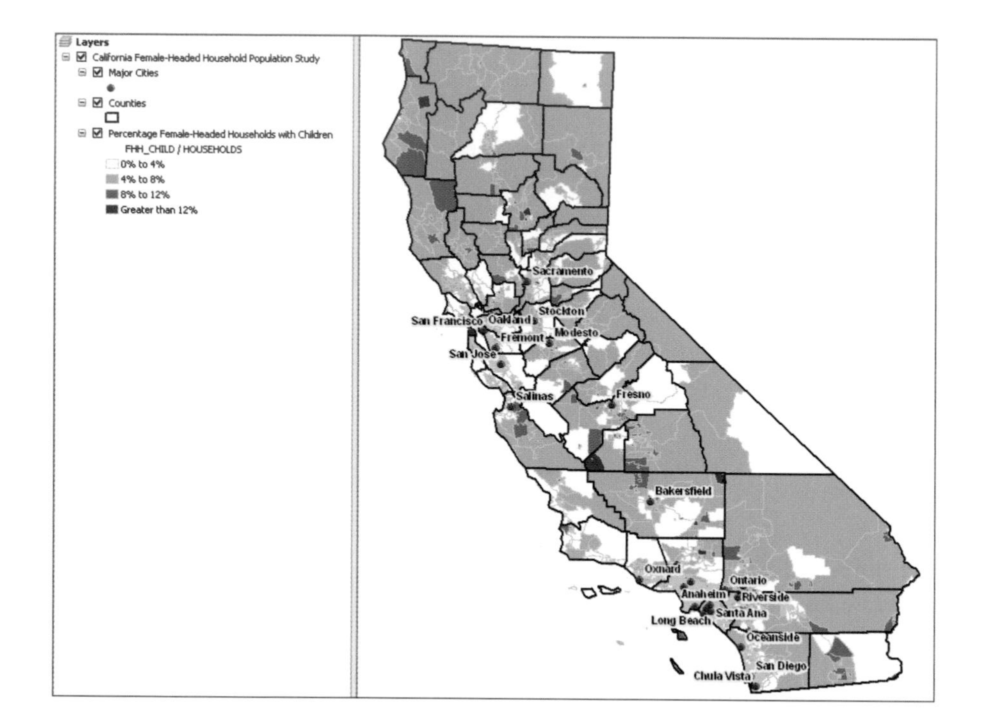

2 **In the table of contents, right-click California Female-Headed Household Population Study and click Create Layer Package.**

3 **In the Layer Package dialog box, select the "Save package to file" option.**

T 1-5

4 **Click the Browse button, browse through MyExercises to your Chapter1 folder, and then click Save.** The layers in this group layer are saved to this folder as the California Female-Headed Household Population Study.lpk file, each symbolized according to the symbols in ArcMap.

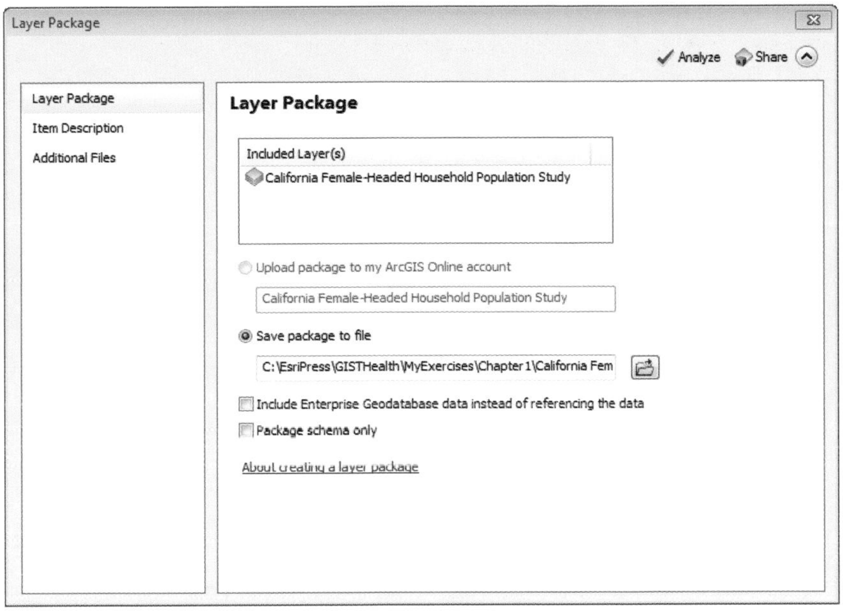

5 **Click Item Description.** Provide a Summary and Tags for your layer package. For Summary, type "California Population Demographic Study." For Tags, type "demographics, obesity, poverty, population, California."

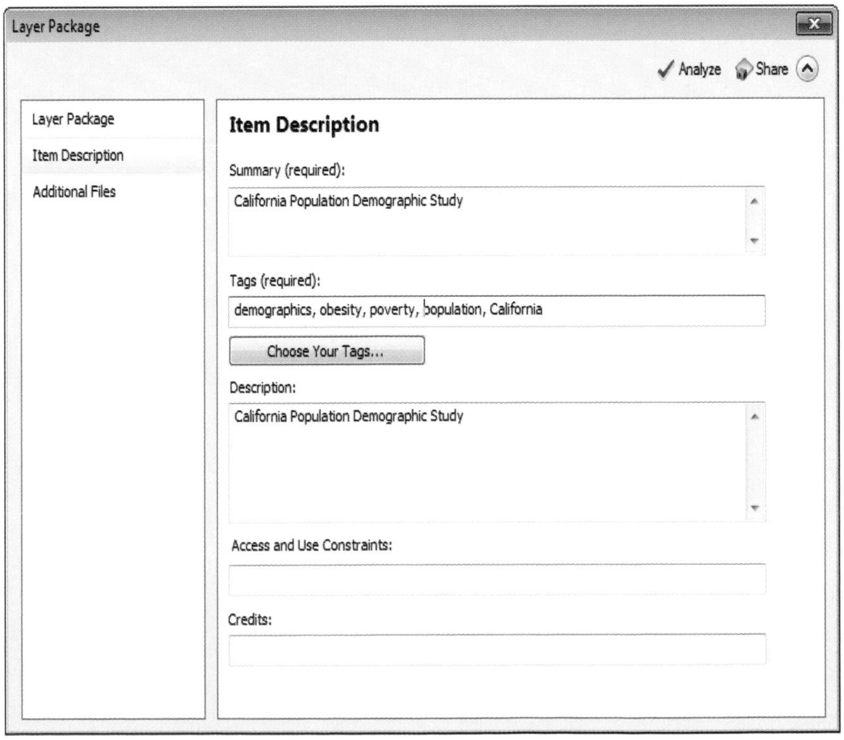

6 **Click the Analyze and Share buttons.** Creating the layer package takes time. Be patient while the layers are exported to the .lpk file.

7 **Click OK.** A message appears once the layer package is complete.

8 **Close ArcMap.**

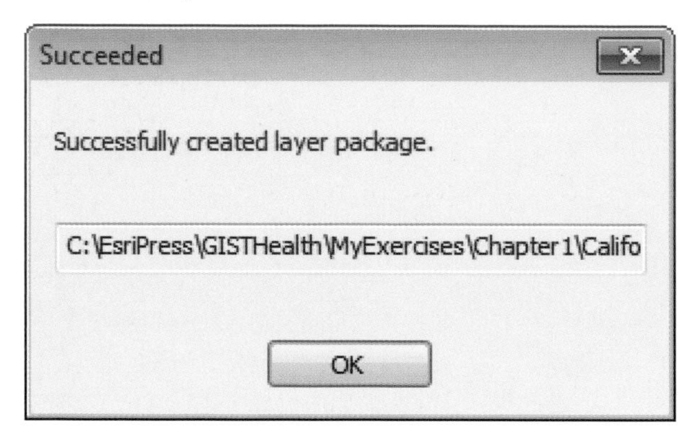

Create an ArcGIS Online account

You are going to post the layer package you just made to ArcGIS Online. To access this capability, you will need an ArcGIS Online account.

1 **In your browser, go to** https://www.arcgis.com/.

2 **Click the Sign In link in the upper right corner of the window.**

3 **Click "Create A Public Account".** Fill out the form and choose Create My Account.

Upload a layer package

1 **Click ArcGIS, and on the ArcGIS Online home page, click the My Content link and then the Add Item button** Add Item **.**

2 **In the Add Item dialog box, click the Browse button, browse through MyExercises to your Chapter1 folder, and then click California Female-Headed Household Population Study.lpk. Click Open.** The title automatically fills in, but you must add at least one tag for the layer.

3 In the Add Item dialog box, type obesity, population, poverty **for tags.**
These layers could be used in these or other similar demographic studies.

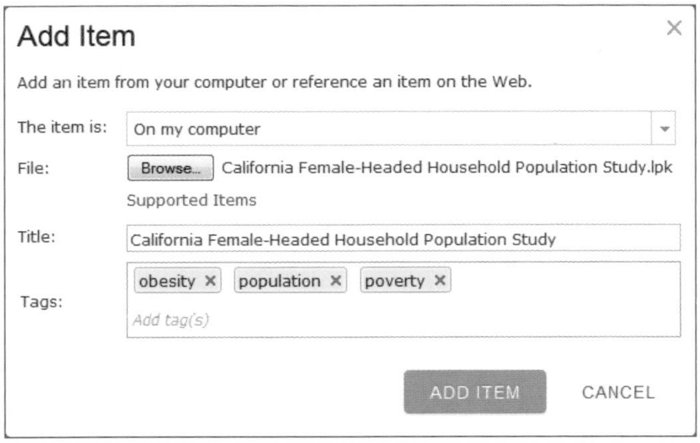

Add Item
Add an item from your computer or reference an item on the Web.
The item is: On my computer
File: Browse... California Female-Headed Household Population Study.lpk
Supported Items
Title: California Female-Headed Household Population Study
Tags: obesity × population × poverty ×
Add tag(s)
ADD ITEM CANCEL

4 Click Add Item. Be patient while your layer package is uploaded. Your layers will appear in your content area.

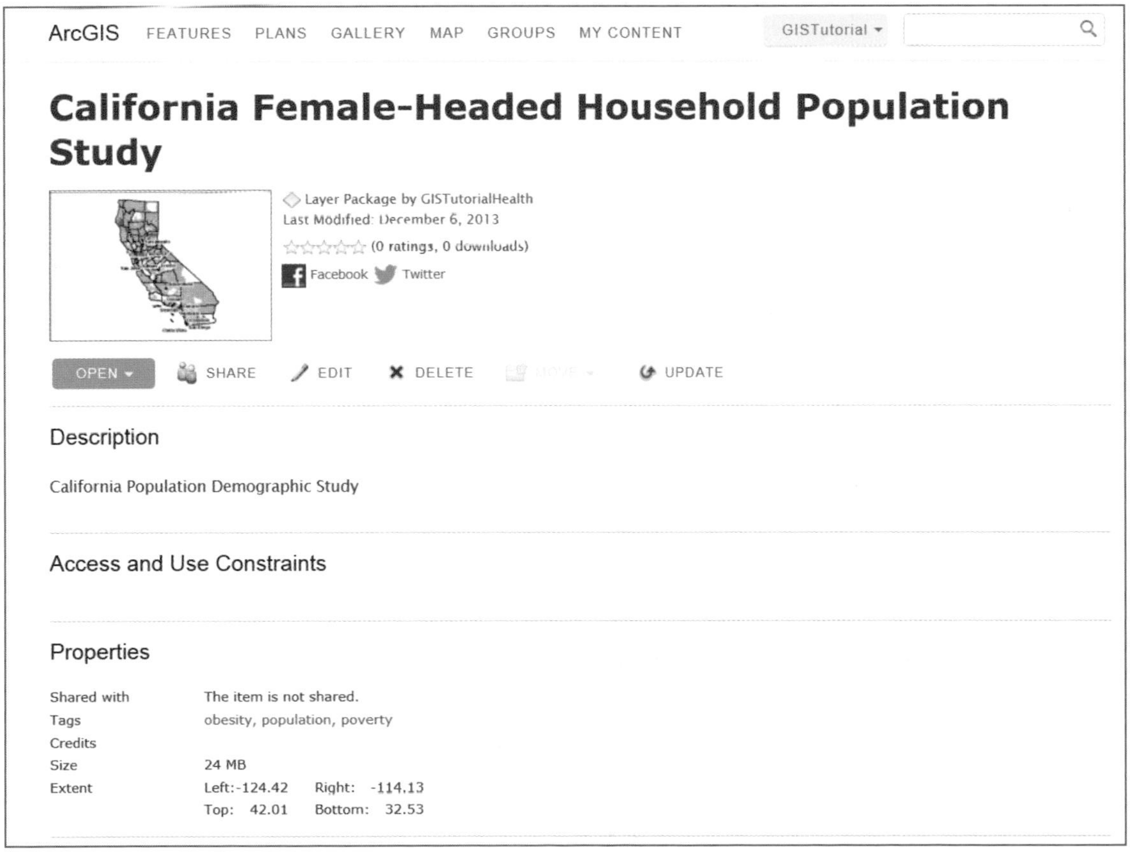

ArcGIS FEATURES PLANS GALLERY MAP GROUPS MY CONTENT GISTutorial

California Female-Headed Household Population Study
Layer Package by GISTutorialHealth
Last Modified: December 6, 2013
(0 ratings, 0 downloads)
Facebook Twitter
OPEN SHARE EDIT DELETE MOVE UPDATE

Description
California Population Demographic Study

Access and Use Constraints

Properties
Shared with The item is not shared.
Tags obesity, population, poverty
Credits
Size 24 MB
Extent Left: -124.42 Right: -114.13
Top: 42.01 Bottom: 32.53

Share a layer package

1 **Click the Share button** Share **.**

2 **In the Share dialog box, click "Everyone (public)" and then OK.** Instead of sharing your uploaded content with everyone, you can limit it to members of a group that you create and ask members to join.

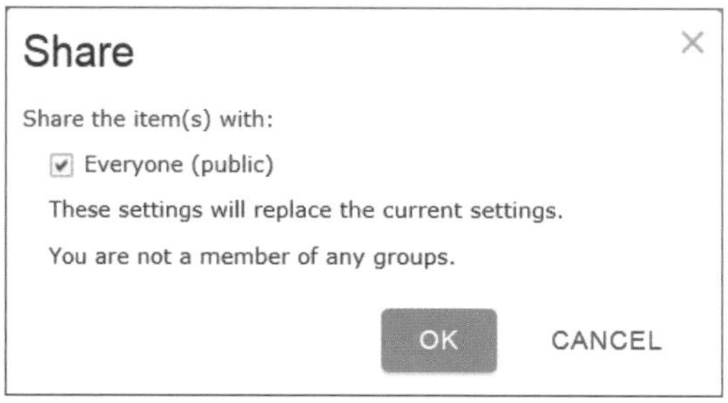

Share

Share the item(s) with:

☑ Everyone (public)

These settings will replace the current settings.

You are not a member of any groups.

OK CANCEL

3 **Click the My Content link.** You will see that your layer package is now available.

4 **Exit the website.**

Tutorial 1-6

Creating health maps using ArcGIS Online content

ArcGIS Online is a website that not only allows you to share maps you create using desktop GIS, but it is also the Esri repository for maps, data, applications, and tools. ArcGIS Online includes content from Esri, its partners, and the GIS community at large. Anyone can share maps and data on ArcGIS Online. In this tutorial, you will create maps showing areas in California where there is a high percentage of overweight children and limited access to supermarkets and farmers' markets.

Add the California Health Indicators layer

1 **In your browser, go to** https://www.arcgis.com/.

2 **Click the Sign In link in the upper-right corner of the window and sign in using your ArcGIS Online Account.**

3 **Click the Map link.**

4 **Click the Basemap button** [Basemap] **and then Terrain with Labels for the basemap.** Notice the other basemap options, including imagery or topographic maps.

5 In the "Find an address or place" box, type California, **and press ENTER. Close the Location pop-up window.** The map zooms to the state of California.

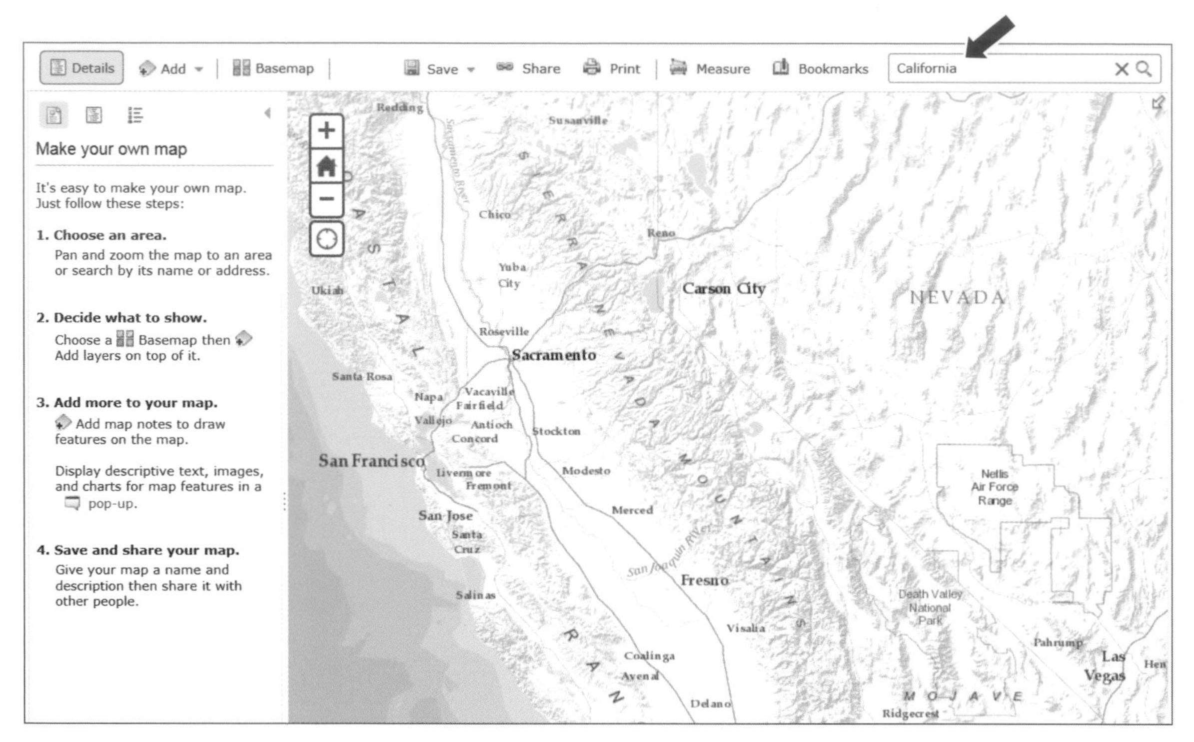

6 Click the Add Content to Map button [Add] **and then Search for Layers.**

7 In the Find box, type health California. In the box, select ArcGIS Online. **Press GO.**

8 Scroll through the results list, click California Health Indicators and then "Add to map". The resulting map shows the percentage of overweight children for grades 5, 7, and 9, reported at the district and school levels. The darker red areas have higher percentages of overweight children. (See facing page.)

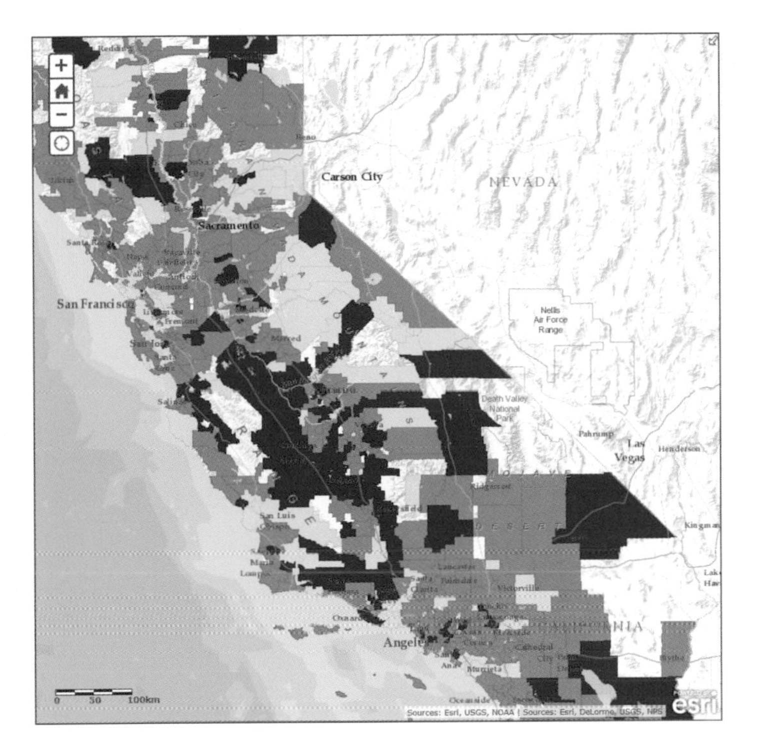

9 Click the Zoom In (+) button and pan the map until you see the bright red area near San Diego, California. The area of focus is southern California near the Mexican border. Be careful not to zoom in too close. Otherwise, your color coded map will appear as point symbols. If this happens, simply zoom out more.

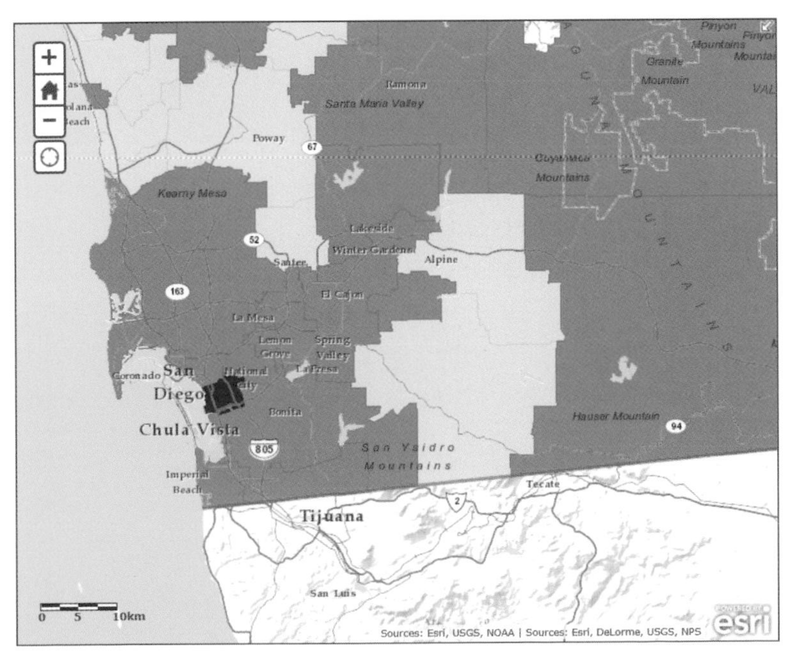

T 1-6

10 **Click Done Adding Layers.**

Change layer transparency

1 **In the Contents area, click the arrow to the right of the California Health Indicators layer, click Transparency, and drag the transparency bar to 50%.** The shaded relief under the health indicator polygons is now visible.

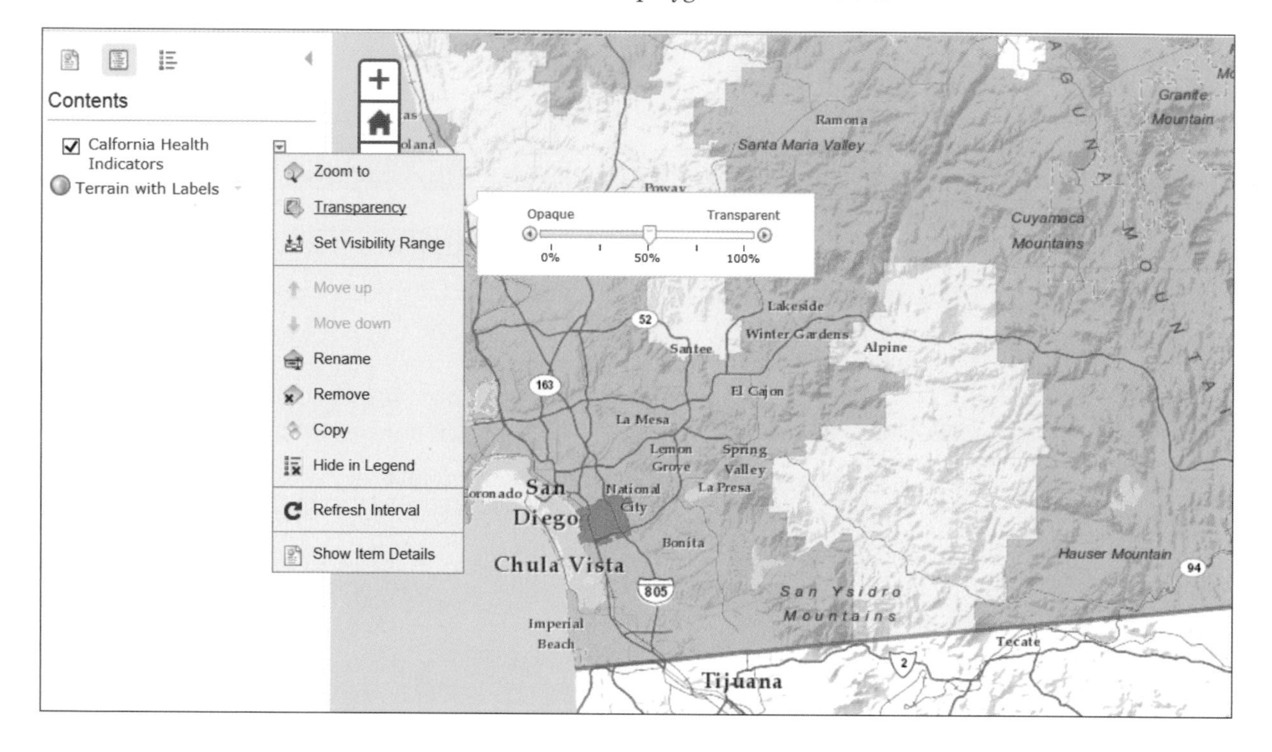

Explore layer content and legends

1 **Select the check box next to the California Health Indicators layer.** This turns the layer off.

2 **Select the check box again to turn the layer on.**

3 **Zoom and pan to San Diego Naval Air Station near San Diego Bay.** The resulting map displays graduated point markers symbolizing the number of overweight children per school.

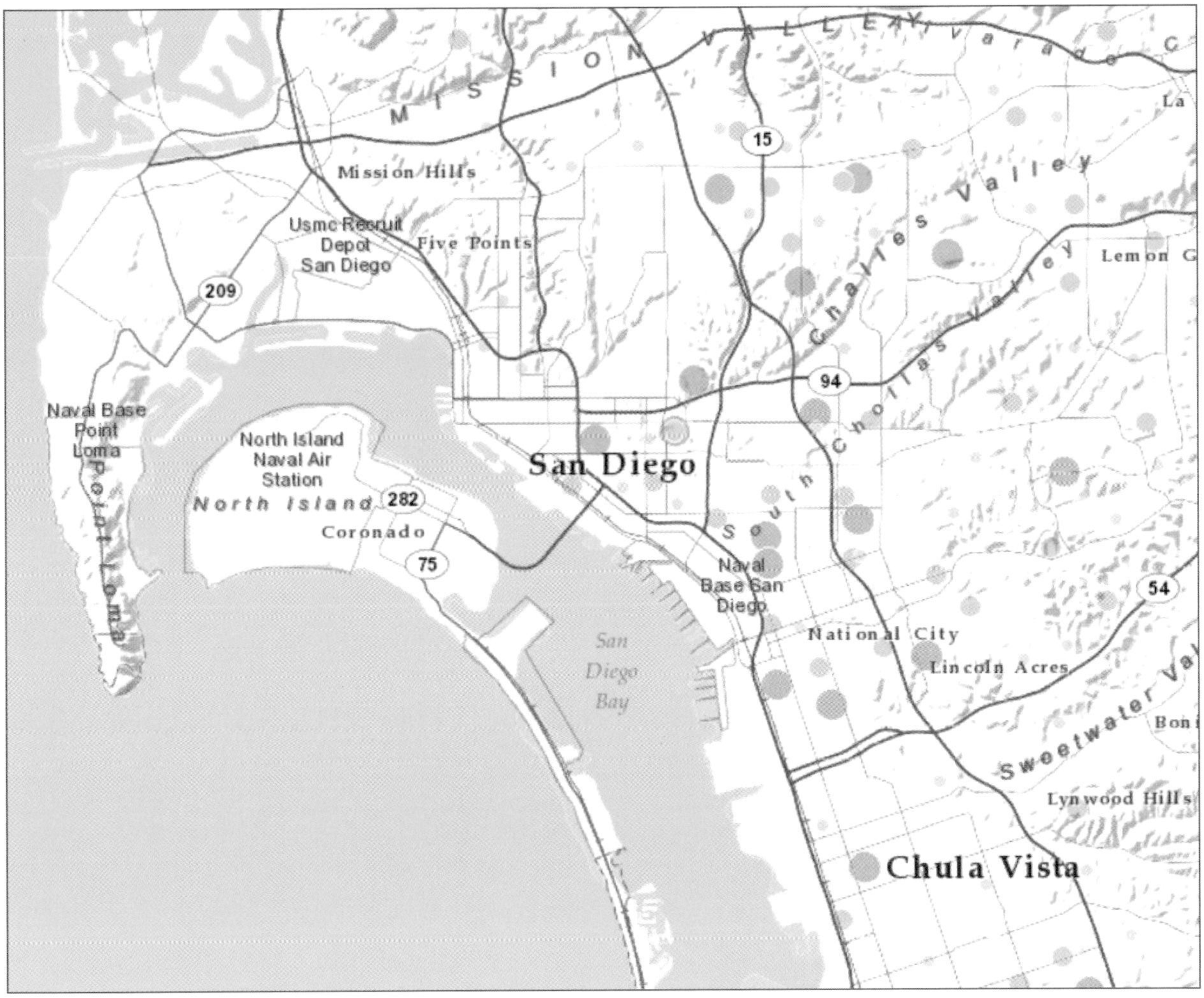

4 **In the Contents list, click California Health Indicators (not its check box) and then % Overweight by School.** The map legend shows the classifications for the number of overweight children by school.

5 Click the Show Map Legend button . The resulting map has a nice legend and is a detailed map.

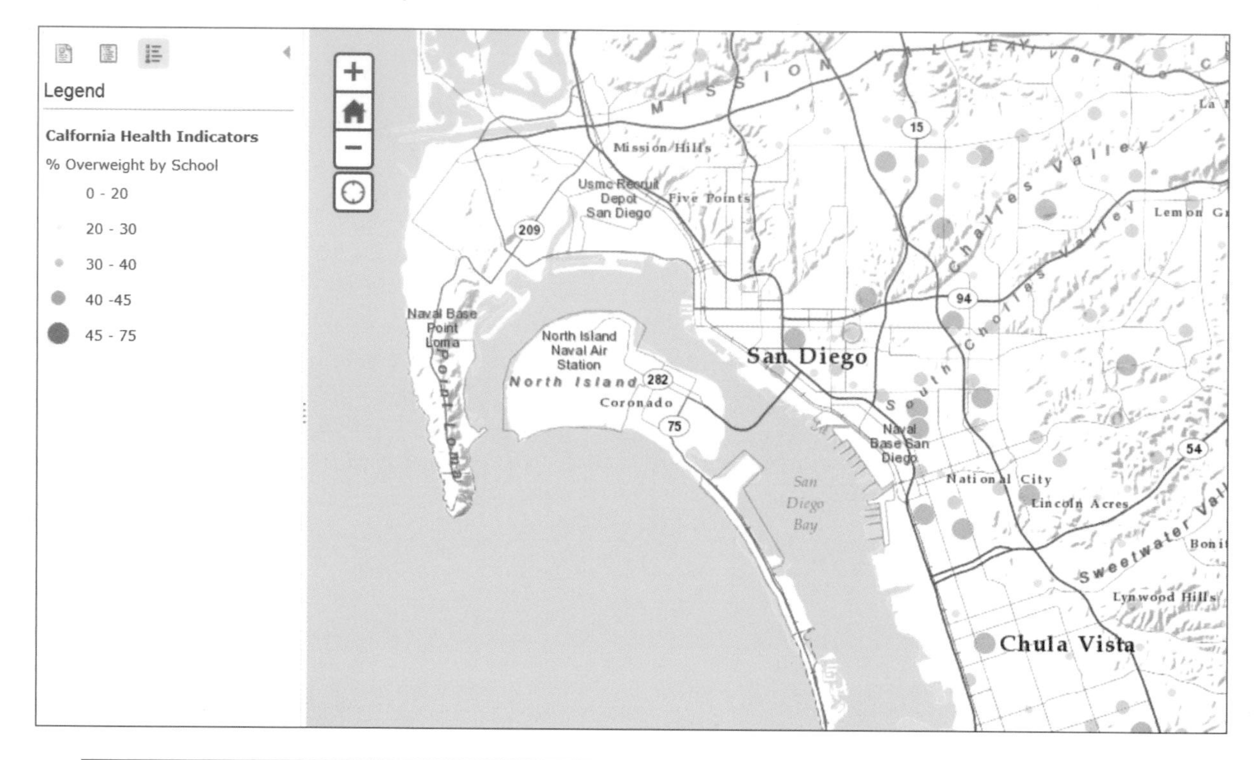

YOUR TURN

Zoom in to see school names displayed on the map. Change the basemap to see street-level details. Zoom back to the San Diego Bay area. Change the basemap back to Terrain with Labels.

Explore a layer description

1 Click the Show Contents of Map button .

2 Click the arrow to the right of the Terrain with Labels layer and select Description. A web page describing the basemap layer appears.

Terrain with Labels

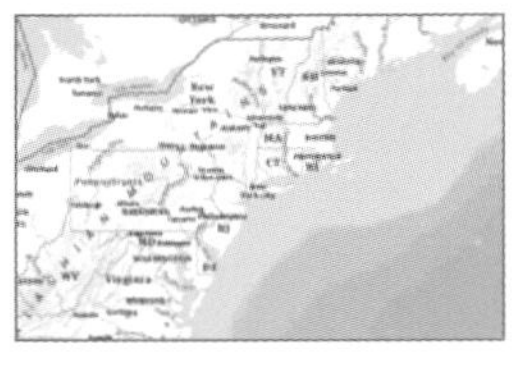

This map features shaded relief imagery, bathymetry and coastal water features that provide neutral background with political boundaries and placenames for reference purposes.

Web Map by esri_en
Last Modified: September 18, 2013

(1 rating, 6,369,159 views)

Facebook Twitter

OPEN SHARE

Description

This map features shaded relief imagery, bathymetry and coastal water features that provide neutral background with political boundaries and placenames for reference purposes. The map is intended to support the ArcGIS Online basemap gallery. For more details on the map, please visit the World Terrain Base and World Reference Overlay map service descriptions.

Access and Use Constraints

This work is licensed under the Esri Master License Agreement.
View Terms of Use

Map Contents

Terrain with Labels:
http://services.arcgisonline.com/ArcGIS/rest/services/World_Terrain_Base/MapServer
Terrain with Labels:
http://services.arcgisonline.com/ArcGIS/rest/services/Reference/World_Reference_Overlay/MapServer

Properties

Tags	basemap	
Credits		
Size	1 KB	
Extent	Left: -180	Right: 180
	Top: 90	Bottom: -90

3 Scroll to read the entire map description. When you are finished, click the Map link to go back to the ArcGIS My Map page.

Save the map

1 On the Map toolbar, click the Save Map button Save **and then Save.**

2 In the Title box, type Overweight Children By School **and for the tag, type** obesity.

3 In the "Save in folder" box, select your ArcGIS Online Account.

4 Click Save Map.

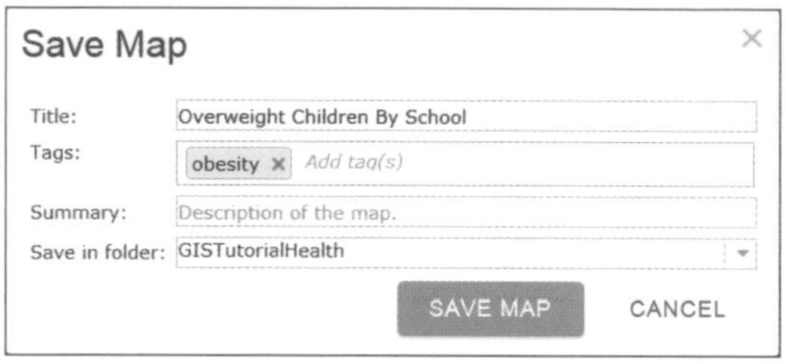

Save Map

Title: Overweight Children By School

Tags: obesity × Add tag(s)

Summary: Description of the map.

Save in folder: GISTutorialHealth

SAVE MAP CANCEL

YOUR TURN

Select Add and Search for Layers. Type **food** as a layer to search for in ArcGIS Online and add the food layers called Supermarket Access Map Service and USA Farmers Markets map service to your map. The latter map service contains locations of farmers' markets as reported to the US Department of Agriculture (USDA). Zoom to various areas of California and see if there is a correlation between overweight children by school and access to supermarkets and farmers' markets. Practice turning layers on and off. Save your map as a new map called **Overweight Children Compared to Food Sources** with the tags **obesity, food**.

Tutorial 1-7

Using maps on a smart phone and tablets

Free ArcGIS apps are available from Google Play, the Apple App Store, Amazon Appstore, and Windows Marketplace. In these exercises you learn how to use the ArcGIS app on the iPhone but similar steps can be used on other smart devices. Open a map in ArcGIS Explorer Online

1 **Search for ArcGIS at the Apple App Store and install Esri ArcGIS on your iPhone.**

2 **Open the Esri ArcGIS app.**

3 **Click the Sign In button.**

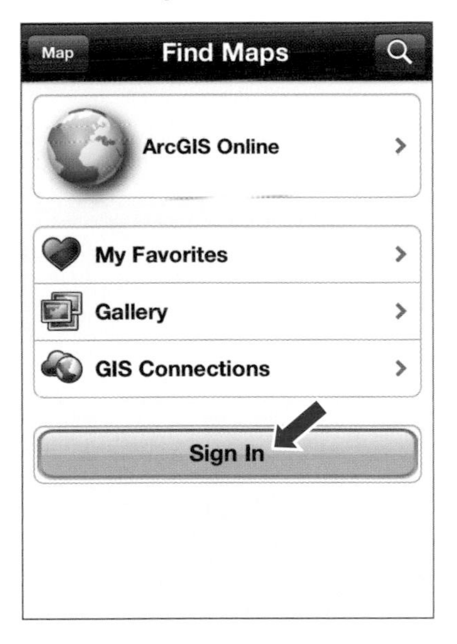

4 Enter your ArcGIS Online (Esri account) username and password.

5 Click the icon in the upper left corner of the app.

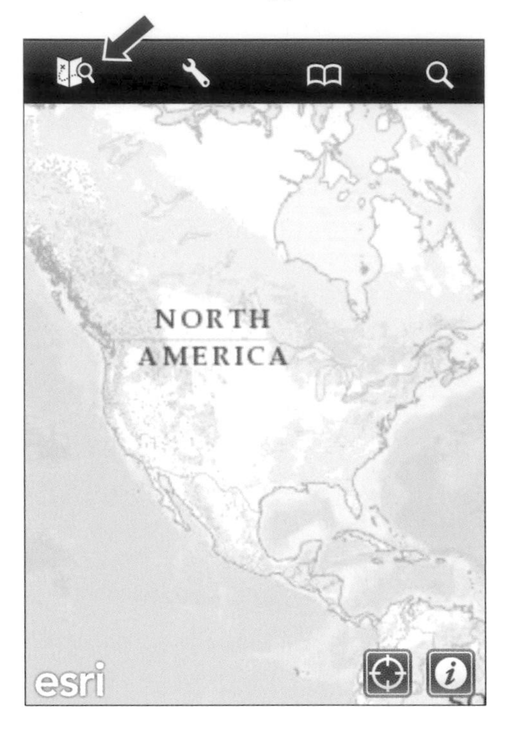

6 Click My Maps.

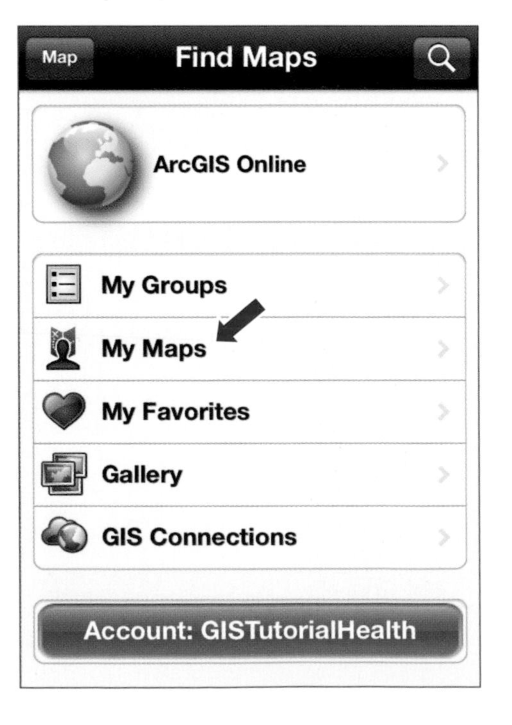

7 **Click the second map, Overweight Children Compared to Food Sources map.** The map opens on your iPhone. ▶

8 **Use usual iPhone gestures to zoom in or out and pan to the Naval Base in San Diego, near the San Diego Bay.**

9 **Click the Identify button on the lower left of the screen.** This provides access to three buttons: Legend for the map legend, Content for the table of contents, and Detail for documentation. ▶

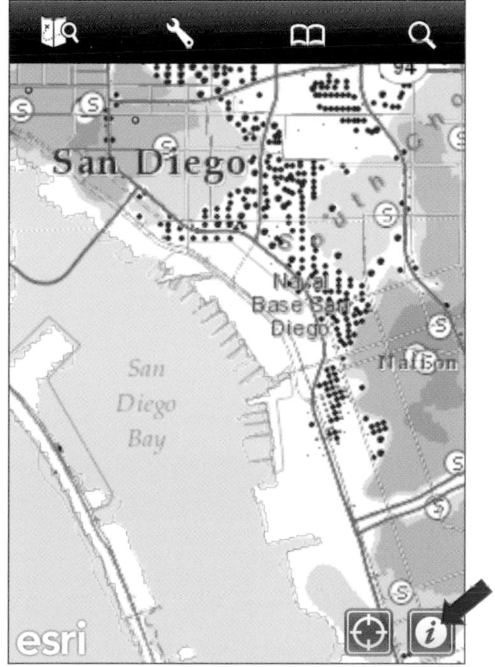

The legend appears by default. ▶

Map Overweight Childr...

Supermarkets

Supermarkets included in analysis

T = Supermarket, included

Supermarkets included in analysis

T = Supermarket, included

People

People in Poverty with Low Access

1 - 4 people

5 - 10

11 - 50

51 - 100

Legend Content Detail

10 Click the Content button. The layers you added in ArcGIS.com appear. You can turn layers on and off and change the basemap. The Detail button will show documentation about the map creation. ▶

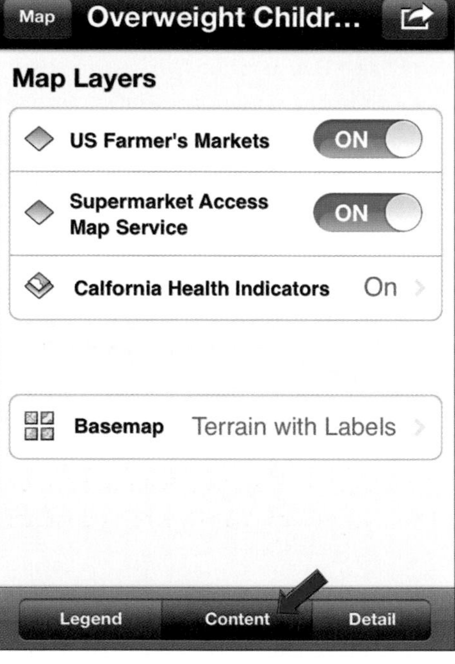

11 Click the Map button at the top left of the screen. You now see your map again.

YOUR TURN

Explore other smart app functions such as Measure Distance, Measure Area, and Bookmarks found on the top bar of the app.

Summary

GIS is a fascinating and valuable information technology, enabling spatial processing and visualization of data in ways never before possible. At the most basic level, GIS makes it easy to quickly compose and render maps from base layers. You can easily turn map layers on and off to study spatial patterns and correlations. You saw how GIS connects visual maps and underlying attribute data when you labeled map features and used choropleth and graduated point marker maps to render numeric scales for variables. In later tutorials, you will discover additional powerful uses for attribute data connected to map features.

Three components make GIS analysis possible for applications such as health care. The first is the national map infrastructure—a collection of basemaps, census and other data, and geocodes for uniquely identifying areas. In the United States, this resource is a public good, paid for by tax dollars and available for use at no or nominal cost. Commercial map layers are also available at reasonable cost and in many cases are essential for applications. This chapter introduced important components of map layers, including geographic and rectangular coordinate systems, projections between the two types of coordinate systems, and map scale.

The second component necessary for applications is user-friendly and powerful GIS software. ArcGIS for Desktop is the software used in this book. This chapter covered the primary uses and interfaces of the two major ArcGIS application packages: the ArcCatalog utility for browsing and maintaining spatial data files and ArcMap for creating maps and analyzing data. This chapter asked you to examine the input map layers and GIS data for studying lung cancer mortality in white males. The spatial patterns you observed suggest possible correlations within the mortality data, including poverty, tobacco growing, and coal mining.

The third component explores online GIS tools developed by Esri—ArcGIS Online. Although the analytic capabilities of these tools are not as advanced as desktop GIS, they are easy to use and enable beginning GIS users to work with, share, and explore existing map layers related to various health conditions such as obesity.

We should probably add a fourth component that is necessary for successful GIS applications: GIS analysts. Knowing how to use GIS is not a common skill, and there is a lot to learn. Nevertheless, this book will help you use GIS productively and efficiently, and make the best use of your limited and valuable time.

Assignment 1-1
Benchmark health GIS websites

Many health organizations make maps and basic GIS functions available online. Examples include the World Health Organization Public Health Mapping and GIS website (http://www.who.int/topics/geographic_information_systems/en/), the Geographic Information Systems (GIS) at the Centers for Disease Control and Prevention (http://www.cdc.gov/gis/), and the National Cancer Institute (http://www3.cancer.gov/atlasplus).

Note: URLs may change. If you cannot access these sites for the World Health Organization, Centers for Disease Control, or National Cancer Institute, try to find similar sites for these organizations.

The objective of this assignment is to investigate the unique capabilities of GIS and its applications to health. Start by studying the aforementioned websites. Then browse the Internet to find an interesting health-related website that uses GIS (excluding the sites already listed).

Create a PowerPoint presentation

Create a Microsoft PowerPoint presentation called **Assignment1-1YourName.pptx** and save it to your Chapter1 folder in MyAssignments. Include the following in your presentation:

- Title page, including title, website URL, and your name
- Purpose of the website and its use of GIS
- Screen captures of the website (about half a dozen), including maps
- A brief analysis of the GIS that includes:
  - GIS content provided
  - GIS functionality provided
  - Effectiveness in providing information
  - Ease of use
- Summary of what makes the website valuable in terms of functionality and content

WHAT TO TURN IN

If your work is to be graded, turn in the following files:

- ***Microsoft PowerPoint presentation:*** \EsriPress\GISTHealth\MyAssignments\Chapter1\Assignment1-1YourName.pptx

Assignment 1-2
Create a map using GIS websites

Many organizations have data in tables or spreadsheets stored as addresses or latitude and longitude points and want to use interactive map viewers to view locations and other GIS layers over the Internet. For example, a health care organization might have street addresses for hospitals or clinics. These can be added to ArcGIS Online, then compared with layers using content provided by Esri, its partners, or the GIS community at large. In this assignment you add an Excel spreadsheet of mammography clinics for one county from your desktop computer, add population or other health layers from ArcGIS Online, and share the results with the public.

Start with the following:

\EsriPress\GISTHealth\Data\Datafiles\Clinics.csv – comma separated files of mammography clinics in Allegheny County, PA and surrounding areas. The file includes clinic addresses and ZIP Codes.

Create an ArcGIS map

Requirements are:

- In ArcGIS.com, add the mammography clinics comma separated file (using addresses) to a new map using the option "Add Layer From File".
- From ArcGIS Online, find and add a population layer displaying the US Median Age.
- From ArcGIS Online, find another interesting related layer (for example, other population or health) and add it to your map.
- Save your map called **Assignment1-2YourName** using tags mammography, clinics, population.
- Share your finished map with the public. Note the URL for the map link created when you shared the map.

Create a PowerPoint presentation

Copy and paste your map image(s) into a Microsoft PowerPoint presentation called Assignment1-2YourName.pptx and save it to your Chapter1 folder in MyAssignments.

Include the following:

- Title slide including your name and the URL link to your map on ArcGIS.com that was created when you shared it.
- Slide explaining the slide(s) to come
- Slide including map of mammography clinics and US Median Age with observations (for example, are mammography clinics in locations where the population is over the age of 40?)
- Slide including map of mammography clinics and other layer found on ArcGIS.com with observations.
- Summary slide describing other data that would be useful for this study.

> ***Hint:*** *To create a screen capture of your slides, use the PRINT SCREEN key to save a graphic image of your map(s). Then use Copy and Paste or CTRL+V to paste the image into your PowerPoint slides. Mac users can press COMMAND+SHIFT+4 to save an image.*

WHAT TO TURN IN

If your work is to be graded, turn in the following files:

- ***Microsoft PowerPoint presentation:*** \EsriPress\GISTHealth\MyAssignments\Chapter1\Assignment1-2YourName.pptx

Assignment 1-3

Create and upload layer packages

Sharing map layers that you create using your ArcGIS for Desktop application will allow others to benefit from your map expertise. In this assignment, you will create additional population and health layers using a map document you used earlier in this chapter.

Create population and health layer packages

Start ArcMap and open map document Tutorial1-4.mxd.

Create layer packages for the following map layers:

- Cities with 250,000 or Greater Population called **MajorUSCities.lpk** and saved to your Chapter1 folder in MyAssignments
- States called **States.lpk** and saved to your Chapter1 folder in MyAssignments
- Percentage Female-Headed Households with Children called **PercentageFHHChildren.lpk** and saved to your Chapter1 folder in MyAssignments
- Lung Cancer Mortality per 100,000 White Males, 1970–1994, called **WhiteMaleLungCancerMortality70_94.lpk** and saved to your Chapter1 folder in MyAssignments

Add these layer packages to your ArcGIS Online account in the My Content section. These layer packages will then be ready to share with others should you choose to do so.

WHAT TO TURN IN

If your work is to be graded, turn in the following files:

- ***Layer packages:***
  - EsriPress\GISTHealth\MyAssignments\Chapter1\MajorUSCities.lpk
  - \EsriPress\GISTHealth\MyAssignments\Chapter1\States.lpk
  - \EsriPress\GISTHealth\MyAssignments\Chapter1\PercentageFHHChildren.lpk
  - \EsriPress\GISTHealth\MyAssignments\Chapter1\WhiteMaleLungCancerMortality70_94.lpk

If instructed to do so, instead of individual files, turn in a compressed file, **Assignment1-3YourName.zip**, that includes all the preceding files. Do not include path information in the compressed file.

References

Clarke, K. C. 2003. *Getting Started with Geographic Information Systems.* 4th ed. Upper Saddle River, NJ: Prentice Hall.

Featherly, K. 2004. "Battling Bioterror." *Healthcare informatics Online.* http://www.healthcare-informatics.com/issues/2004/02_04/cover.htm#disease (no longer available).

Hagland, M. 2004. "Harnessing Efficiency." *Healthcare Informatics Online.* http://www.healthcare-informatics.com/issues/2004/02_04/cover.htm#workflow (no longer available).

Johnson, M., W. L. Gorr, and S. Roehrig. 2005. "Location of Service Facilities for the Elderly." *Annals of Operations Research* 136, no. 1: 329–49.

Kennedy, E. 2004. "Statement on the Introduction of the Health Care Modernization, Cost Reduction, and Quality Improvement Act". http://kennedy.senate.gov/~kennedy/statements/04/05/2004513C28.html (no longer available).

Protti, D. J. 2005. "The Use of Computers in Health Care Can Reduce Errors, Improve Patient Safety, and Enhance the Quality of Service: There is Evidence." Special Report: IT in the Health-Care Industry. *The Economist* 65 (April 30, 2005). http://www.connectingforhealth.nhs.uk/worldview/protti2 (no longer available).

Chapter 2

Visualizing health data

Objectives

- Visualize breast cancer mortality by US county
- Understand the composition of GIS map layers
- Learn how to navigate using zooming, panning, and bookmarks
- Understand the connection between visual map features and tabular data
- Learn how to select subsets of map features for processing
- Learn how to find map features
- Use data sorting and labeling to produce information

Health-care scenario

According to the National Cancer Society, breast cancer remains the most frequently diagnosed cancer in women in the United States. Determining top geographic areas where breast cancer deaths occur may lead health officials to provide better targeted screening or interventions.

Solution approach

You are just starting to use ArcGIS, so this chapter focuses on the basics of understanding and using GIS. To begin, you will work with an existing GIS document that you will open in ArcMap and modify by adding and symbolizing a map layer. Once the map document is in usable form, you will explore the map and associated attribute data using several GIS tools to do the following:

- Zoom, pan, and set spatial bookmarks to get close-up views of the map in selected areas of the United States
- Find and identify features and access feature attribute data to get information
- Select subsets of map layers to work with them and sort records to identify top cancer counties
- Label and annotate to add information to maps

Tutorial 2-1
Manipulating layers in a map document

In the first part of this chapter, you will learn the basics of the ArcMap software package. You will begin by opening an existing map document, and then learn how to add and manipulate map layers.

Start ArcMap and open an existing map document

1 **On the taskbar, click Start and then All Programs > ArcGIS > ArcMap 10.2**

2 **Browse through the Maps folder, select Tutorial2-1.mxd, click Open, and click OK if prompted by a warning on VBA code.** This map of US cities and states has two map layers already included, renamed, and symbolized. The first layer is Major US Cities (with population over 100,000). The second layer is Breast Cancer Deaths by State. We downloaded this data from the National Cancer Institute's Cancer Mortality Maps website, http://www3.cancer.gov/atlasplus. This site provides valuable information about cancer mortality in the United States during the time period 1950–2004, based on data obtained from the National Center for Health Statistics (NCHS), the federal government's principal vital- and health-statistics agency. If you wish to obtain other cancer statistics, visit this site or other websites such as http://www.cancer.gov/, http://seer.cancer.gov/, and http://wonder.cdc.gov/ (See facing page.)

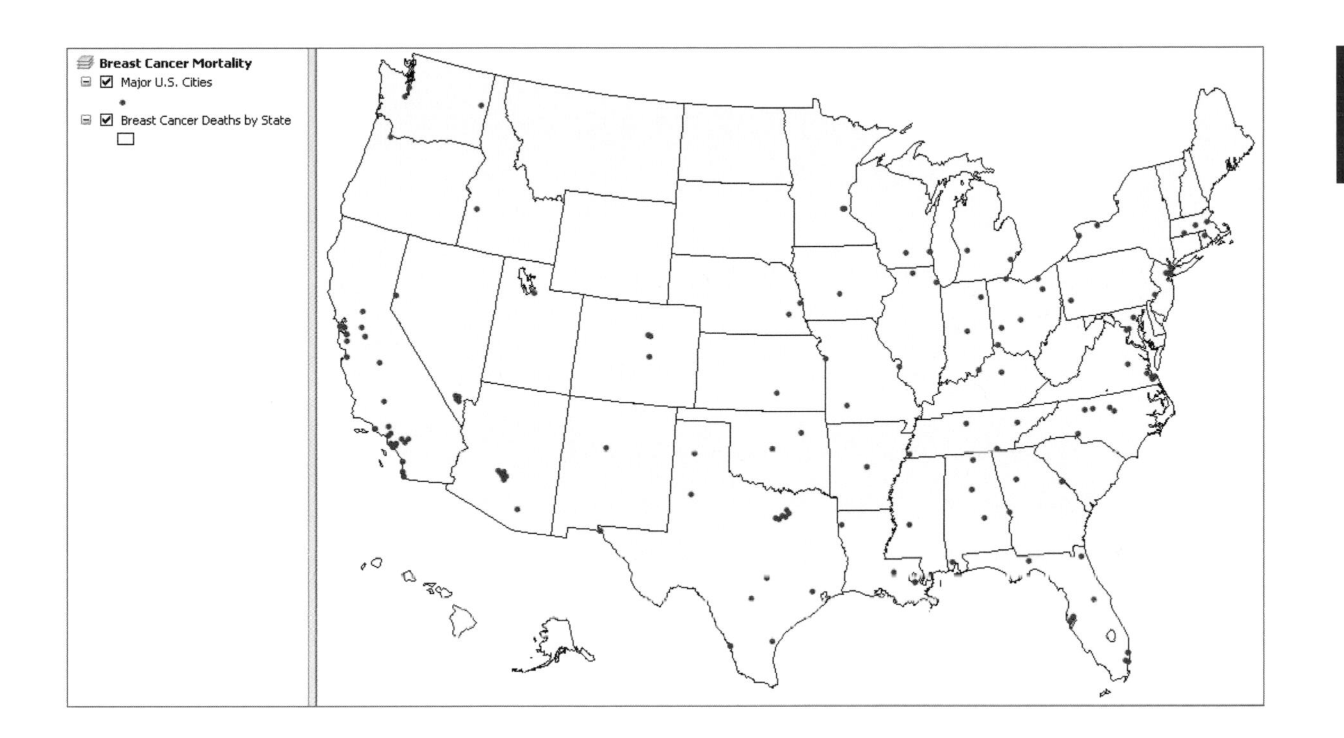

Add a layer

You can add additional map layers to your map for more detailed analysis. For example, the National Cancer Institute collects cancer data by county as well as by state. You can add a layer of data showing the breast cancer mortality rates and the number of deaths per county. This data was saved by the authors as a file geodatabase feature class, which contains polygons for counties and related data on death rates.

1 Click the Add Data button .

2 In the Add Data dialog box, click the Connect To Folder button .

3 In the Connect to Folder dialog box, browse to Computer, click the drive where you installed the GISTHealth data (for example, C:\), and click OK.
You only need to browse to the root drive and not go beyond this point. Once this connection is made, you can easily browse to any folder on this computer drive. If your data is stored on an external drive such as a jump drive, you will need to connect to that drive.

4 In the Add Data dialog box, browse to \EsriPress\GISTHealth\Data\NCI.gdb, click the BreCounty layer, and click Add.

Add Data
Look in: NCI.gdb
BreCounty
BreState
LungCounty
LungState
Name:
Show of type: Datasets, Layers and Results
Add
Cancel

ArcMap chooses a random color for the counties layer. You will change the color later.

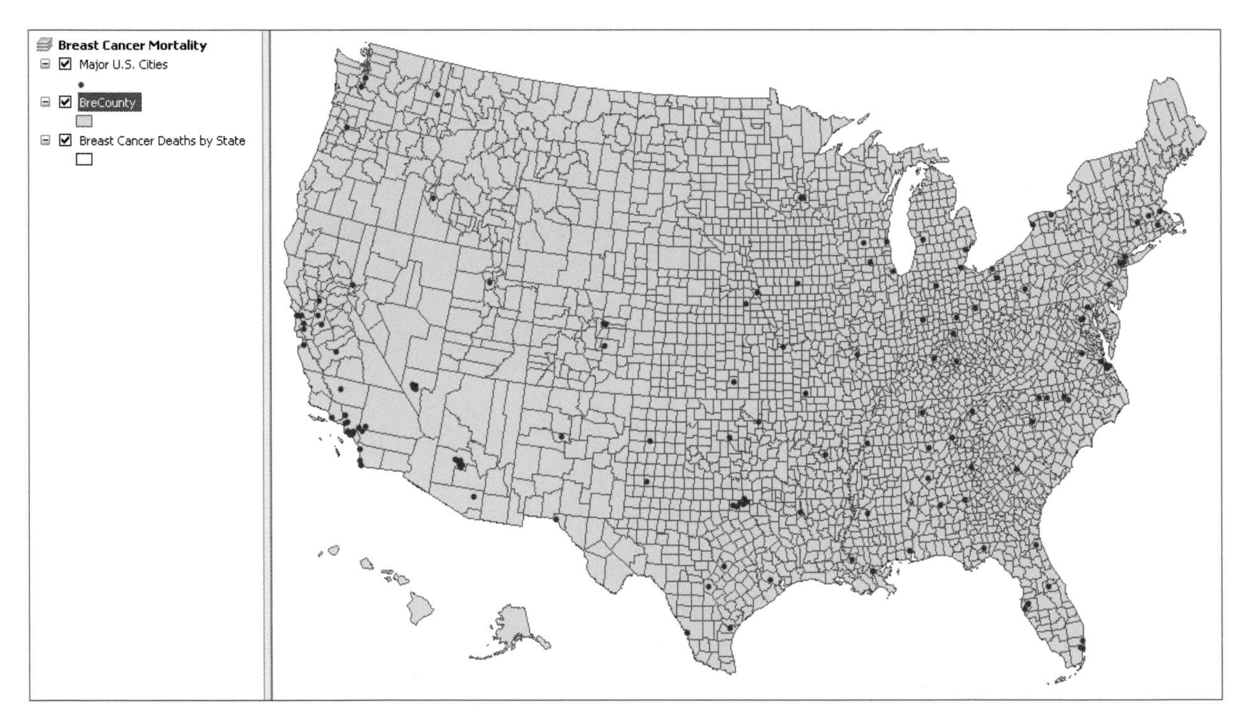

Change the layer display order

Changing a layer's display order is important because features may be covered up by other features in your map. ArcMap draws map layers from the bottom up, so if larger features are on top of smaller features, the smaller ones will not display.

1 Click the List By Drawing Order button, and then in the table of contents, press and hold the left mouse button on the Major U.S. Cities layer.

2 **Drag the Major U.S. Cities layer to the bottom of the table of contents.**
Because the cities layer is now drawn first, its points are covered up by the states and counties layers and cannot be seen.

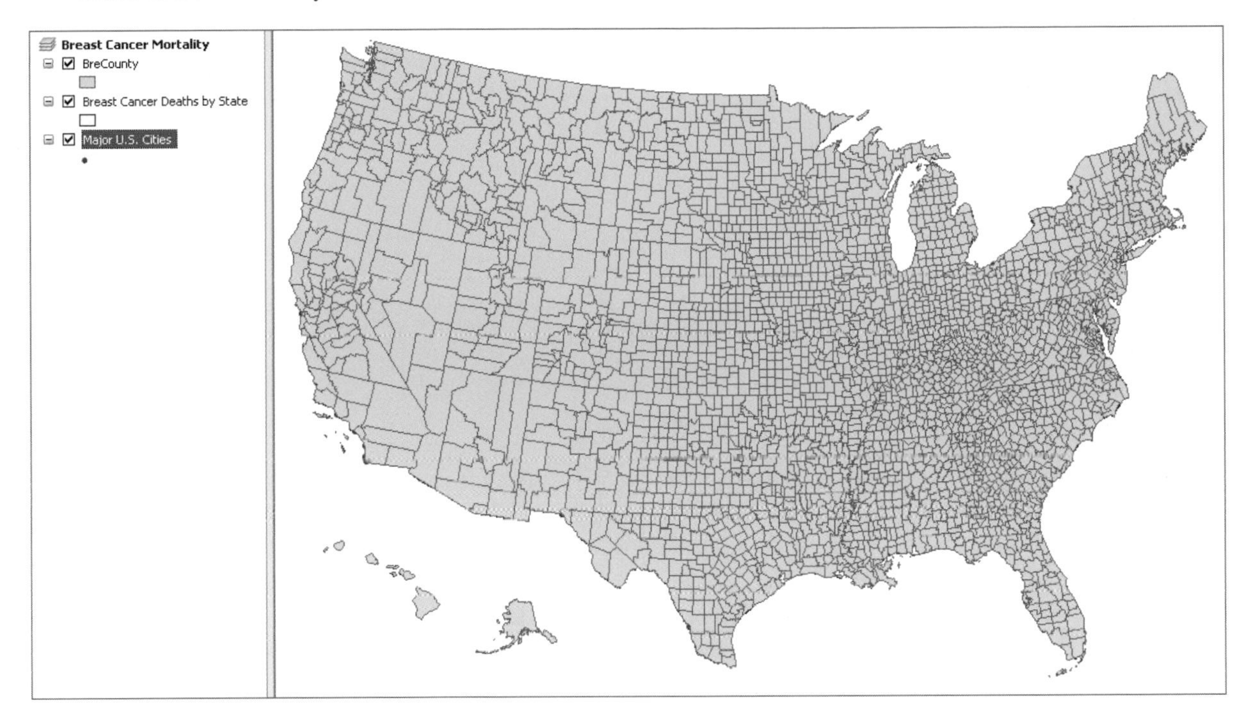

3 **Drag the Major U.S. Cities layer back to the top of the table of contents.**
Because the cities layer is now drawn last, its points can again be seen.

YOUR TURN

Drag the BreCounty layer to the bottom of the list and observe what happens. Then drag it back to the middle of the three layers.

Rename a layer

You will notice that when you initially add a layer, ArcMap uses the name of the feature class as the default name of the layer in the table of contents. You will often want to change the name of the layer to a label that is easier to understand.

1 **In the table of contents, right-click the BreCounty layer and select Properties.**

2 **Click the General tab, and in the Layer Name box, type** Breast Cancer Deaths by County **and then click OK.** The layer name is now changed in the table of contents.

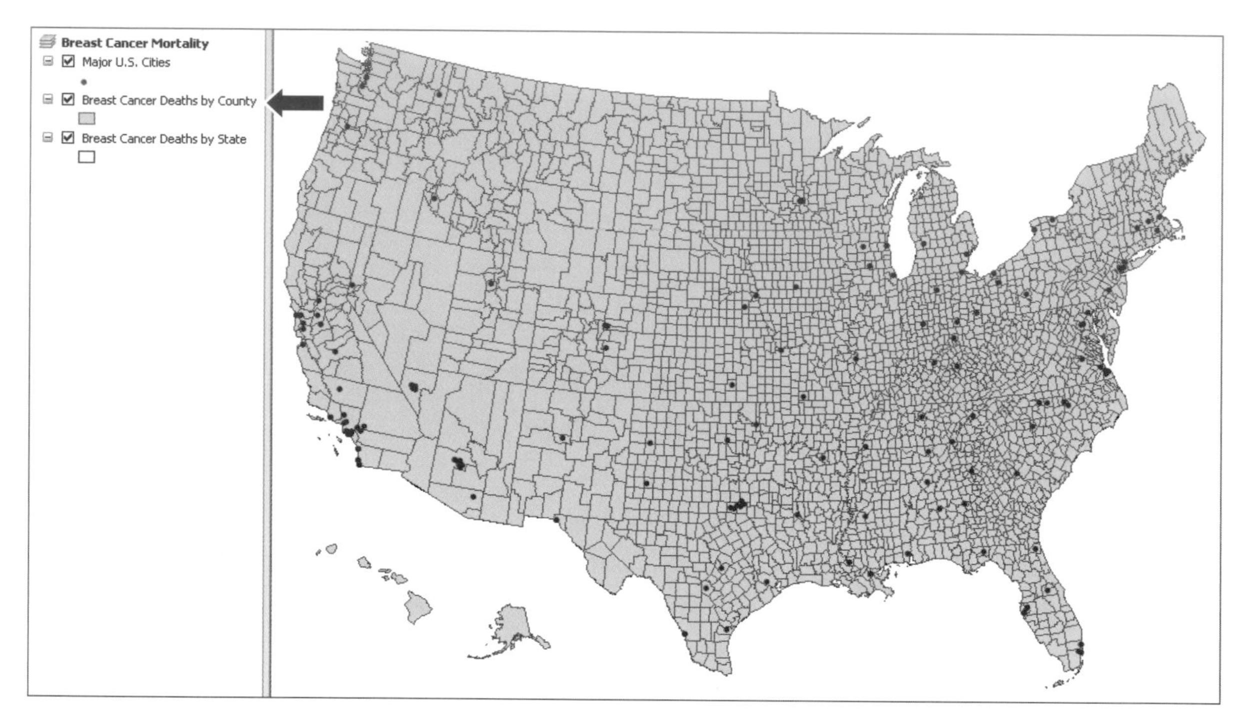

Change the boundary-layer fill color

To better see the counties for the Breast Cancer Deaths by County layer, you will want to change the color properties of both the county and the state layers. First, you will change the counties to a white fill color with a light-gray outline.

1 **In the table of contents, click the layer symbol for Breast Cancer Deaths by County.** The layer symbol is the rectangle below the layer name in the table of contents.

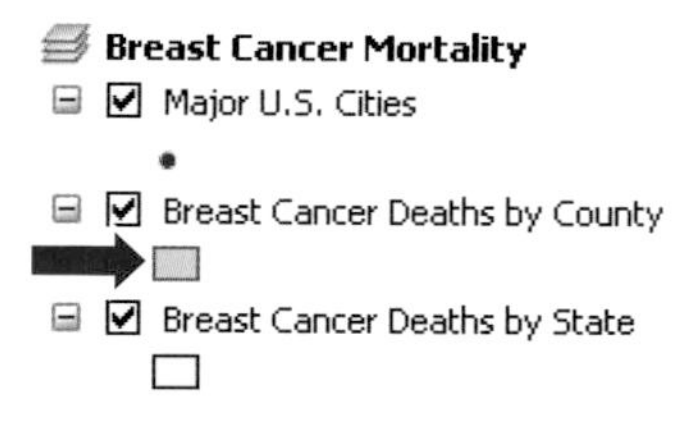

2 In the resulting Symbol Selector dialog box, click the Fill Color arrow.

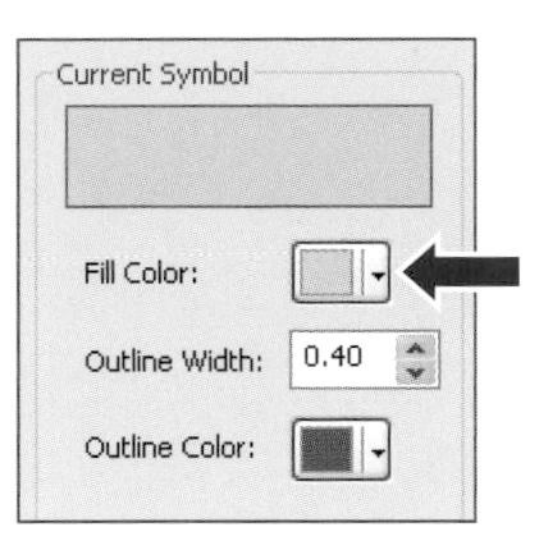

3 In the color palette, click the Arctic White tile.

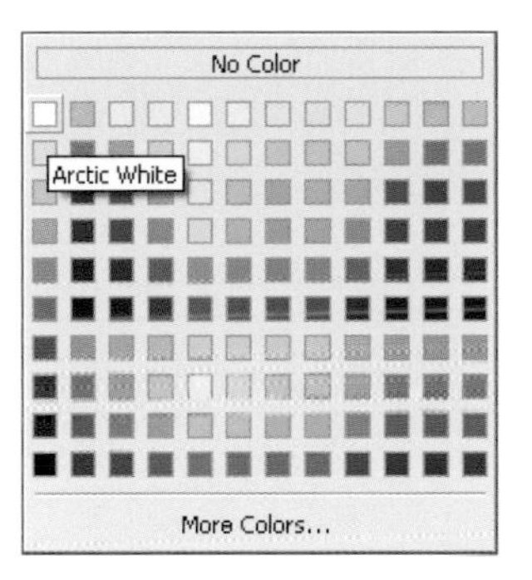

4 Click OK. On the map, the fill color of the layer changes to Arctic white.

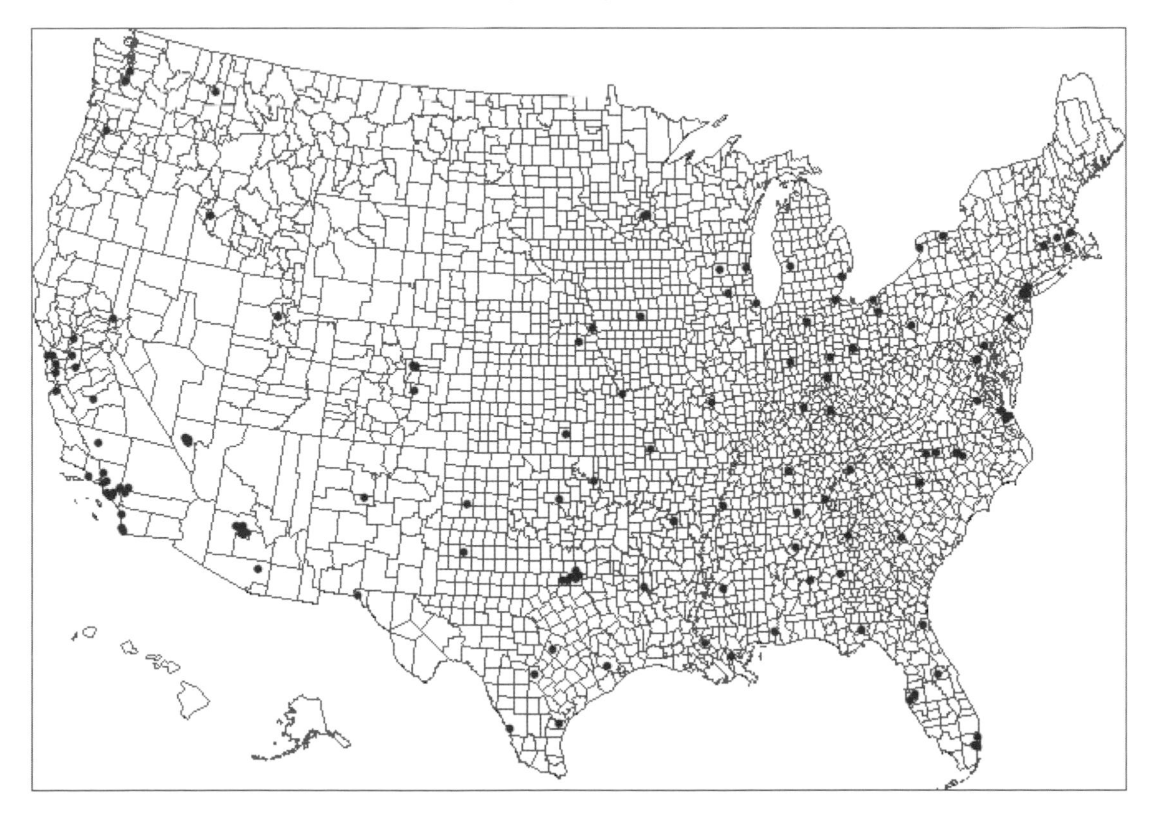

Change the layer outline color

1 **In the table of contents, click the layer symbol for Breast Cancer Deaths by County.**

2 **In the Symbol Selector dialog box, click the Outline Color arrow.**

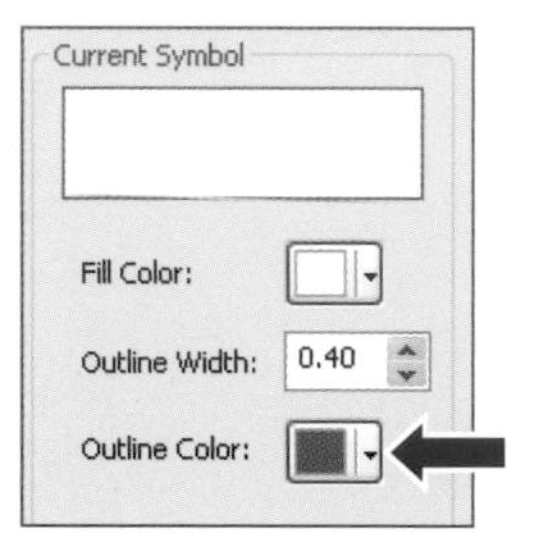

3 **In the color palette, click the Gray 20% tile.**

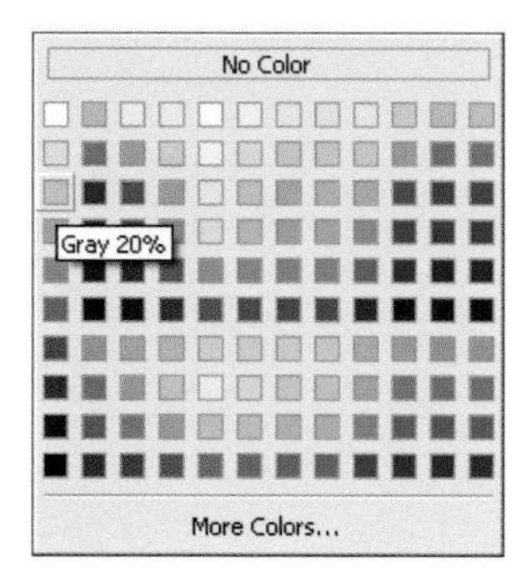

4 **Click OK.** On the map, the outline color of the layer changes to light gray.

Change the layer outline width

Because county and state boundaries share some of the same lines, it is useful to display the Breast Cancer Deaths by State layer using a Hollow fill and a dark, thick outline so you can see the county polygons above it.

1 **In the table of contents, click the layer symbol for Breast Cancer Deaths by State.**

2 **In the Symbol Selector dialog box, click Hollow.**

3 **In the Outline Width box, type** 1.25, **and click OK.** (See facing page.)

4 **In the table of contents, drag the Breast Cancer Deaths by State layer so it is just above Breast Cancer Deaths by County.** The resulting map is much easier to read. The layer names are self-descriptive, and it is easy to distinguish between the county and state outlines.

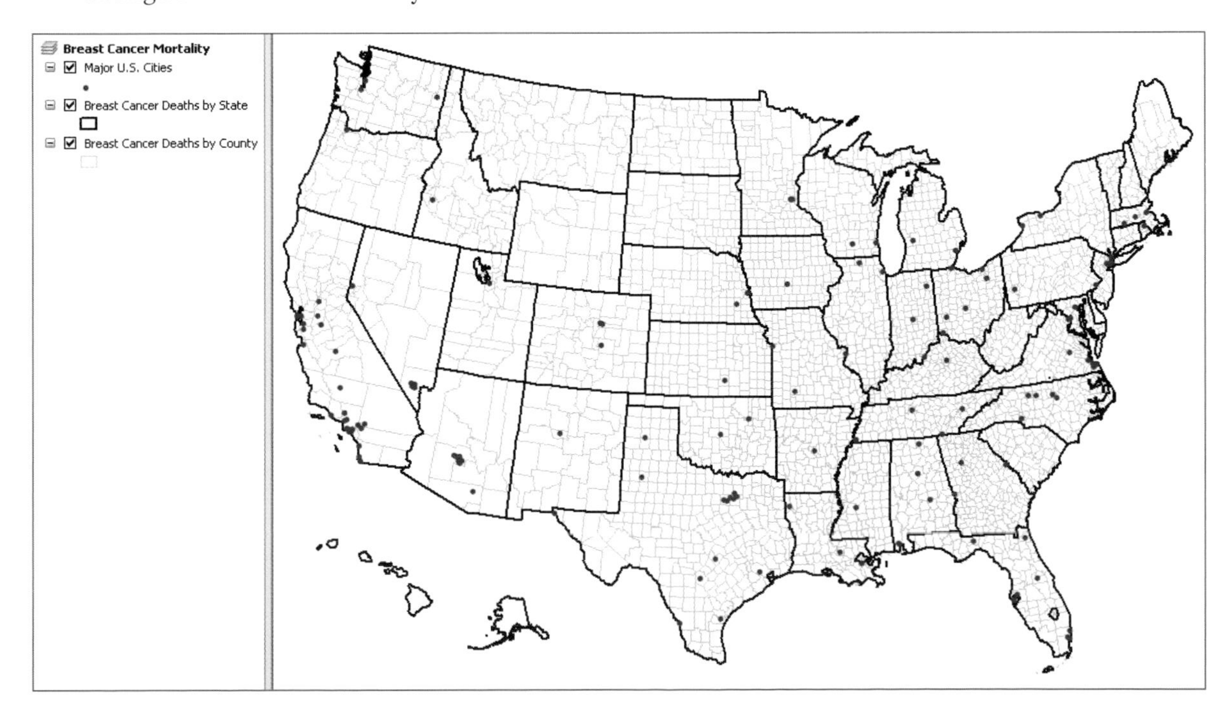

Drag a layer from the Catalog window into the table of contents

The Catalog window allows you to explore, maintain, and use GIS data through its many ArcCatalog utility functions. From Catalog, you will drag a map layer into the table of contents as an alternative method to add data.

1 **Click Windows > Catalog.**

2 **In the Catalog window, browse through the Data folder to UnitedStates.gdb.**

3 **Drag USLakes from UnitedStates.gdb in the Catalog window to the top of the table of contents. If you get a warning about the coordinate system, click yes to "use this coordinate system anyway."** The map layers in the table of contents draw in order from the bottom up, so if you dropped USLakes at the bottom of the table of contents, the states would cover the lake features.

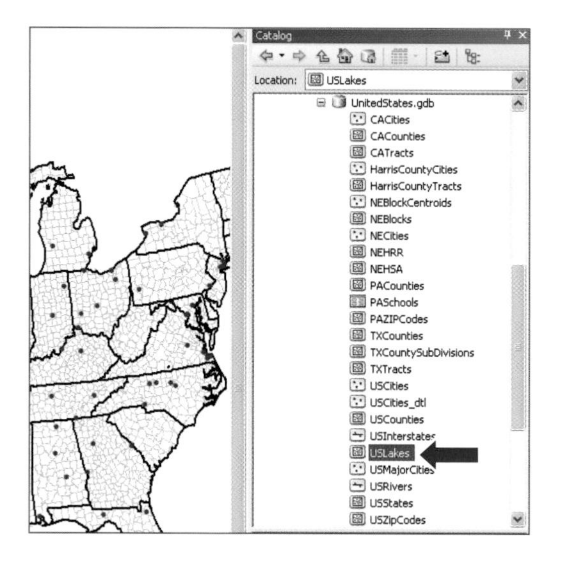

Remove a layer

1 **In the table of contents, right-click USLakes and click Remove.** This action removes a map layer from the map document, but it does not delete it from its storage location—in this case, the United States geodatabase.

YOUR TURN

From the Catalog window, add USRivers and USInterstates from the United States geodatabase. Practice changing the layer colors and outlines, drag the layers to the top and the bottom of the table of contents, and remove the layers when you are finished.

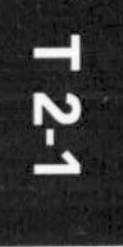

Use Auto Hide for the Catalog window

Notice that when you opened the Catalog window, it opened in pinned-open mode, which keeps the window open and handy for use but also covers part of your map. The Auto Hide feature of this application window, along with other application windows such as the Table Of Contents and Search windows, keeps the windows available for immediate use but hides them between uses so that you have more room for your map.

1 **Click the Auto Hide button at the top of the Catalog window.** The window closes but leaves a Catalog button on the right side of the ArcMap window Catalog .

2 **Click the Catalog button.** The Catalog window opens.

Next, you will simulate completing a Catalog task by clicking the map document. The window will automatically hide.

3 **Click any place on the map or in the table of contents.**

You can pin the window open again, which you will do next.

4 **Click the Catalog button and then the Unpinned Auto Hide button .** This action pins the Catalog window open until you click the pin again to automatically hide or close the window. Try clicking the map or the table of contents to see the Catalog window remain open.

5 **Close the Catalog window.**

Use relative paths

When you add a layer to a map, ArcMap stores the path to its location in the map document. When you open a map, ArcMap locates the layer data it needs by using this stored path. If ArcMap cannot find the data for a layer, the layer still appears in the ArcMap table of contents, but of course it does not appear on the map. Instead, ArcMap places a red exclamation mark (**!**) next to the layer name to indicate that its path needs repair. You can view information about the data source for a layer and repair it by clicking the Source tab in the Layer Properties dialog box.

Paths can be absolute or relative. An example of an absolute path is C:\EsriPress\GISTHealth\Data\UnitedStates.gdb\USLakes. To share map documents saved with absolute paths, everyone who uses the map must have exactly the same paths to map layers on their computer. That is why rather than absolute paths, the relative path option is favored.

Relative paths in a map specify the location of the layers relative to the current location on the disk of the map document (.mxd file). Because relative paths do not contain drive letter names, the map and its associated data can point to the same directory structure, regardless of the drive or folder in which the map resides. If a project is moved to a new drive, ArcMap will still be able to find the maps and their data by traversing the relative paths.

1 **On the Menu bar, click File > Map Document Properties.** Notice that the check box is selected to "Store relative pathnames to data sources." This option should be set for all map documents in the tutorials and the end-of-chapter assignments in this book.

Map Document Properties
General
File: THealth\MyAssignments\Chapter2\Assignment2-1.mxd
Title: Assignment2-1.mxd
Summary:
Description:
Author: Kurland and Gorr
Credits:
Tags:
Hyperlink base:
Last Saved: 6/17/2011 9:18:18 AM
Last Printed:
Last Exported: 5/3/2011 6:37:47 PM
Default Geodatabase: C:\Documents and Settings\Kristen Kurland\My D
Pathnames: Store relative pathnames to data sources
Thumbnail: Make Thumbnail Delete Thumbnail
OK Cancel Apply

2 **Click OK.**

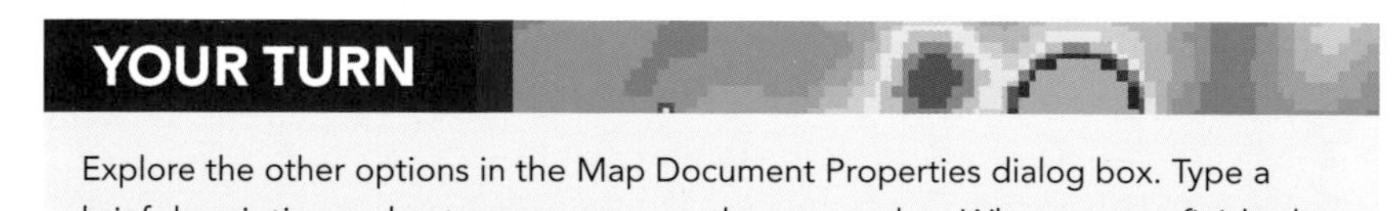

Explore the other options in the Map Document Properties dialog box. Type a brief description and enter your name as the map author. When you are finished, click OK.

Save the map document

1 **On the Menu bar, click File > Save As.**

2 **Save your map document as** Tutorial2-1YourName.mxd **to your Chapter2 folder in MyExercises. If you get a VBA code warning, click OK.** Do not close ArcMap.

Tutorial 2-2

Zooming to and panning health features on a map

Sometimes you will want to concentrate on a particular area of a map. You will also quickly learn that some geographic features are too small to see when viewing an entire map. If you enlarge a particular area, you can see the details more easily. Zooming and panning enlarges or reduces the display and shifts it to reveal different areas of the map. You will find zoom and pan buttons on the Tools toolbar.

Zoom in

1 On the Tools toolbar, click the Zoom In button.

2 Press and hold the mouse button on a point above and to the left of the state of Illinois.

3 Using the mouse, drag the pointer to draw a box around the state of Illinois. Then release the mouse button.

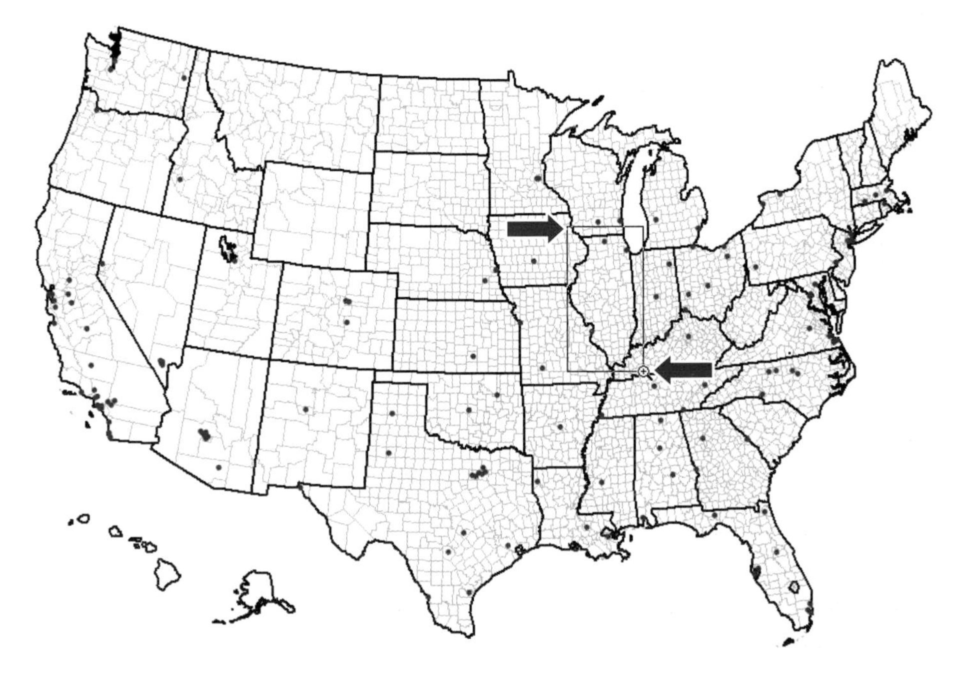

The resulting map is a zoomed area of the state of Illinois.

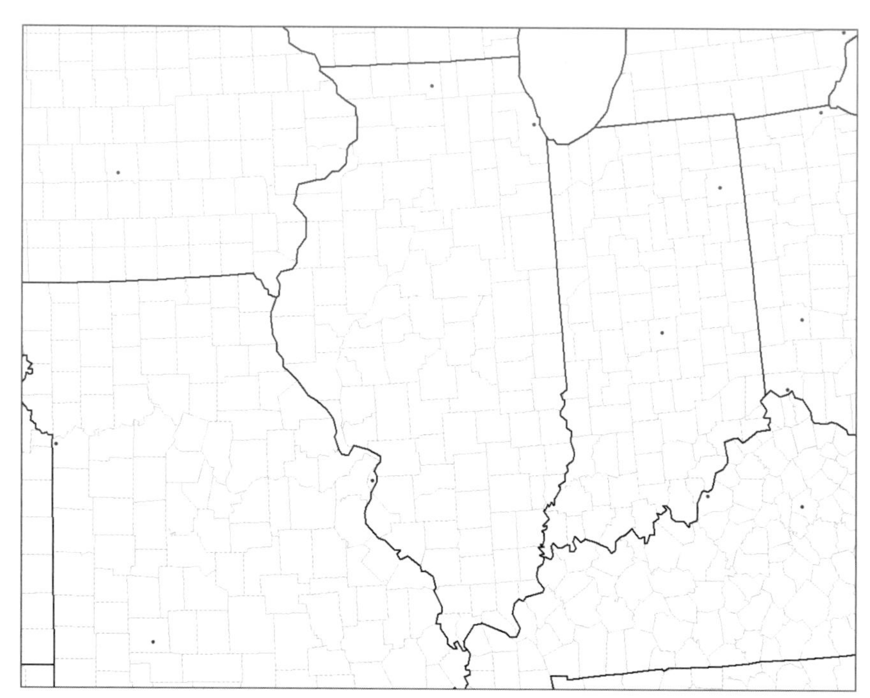

4 **Click the screen to zoom in, centered on the point you clicked.** This is an alternative to drawing a rectangle for zooming in.

Pan

If you want to see a neighboring state without zooming out, use the Pan button.

1 **On the Tools toolbar, click the Pan button .**

2 **Move the pointer anywhere into the map view.**

3 **Pressing the left mouse button, drag the pointer in any direction.**

4 **Release the mouse button.** Panning shifts the current map display to the left or right, up or down, without changing the current scale. In the figure, you can see Illinois, Indiana, and Ohio. (See facing page.)

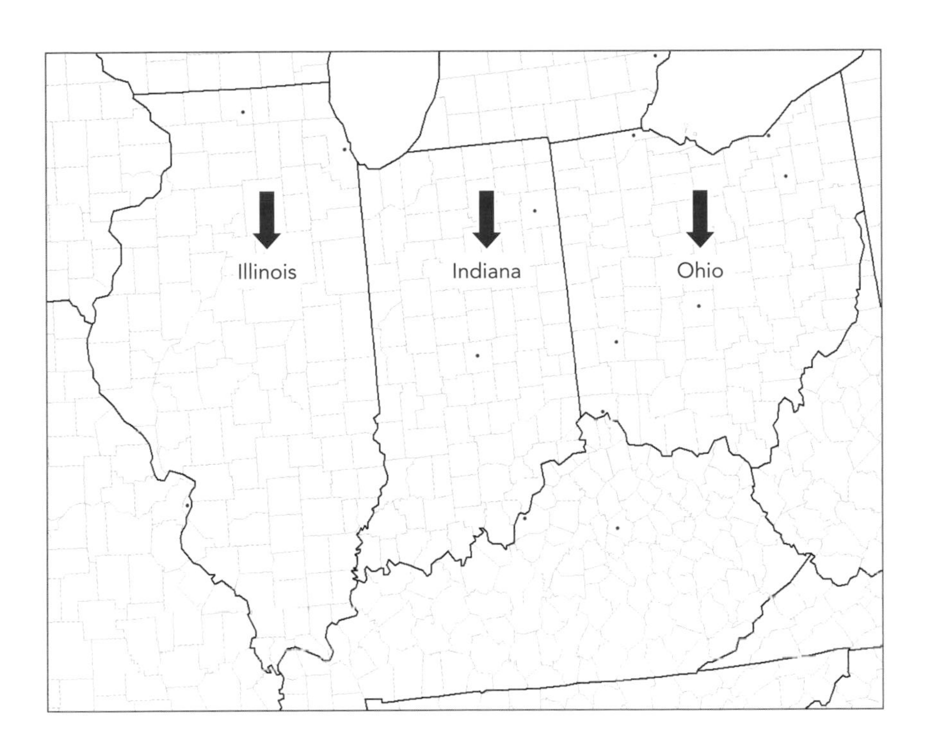

Zoom to the full extent

If you want to zoom out to view the entire map, use the Full Extent button.

1 **On the Tools toolbar, click the Full Extent button** . The map zooms out to the outermost extent of all features.

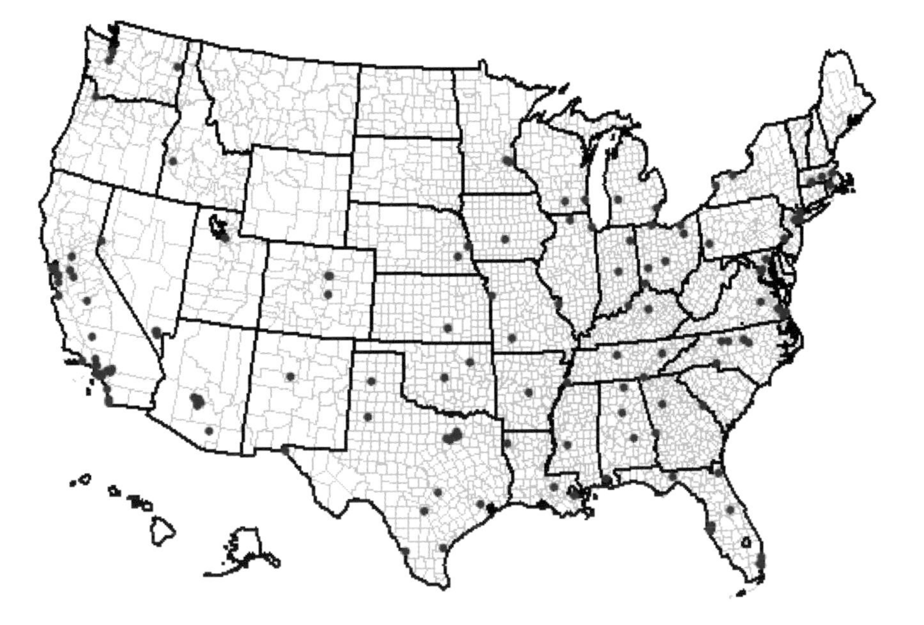

YOUR TURN

Practice using the other zoom functions such as Fixed Zoom In and Fixed Zoom Out, which zoom by a fixed percentage at each click. You can zoom back to the previous extent by using the blue arrow on the Tools toolbar. Zoom to the full extent of the map when you are finished.

Save the map document

1. **On the Menu bar, click File > Save As.**

2. **Save your map document as** Tutorial2-2YourName.mxd **to your Chapter2 folder in MyExercises.** Do not close ArcMap.

T 2-3

Tutorial 2-3
Creating spatial bookmarks

Spatial bookmarks save the current display, at its current zoom status, with a name. You can then easily return to the saved area by accessing the bookmark. This is useful if you use GIS in presentations or if you want to move quickly to a study area or region of interest.

Create a bookmark

1 **With the Zoom In button selected, drag the pointer to draw a rectangle around Florida to zoom to the state of Florida.** This will zoom in to the extent of the state of Florida.

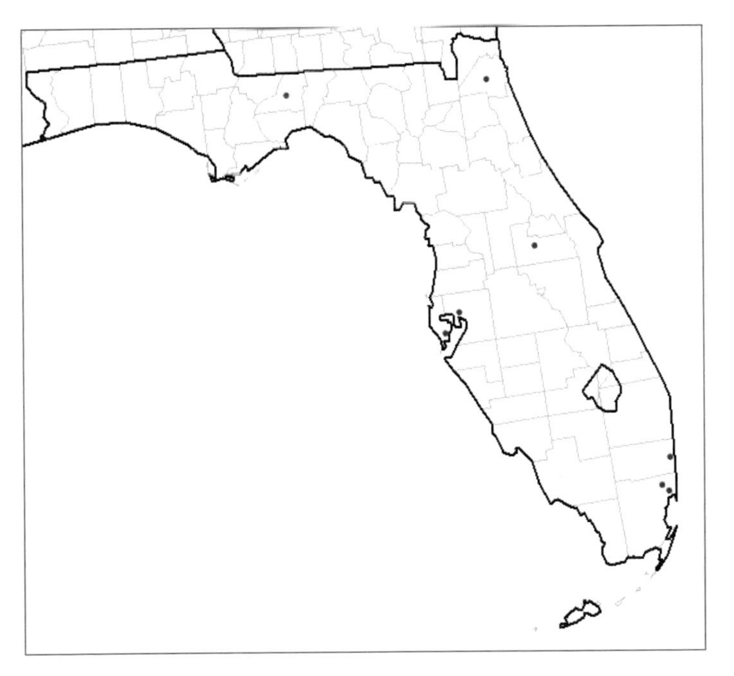

2 **On the Menu bar, click Bookmarks > Create Bookmark, type** Florida **for Bookmark Name, and click OK.**

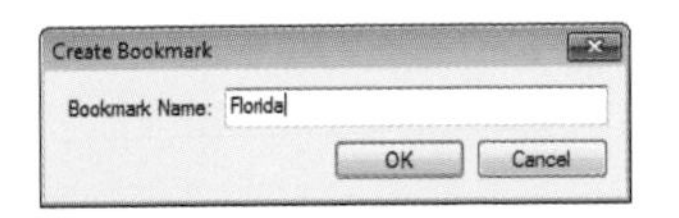

3 **On the Tools toolbar, click Full Extent.**

4 **On the Menu bar, click Bookmarks > Florida.** ArcMap zooms to the extent of the saved bookmark for Florida, which can be helpful if you frequently zoom to this extent.

YOUR TURN

Zoom to and create spatial bookmarks for California, New York, and Texas or other states that may be familiar to you. Try out your new bookmarks. On the Bookmarks menu, click Manage Bookmarks and remove the California bookmark. Zoom to the full extent when you are finished.

Save the map document

1 **On the Menu bar, click File > Save As.**

2 **Save your map document as** Tutorial2-3YourName.mxd **to your Chapter2 folder in MyExercises.** Do not close ArcMap.

Tutorial 2-4

Identifying breast cancer mortality rates and deaths by state

Using GIS, you can interact with map layers to get information. The Identify tool is a commonly used point-and-click tool for browsing through attribute data associated with a map feature. In this section, you will use the Identify tool to learn about mortality rates and the number of breast cancer deaths per state and per county.

Identify features

1 Turn off all layers except Breast Cancer Deaths by State.

2 On the Tools toolbar, click the Identify button .

3 Click inside the state of Texas. ▶

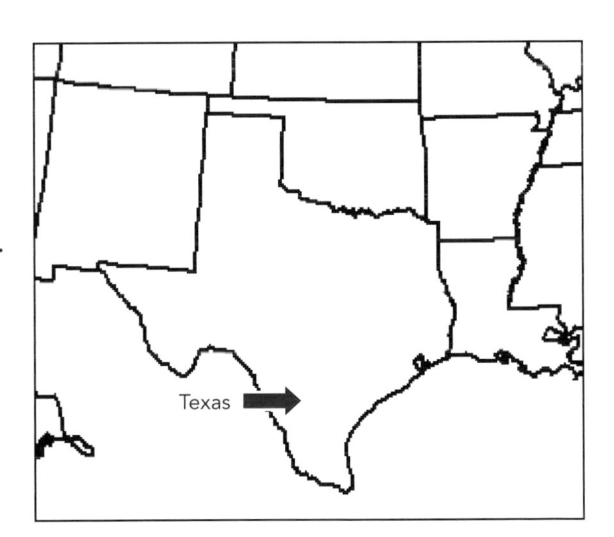

The state of Texas temporarily flashes and the results appear in the resulting Identify dialog box. The names of attributes use the following codes: R = Mortality rate per 100,000 people, C = Number of deaths, WM = White Male, WF = White Female, BM = Black Male, and BF = Black Female. Date ranges are also shown: 95_99 = 1995–1999 and 00_04 = 2000–2004. So, if you are interested in the mortality rate for white females from 2000 to 2004, you would look for the field RWF00_04. You can see that this mortality rate is 23.579. The rate for all ages by state per 100,000 persons is age-adjusted using the US population in 2000. ▶

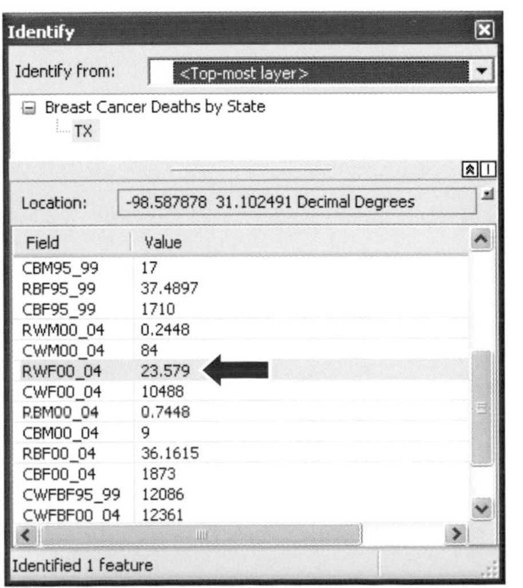

4 Click another state to see the breast cancer mortality rates for white females from 2000 to 2004.

5 Close the Identify dialog box.

Restrict layers to identify

If you have many layers turned on, you may have difficulty selecting the appropriate feature to identify. For example, if both layers are turned on, you may select a county instead of a state. To solve this problem, you can restrict the identify selection to one layer only, ignoring the features in other layers.

1. **In the table of contents, click the Breast Cancer Deaths by County layer to turn it on.**

2. **On the Tools toolbar, click the Identify button.**

3. **Click any state or county polygon feature.**

4. **In the Identify dialog box, click the "Identify from" arrow and select Breast Cancer Deaths by County.** This restricts the identify selection to features in this layer only, ignoring the features in other layers. ▶

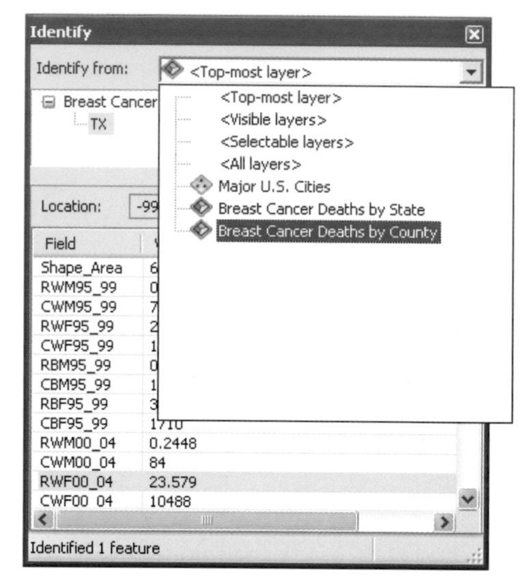

5. **Zoom to the state of Texas.** Use your spatial bookmark if you created one.

6. **Click any county polygon feature in Texas.** Observe the attribute values in the Identify dialog box. Notice that another date range (1990–1994) for breast cancer counts and rates is available for counties. ▶

Identify

Identify from: Breast Cancer Deaths by County

Breast Cancer Deaths by County

Location: -97.859592 30.381409 Decimal Degrees

Field	Value
RWF90_94	26.6808
CWF90_94	284
RBM90_94	0
CBM90_94	0
RBF90_94	37.394
CBF90_94	46
RWM95_99	0.1066
CWM95_99	1
RWF95_99	26.3071
CWF95_99	308
RBM95_99	0
CBM95_99	0
RBF95_99	42.9963
CBF95_99	59
RWM00_04	0
CWM00_04	0
RWF00_04	24.2819

Identified 1 feature

7. **Close the Identify dialog box.**

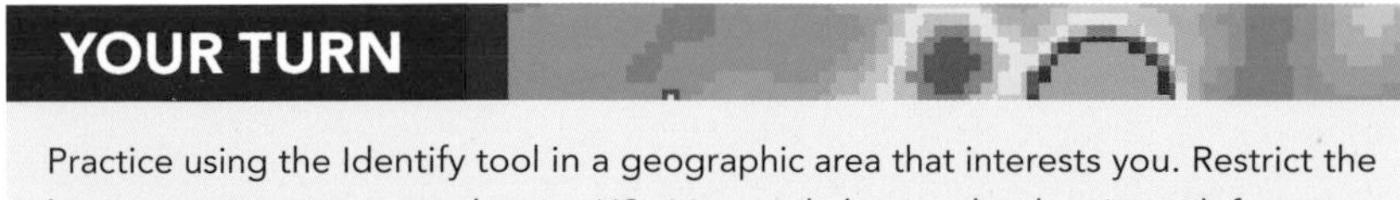

Practice using the Identify tool in a geographic area that interests you. Restrict the layers to state, county, and major US cities, and observe the data in each feature class. Are you able to observe any health-care trends for breast cancer?

Use advanced Identify tool capabilities

You can use the Identify tool to navigate and create spatial bookmarks.

1. **Zoom to the full extent and turn off all layers except Breast Cancer Deaths by State.**
2. **Click the Identify button, click inside any feature, and in the "Identify from" list, click Breast Cancer Deaths by State.**
3. **Click inside the state of Illinois.**

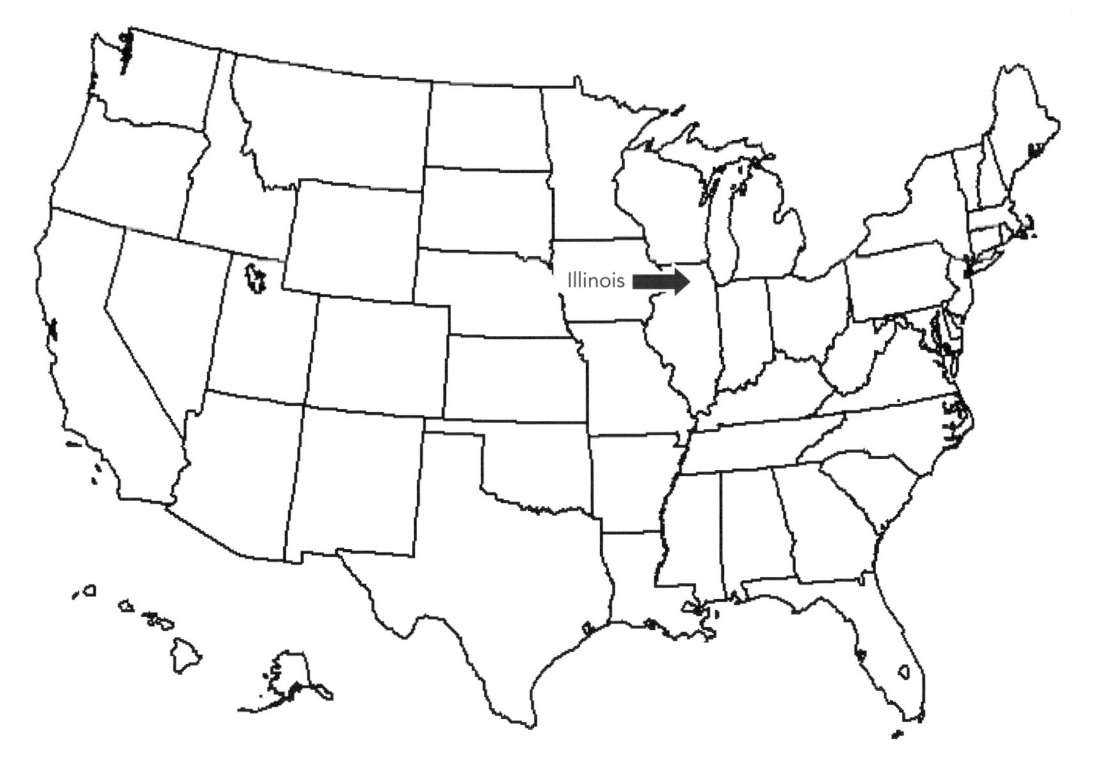

4 **In the Identify dialog box, right-click the state abbreviation name (IL) and click Zoom To.** The map display zooms to the extent of the state of Illinois.

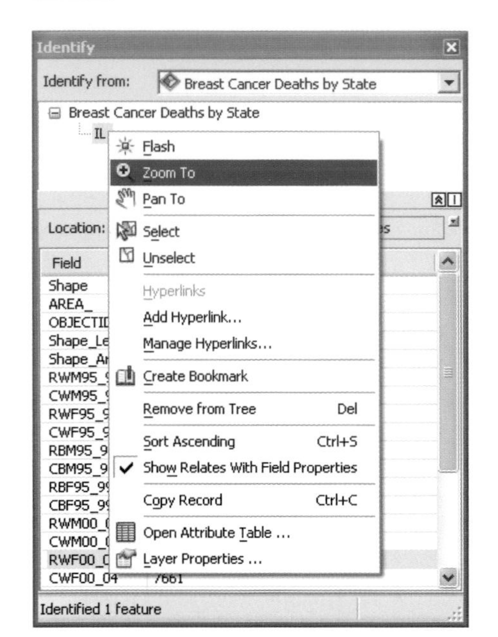

5 **Right-click the state abbreviation name again and click Create Bookmark.**

6 **Close the Identify dialog box.**

7 **Click Full Extent.**

8 **Click Bookmarks > IL.**

Save the map document

1 **On the Menu bar, click File > Save As.**

2 **Save your map document as** Tutorial2-4YourName.mxd **to your Chapter2 folder in MyExercises.** Do not close ArcMap.

Tutorial 2-5
Selecting map features

GIS links graphic features of a map layer to associated attribute records in a table. When you select features on a map, you can correlate them with the records in the table. That way, you can perform functions on a subset of features and records, including generating statistics, making new layers, or doing analysis.

Select a single feature

1. **In the table of contents, turn on the Major U.S. Cities layer.**
2. **Click Full Extent.**
3. **On the Tools toolbar, click the Select Features button.**
4. **Click inside Texas.** The selected state feature is highlighted on the map.

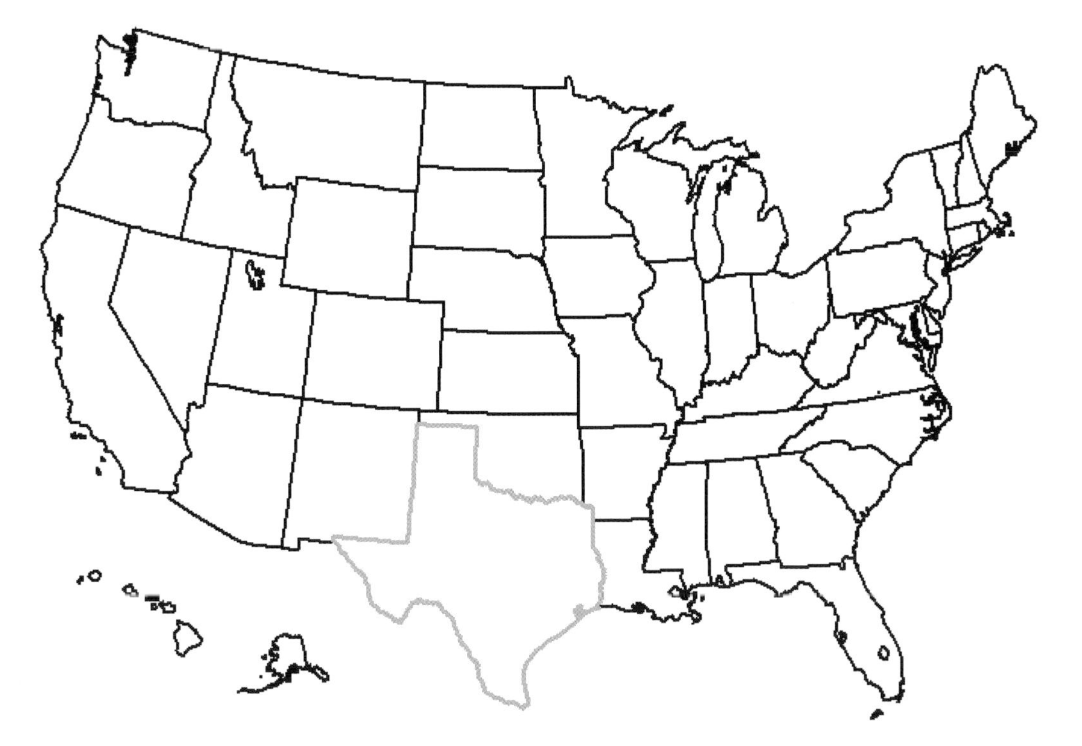

Select multiple features

1 To make multiple selections, hold the SHIFT key and click inside each of the states surrounding Texas.

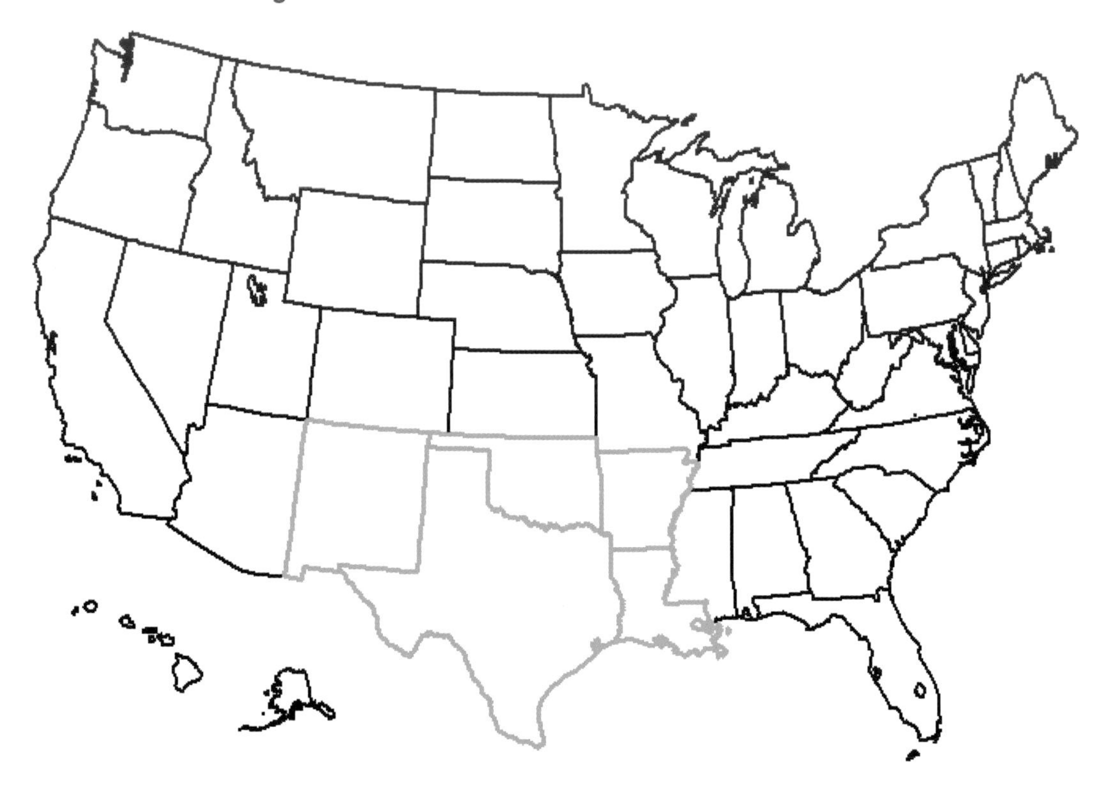

T 2-5

Change the selection color and clear a selection

Sometimes you will want to produce a map that has certain features selected. Then you'll want to be able to change the selection color for the purpose at hand. For example, a bright red color might be better for drawing attention to map features.

1 On the Menu bar, click Selection > Selection Options.

2 In the Selection Options dialog box, click the color box under Selection Tools Settings.

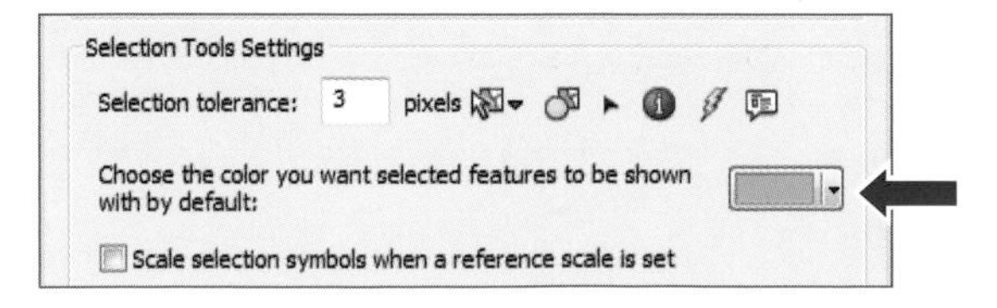

3 **Select Mars Red as the new selection color and click OK.**

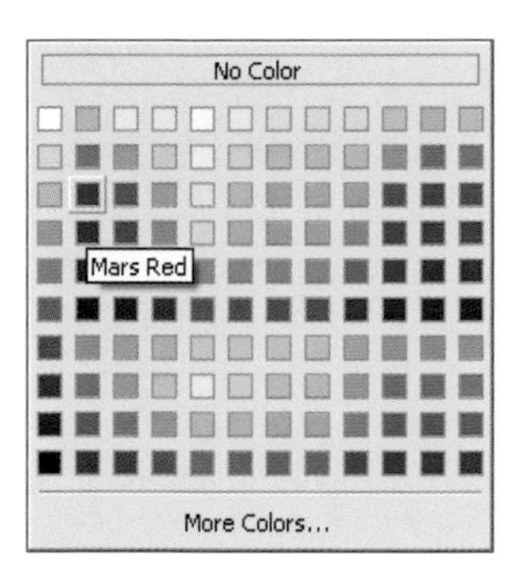

The selection color for map features is now bright red.

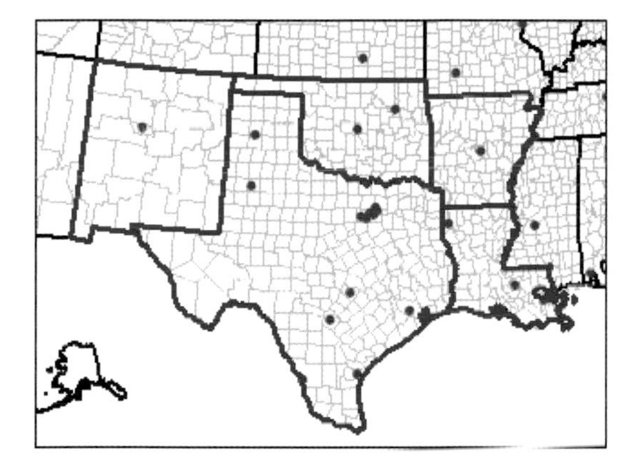

4 **On the Selection menu, click Selection > Clear Selected Features.**

Set selectable layers

When there are many layers in a map document, you may want to restrict which ones are selectable. This simplifies the selection process.

1 **In the table of contents, turn on all three map layers.**

2 **At the top of the table of contents, click the List By Selection button .**

3 **Click to clear the check boxes for Breast Cancer Deaths by State and Breast Cancer Deaths by County to make only Major U.S. Cities selectable.** Now only cities will be selected.

Selectable (no features selected)
Major U.S. Cities 0
Not Selectable
Breast Cancer Deaths by State 0
Breast Cancer Deaths by County 0

4 Click the Select Features button and click a city. The selected city gets the selection color you chose previously and is listed in the table of contents. The name of the city is also displayed in the table of contents.

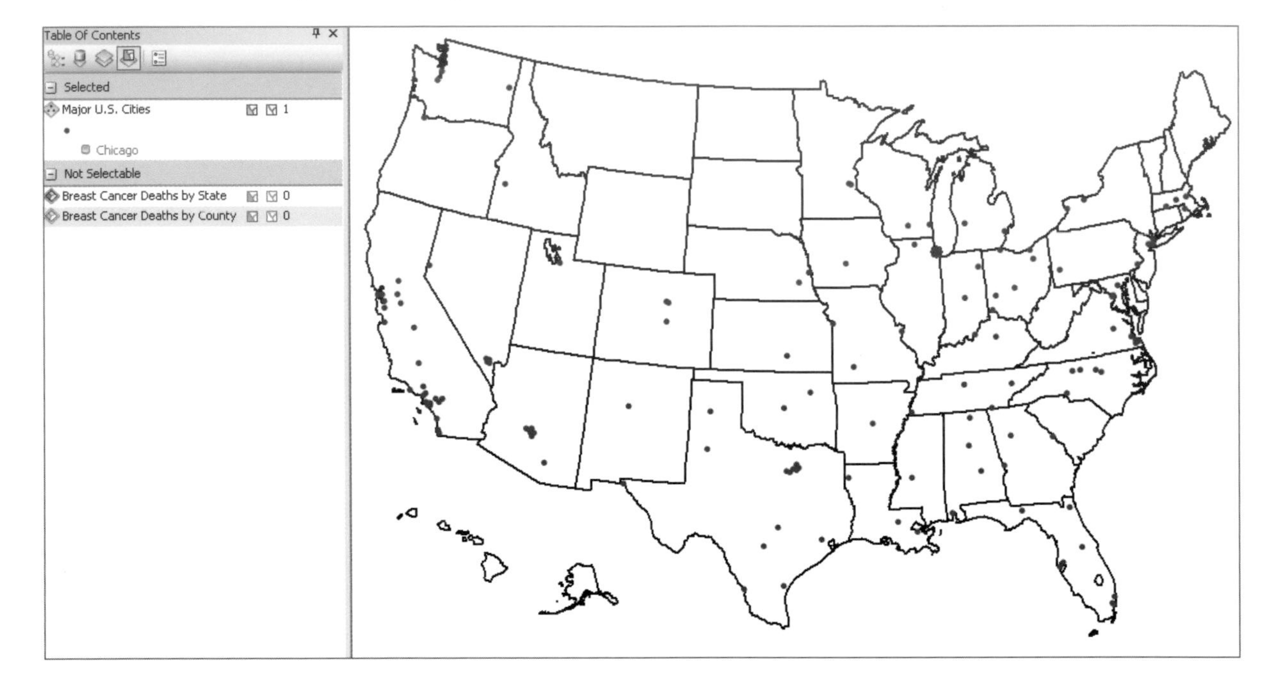

5 On the Tools toolbar, click the Clear Selected Features button.

Select features by graphic

Selecting features by using graphics is a faster way to select multiple features.

1 Click Bookmarks > Florida.

2 Click the Select Features arrow and then Select by Circle.

Select by Rectangle
Select by Polygon
Select by Lasso
Select by Circle
Select by Line

3 Click inside the state of Florida and drag the pointer to draw a circle that includes five cities in the central and northern parts of Florida.
The resulting map shows multiple cities selected and the resulting names included in the table of contents.

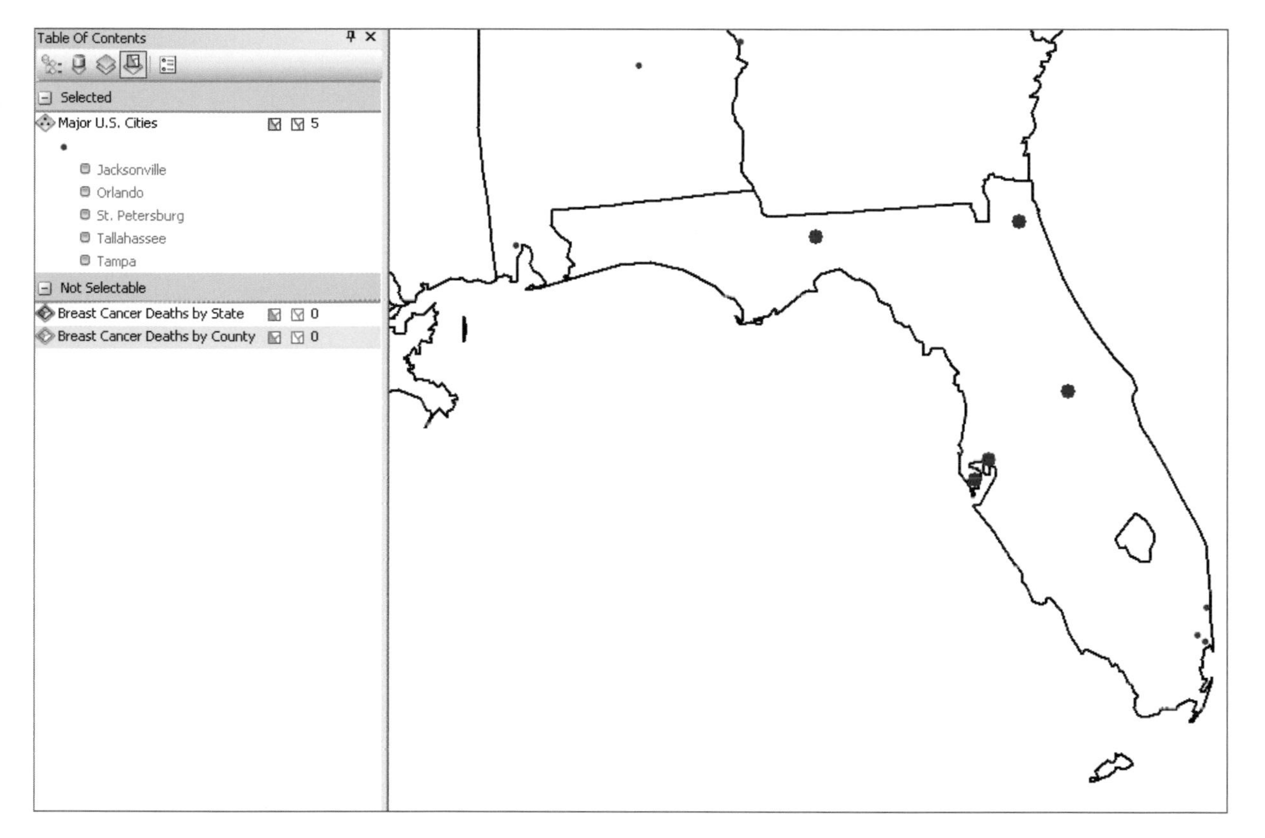

Zoom to selected features

1 **Click Selection > Zoom To Selected Features.** ArcMap zooms to the features selected.

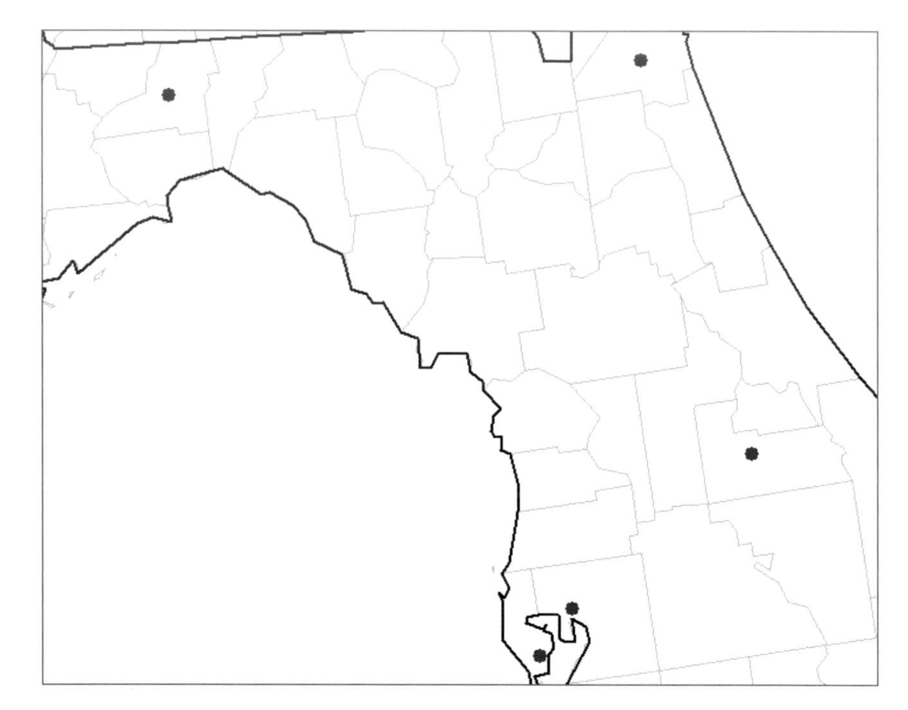

Change the selection symbol

In addition to changing the color of selected features, you can change the symbol either for the entire map or for individual layers.

1 **In the table of contents, right-click the Major U.S. Cities layer and click Properties.**

2 **Click the Selection tab and click the Symbol button.**

Layer Properties

General | Source | Selection | Display | Symbology | Fields | Definition Query | Labels | Joins & Relates | Time | HTML Popup

Show selected features:

using the selection color specified in Selection Options

with this symbol

with this color

OK | Cancel | Apply

3 Click Square 1, Dark Amethyst, and size 12 **as the new selection symbol and click OK twice.**

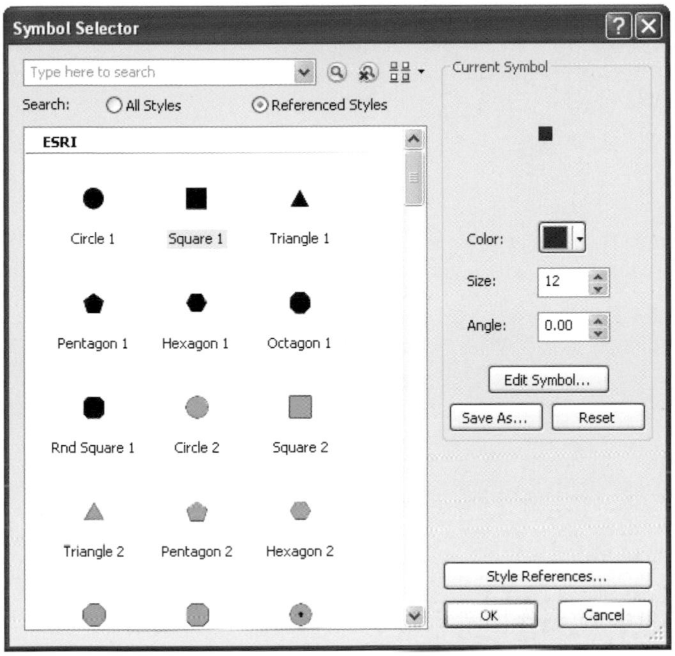

4 The cities will be displayed with the new selection symbol.

5 Clear the selected features and zoom to full map extent.

YOUR TURN

Zoom to Texas. Click the Select Features arrow and click Select by Lasso. Select multiple cities in the state of Texas. Clear the selected features.

In the table of contents, make Breast Cancer Deaths by County the only selectable layer. Select features for five counties in Texas, zoom to those selected features, and then clear the selection.

Save the map document

1 On the Menu bar, click File > Save As.

2 Save your map document as Tutorial2-5YourName.mxd **to your Chapter2 folder in MyExercises.** Do not close ArcMap.

Tutorial 2-6
Finding map features

The connection between GIS features and their attributes provides several ways to locate features in the map. In cases where you know what you're looking for but don't know its location, you can use the Find tool.

Use the Find tool

1 Zoom to full map extent and make all map layers selectable.

2 On the Tools toolbar, click the Find button .

3 In the Find dialog box, in the Find box, type Philadelphia**; for In, select <All layers>; and for Search, select the "Find features that are similar to or contain the search string" check box.**

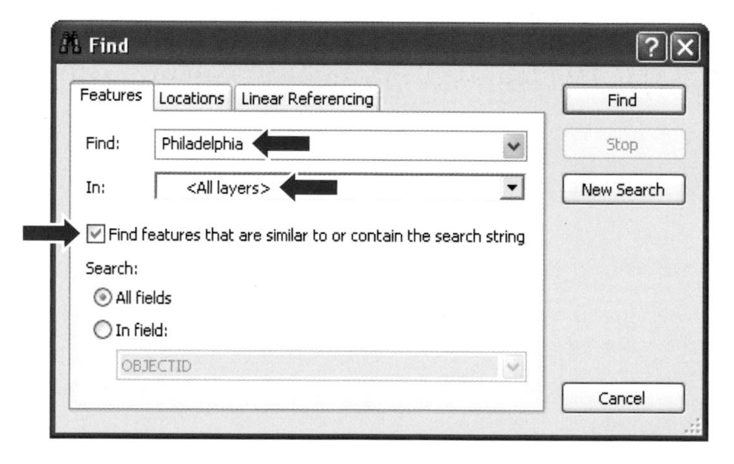

4 Click Find. The results appear in the bottom section of the Find dialog box. Note that ArcMap finds both the city and the county of Philadelphia. Both these records were located because the software searches all visible layers. You can restrict the Find tool to a specific layer by using the In list seen in step 3.

Value	Layer	Field
Philadelphia	Major U.S. Cities	NAME
PHILADELPHIA	Breast Cancer Deaths by County	NAME2_

5 Right-click the city name and click Zoom To.

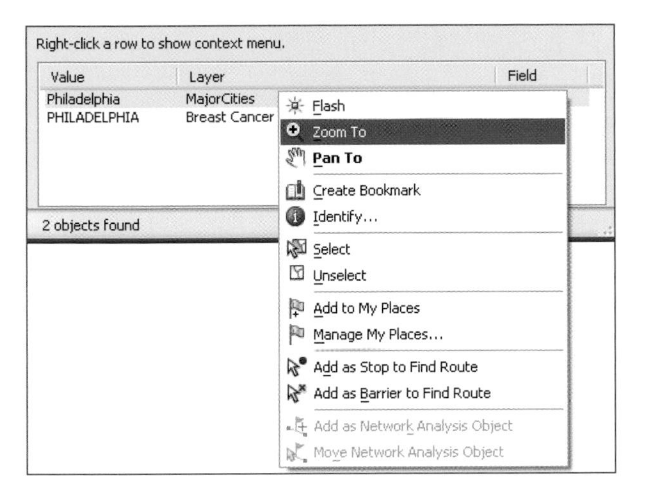

The resulting map zooms to the city of Philadelphia.

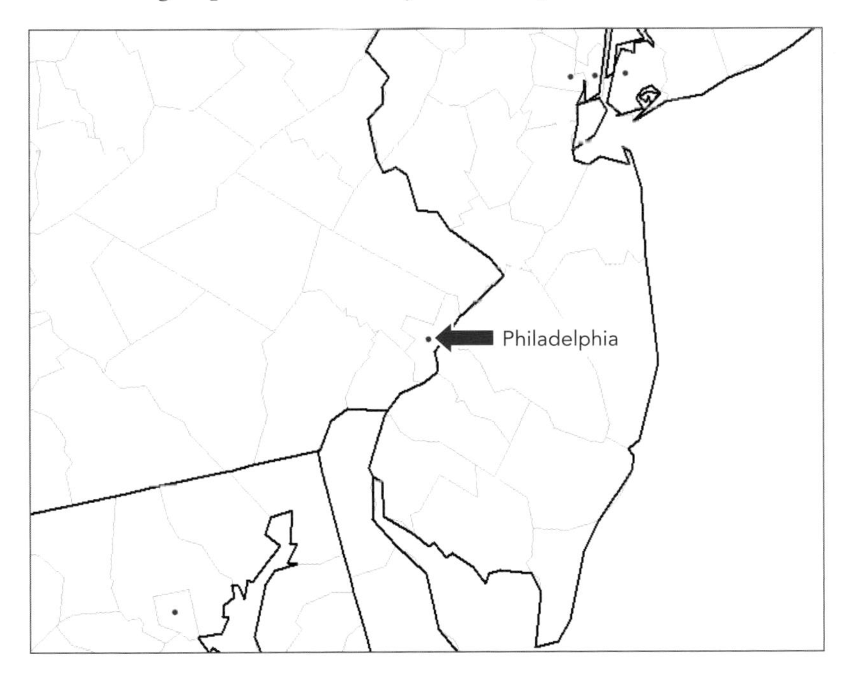

6 Close the Find dialog box.

Save the map document

1 On the Menu bar, click File > Save As.

2 Save your map document as Tutorial2-6YourName.mxd **to your Chapter2 folder in MyExercises.** Do not close ArcMap.

Tutorial 2-7
Using an attribute table to select counties with high breast cancer rates

Each map layer has an associated feature attribute table that contains the data associated with every feature in the layer. Open the attribute table to explore the attributes for the layer on a map. The attribute table provides information you can use to query the data. In this section, you will use attribute tables to determine which US counties had the highest counts and rates of female breast cancer deaths.

Show the connection between layers and tables

1 **Zoom to full map extent.**

2 **In the table of contents, click the List By Drawing Order button.**

3 **Right-click the Breast Cancer Deaths by County layer and click Open Attribute Table.** The table, which contains one record for each county feature, appears. Each layer has this table, which contains one record per geographic feature.

4 **Resize or move the Breast Cancer Deaths by County attribute table so that both the map and the table can be viewed simultaneously on the screen.**

5 Click the record selector (gray box) at the far left of the table for the first county (Autauga, Alabama) to select that record. Notice that the county is also highlighted on the map.

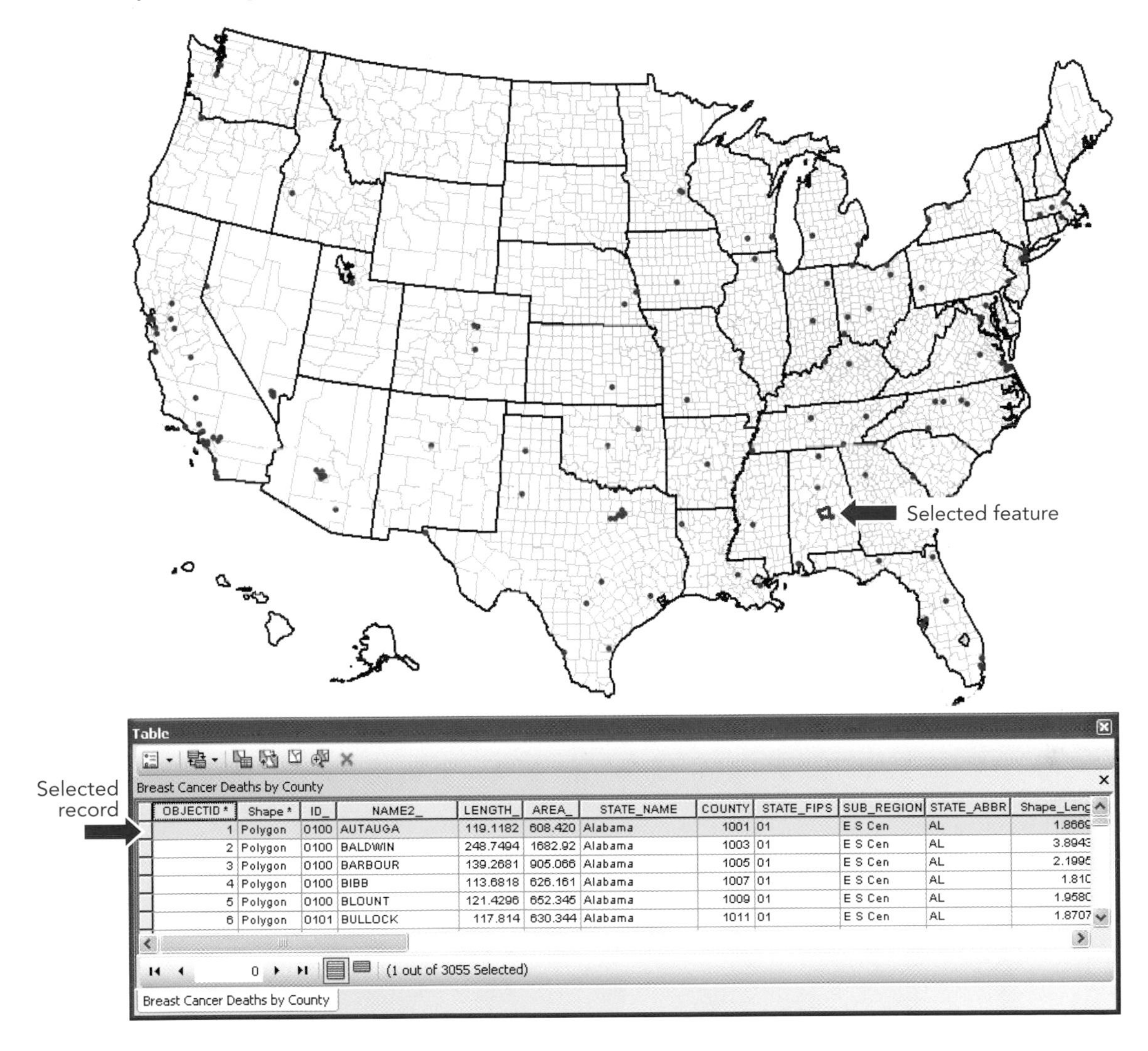

OBJECTID *	Shape *	ID_	NAME2_	LENGTH_	AREA_	STATE_NAME	COUNTY	STATE_FIPS	SUB_REGION	STATE_ABBR	Shape_Leng
1	Polygon	0100	AUTAUGA	119.1182	608.420	Alabama	1001	01	E S Cen	AL	1.866
2	Polygon	0100	BALDWIN	248.7494	1682.92	Alabama	1003	01	E S Cen	AL	3.894
3	Polygon	0100	BARBOUR	139.2681	905.066	Alabama	1005	01	E S Cen	AL	2.199
4	Polygon	0100	BIBB	113.6818	626.161	Alabama	1007	01	E S Cen	AL	1.81
5	Polygon	0100	BLOUNT	121.4296	652.345	Alabama	1009	01	E S Cen	AL	1.958
6	Polygon	0101	BULLOCK	117.814	630.344	Alabama	1011	01	E S Cen	AL	1.8707

6 Scroll to the right in the attribute table to see the breast cancer rates and counts for this county.

YOUR TURN

Click the record selector for various counties in the attribute table to highlight them on the map. Click various counties on the map to highlight them in the feature attribute table. Find the county where you live or one that is familiar to you. Select your county in the attribute table and see the county highlighted on the map. Clear your selected features when you are finished.

Dock the attribute table

In ArcGIS, you can move a window to a new location and dock it or make it stationary. When you move the attribute table window, blue targets appear representing the different locations where you can dock the window. You can drag the window to the target of your choice and drop it there to secure it.

1 **Drag the attribute window by its title bar to a new location.** You will see blue target arrows indicating where you can "drop" the attribute window. Pause over a target to get a preview of where the window will be located if you drop it on that target.

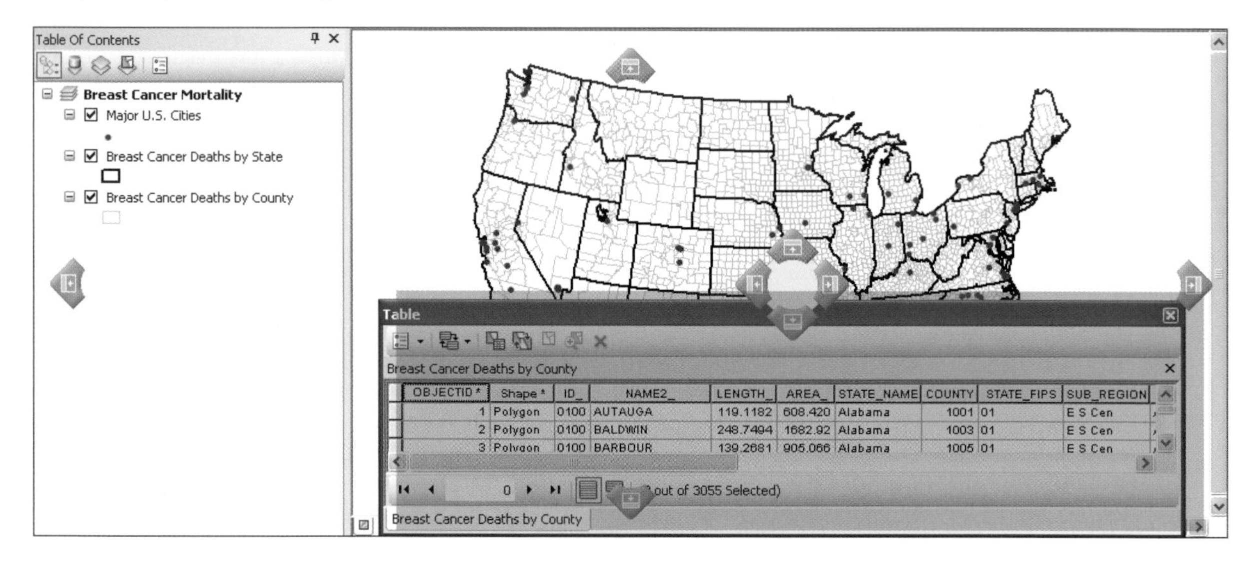

2 **Drop the window on the target at the bottom of the screen.** The attribute table appears at the bottom of the window, and the table of contents and the map are at the top of the screen.

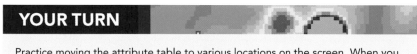

Practice moving the attribute table to various locations on the screen. When you are finished, leave the table floating in the map document.

Move a field

Next you will move and sort fields in the feature attribute table. In particular, you will sort fields in descending order by the total deaths in each county, and then select the highest number of deaths for the entire United States or for a selected state.

1 **On the Tools toolbar, click Clear Selected Features.**

2 In the Breast Cancer Deaths by County table, click the column heading (known as the field name) of the STATE_NAME field, and then press and drag it to the left of the NAME2_ (county name) field.

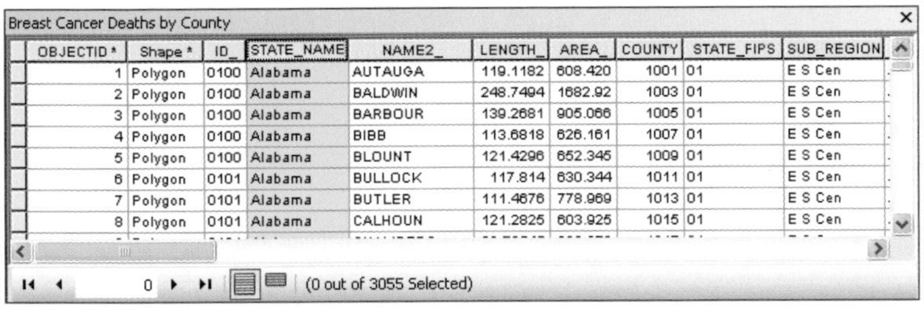

Breast Cancer Deaths by County

OBJECTID *	Shape *	ID_	STATE_NAME	NAME2_	LENGTH_	AREA_	COUNTY	STATE_FIPS	SUB_REGION
1	Polygon	0100	Alabama	AUTAUGA	119.1182	608.420	1001	01	E S Cen
2	Polygon	0100	Alabama	BALDWIN	248.7494	1682.92	1003	01	E S Cen
3	Polygon	0100	Alabama	BARBOUR	139.2681	905.066	1005	01	E S Cen
4	Polygon	0100	Alabama	BIBB	113.6818	626.161	1007	01	E S Cen
5	Polygon	0100	Alabama	BLOUNT	121.4296	652.345	1009	01	E S Cen
6	Polygon	0101	Alabama	BULLOCK	117.814	630.344	1011	01	E S Cen
7	Polygon	0101	Alabama	BUTLER	111.4676	778.969	1013	01	E S Cen
8	Polygon	0101	Alabama	CALHOUN	121.2825	603.925	1015	01	E S Cen

(0 out of 3055 Selected)

3 Move the CWFBF00_04, RWF00_04, and RBF00_04 fields until they are to the immediate right of NAME2_. Notice that the field CWFBF00_04 combines both white and black females. In chapter 5, you will learn how to combine multiple fields using a field calculator.

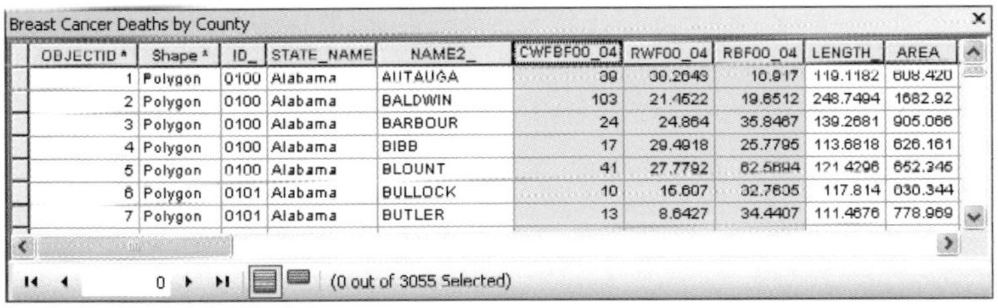

Breast Cancer Deaths by County

OBJECTID *	Shape *	ID_	STATE_NAME	NAME2_	CWFBF00_04	RWF00_04	RBF00_04	LENGTH_	AREA
1	Polygon	0100	Alabama	AUTAUGA	39	30.2043	10.917	119.1182	608.420
2	Polygon	0100	Alabama	BALDWIN	103	21.4522	19.6512	248.7494	1682.92
3	Polygon	0100	Alabama	BARBOUR	24	24.864	35.8467	139.2681	905.066
4	Polygon	0100	Alabama	BIBB	17	29.4918	25.7795	113.6818	626.161
5	Polygon	0100	Alabama	BLOUNT	41	27.7792	62.5884	121.4296	652.346
6	Polygon	0101	Alabama	BULLOCK	10	16.607	32.7605	117.814	630.344
7	Polygon	0101	Alabama	BUTLER	13	8.6427	34.4407	111.4676	778.969

(0 out of 3055 Selected)

Sort a single field

1 In the Breast Cancer Deaths by County attribute table, right-click the CWFBF00_04 field name and click Sort Descending. This sorts the table from the largest number to the smallest number of breast cancer deaths for all females in each US county from 2000 to 2004.

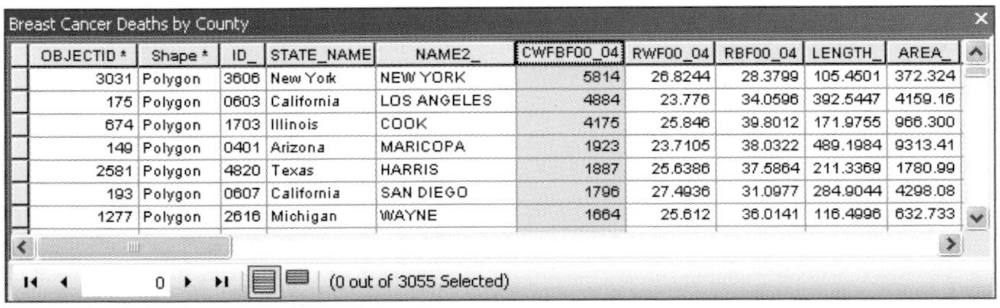

Breast Cancer Deaths by County

OBJECTID *	Shape *	ID_	STATE_NAME	NAME2_	CWFBF00_04	RWF00_04	RBF00_04	LENGTH_	AREA_
3031	Polygon	3606	New York	NEW YORK	5814	26.8244	28.3799	105.4501	372.324
175	Polygon	0603	California	LOS ANGELES	4884	23.776	34.0596	392.5447	4159.16
674	Polygon	1703	Illinois	COOK	4175	25.846	39.8012	171.9755	966.300
149	Polygon	0401	Arizona	MARICOPA	1923	23.7105	38.0322	489.1984	9313.41
2581	Polygon	4820	Texas	HARRIS	1887	25.6386	37.5864	211.3369	1780.99
193	Polygon	0607	California	SAN DIEGO	1796	27.4936	31.0977	284.9044	4298.08
1277	Polygon	2616	Michigan	WAYNE	1664	25.612	36.0141	116.4996	632.733

(0 out of 3055 Selected)

Select the counties with the highest counts of breast cancer

Now that you have prepared the attribute table to sort by the highest number of breast cancer deaths, you can select records to isolate top cancer counties on the map.

T 2-7

1 **In the Breast Cancer Deaths by County table, press CTRL and click the row selectors for the first five records in descending order.** Notice that the corresponding features are highlighted on the map. The areas selected as having the highest number of breast cancer deaths might not be surprising because these are some of the most populated counties in the country.

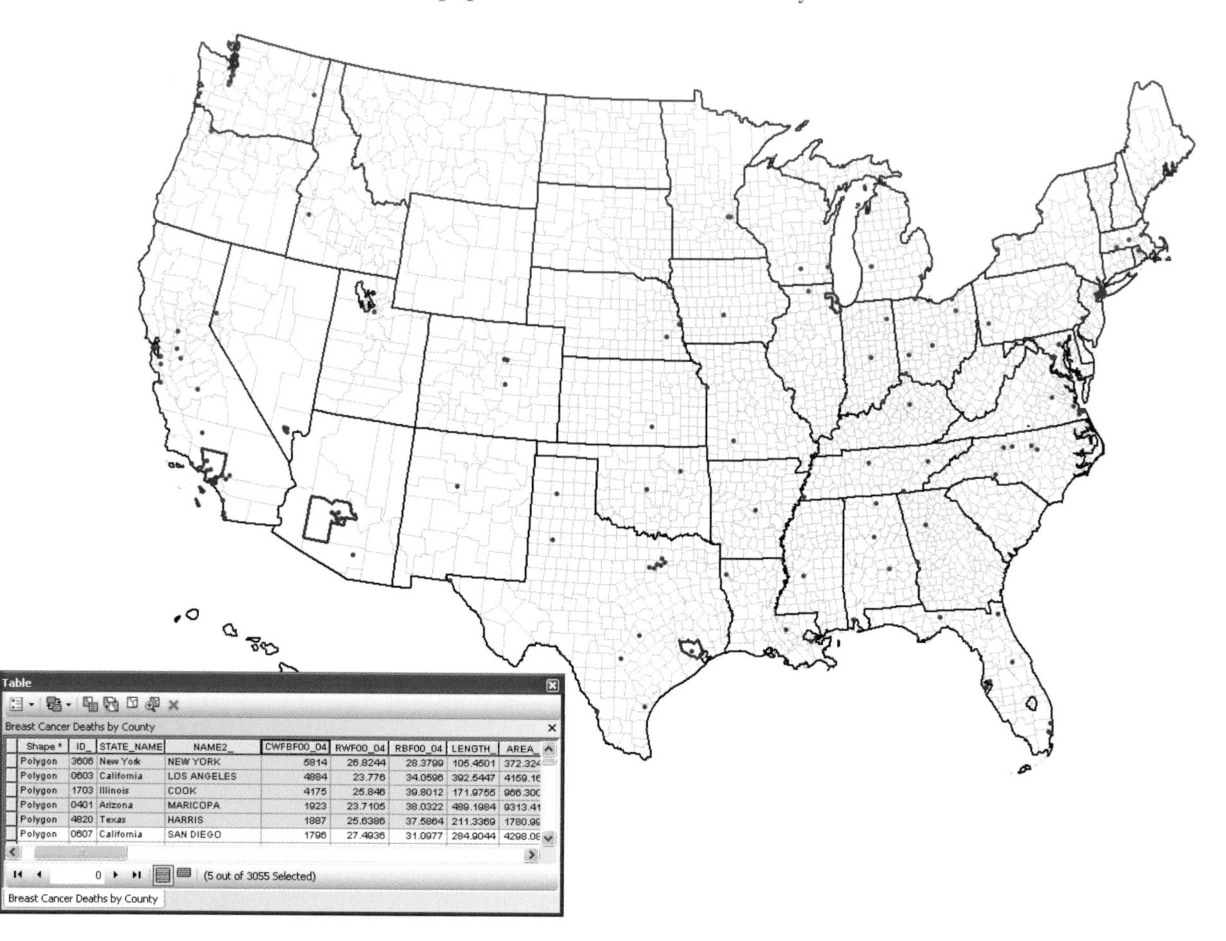

Shape *	ID_	STATE_NAME	NAME2_	CWFBF00_04	RWF00_04	RBF00_04	LENGTH_	AREA_
Polygon	3606	New York	NEW YORK	5814	26.8244	28.3799	105.4501	372.32
Polygon	0603	California	LOS ANGELES	4884	23.776	34.0596	392.5447	4159.1
Polygon	1703	Illinois	COOK	4175	25.846	39.8012	171.9755	966.30
Polygon	0401	Arizona	MARICOPA	1923	23.7105	38.0322	489.1984	9313.41
Polygon	4820	Texas	HARRIS	1887	25.6386	37.5864	211.3369	1780.9
Polygon	0607	California	SAN DIEGO	1796	27.4936	31.0977	284.9044	4298.0

Select the counties with the highest breast cancer rates

A better indicator of breast cancer is the mortality rate per county.

1 **In the Breast Cancer Deaths by County attribute table, right-click the RWF00_04 field name and click Sort Descending.**

2 **Press CTRL and click the row selectors for the first five records in descending order.** Notice that the corresponding features highlighted on the map for the rate of breast cancer deaths for white females are much different from those for the highest count of breast cancer deaths for white females. (See facing page.)

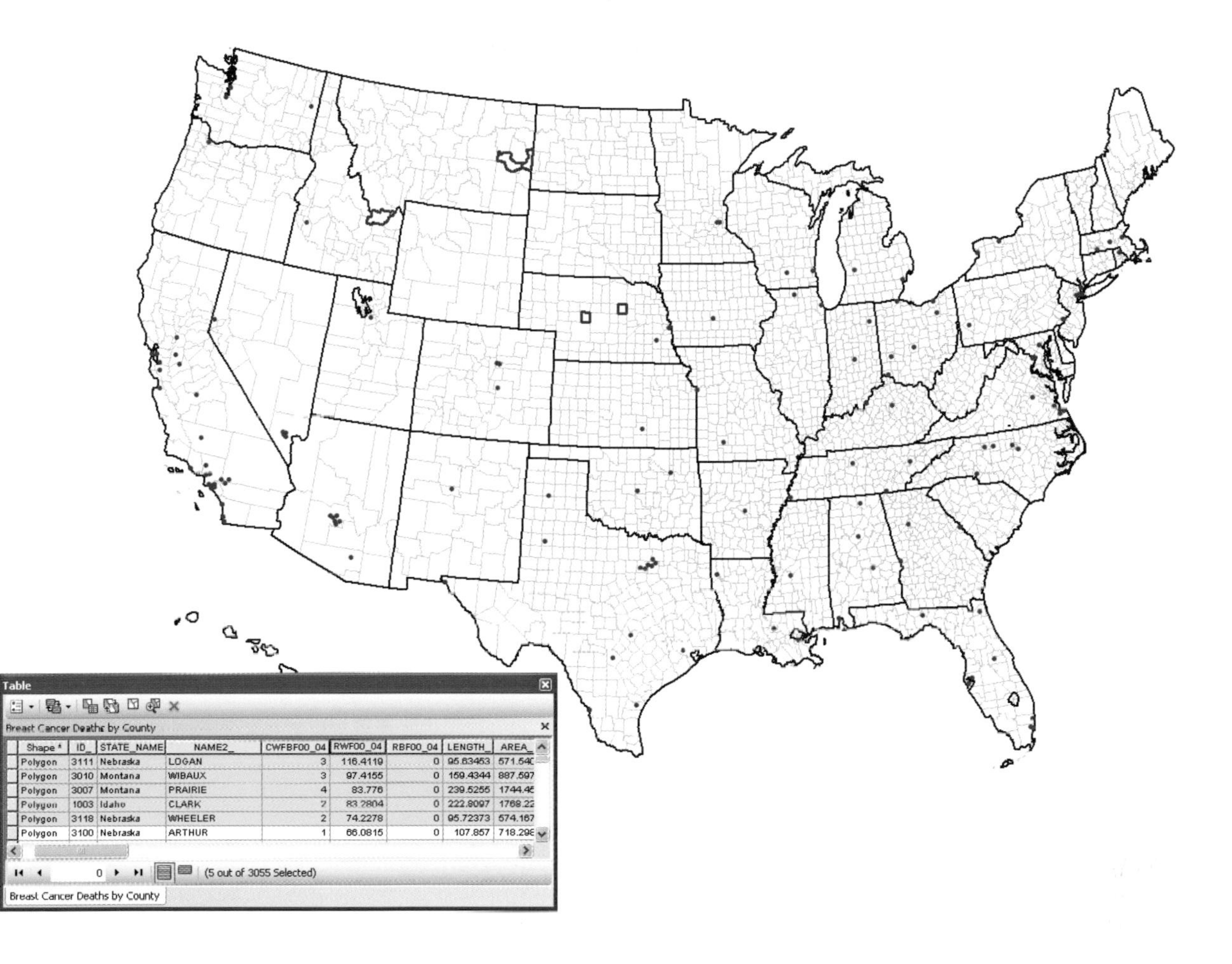

Shape *	ID_	STATE_NAME	NAME2_	CWFBF00_04	RWF00_04	RBF00_04	LENGTH_	AREA_
Polygon	3111	Nebraska	LOGAN	3	116.4119	0	95.63453	571.540
Polygon	3010	Montana	WIBAUX	3	97.4155	0	159.4344	887.597
Polygon	3007	Montana	PRAIRIE	4	83.776	0	239.5255	1744.4
Polygon	1003	Idaho	CLARK	7	83.2804	0	222.8097	1768.22
Polygon	3118	Nebraska	WHEELER	2	74.2278	0	95.72373	574.167
Polygon	3100	Nebraska	ARTHUR	1	66.0815	0	107.857	718.29

YOUR TURN

Find the counties that had the highest rates of breast cancer deaths from 2000 to 2004 for black females. Clear your selections when you are finished.

Sort multiple fields

Sorting by the number of cancer deaths was useful for finding the counties that had the highest number of breast cancer deaths and death rates across the United States, but what if you wanted to examine the number of deaths for one state? To do this, you would need to sort the records by two fields: state and number of deaths.

1 **Right-click the STATE_NAME field and click Advanced Sorting.**

2 **In the Advanced Table Sorting dialog box, click the "Sort by" arrow, select STATE_NAME, and select the Ascending option if it is not already selected.** This sets up the first sort order to sort alphabetically by state.

3 **In the Advanced Table Sorting dialog box, click the "Then sort by" arrow, select CWFBF00_04, and select the Descending option. Click OK.** This sets up the second sort order to sort for highest-to-lowest female deaths between 2000 and 2004.

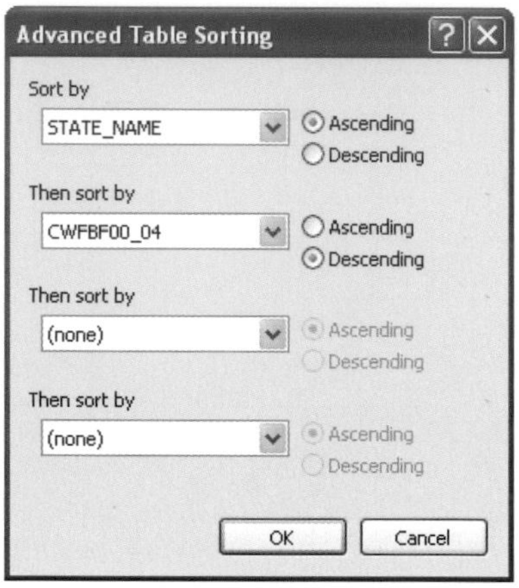

Advanced Table Sorting

Sort by: STATE_NAME — Ascending (selected) / Descending

Then sort by: CWFBF00_04 — Ascending / Descending (selected)

Then sort by: (none) — Ascending / Descending

Then sort by: (none) — Ascending / Descending

OK Cancel

4 **Scroll through the list until you find the records for Texas.**

5 **Select the first five records for Texas.** This selects the five counties that had the highest number of breast cancer deaths for all females.

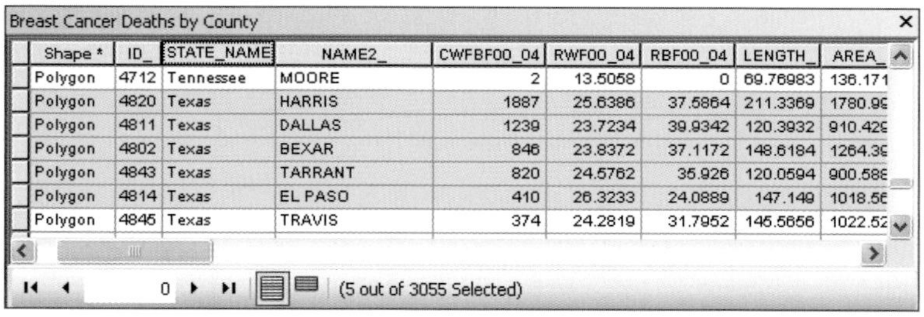

Breast Cancer Deaths by County

Shape *	ID_	STATE_NAME	NAME2_	CWFBF00_04	RWF00_04	RBF00_04	LENGTH_	AREA_
Polygon	4712	Tennessee	MOORE	2	13.5058	0	69.76983	136.171
Polygon	4820	Texas	HARRIS	1887	25.6386	37.5864	211.3369	1780.9
Polygon	4811	Texas	DALLAS	1239	23.7234	39.9342	120.3932	910.42
Polygon	4802	Texas	BEXAR	846	23.8372	37.1172	148.6184	1264.3
Polygon	4843	Texas	TARRANT	820	24.5762	35.926	120.0594	900.58
Polygon	4814	Texas	EL PASO	410	26.3233	24.0889	147.149	1018.5
Polygon	4845	Texas	TRAVIS	374	24.2819	31.7952	145.5656	1022.5

0 (5 out of 3055 Selected)

6 **Close the attribute table.**

7 **Click Bookmarks > Texas or zoom to Texas.** The resulting map shows the locations of the five counties that had the highest number of female breast cancer deaths in Texas. (See facing page.)

T 2-7

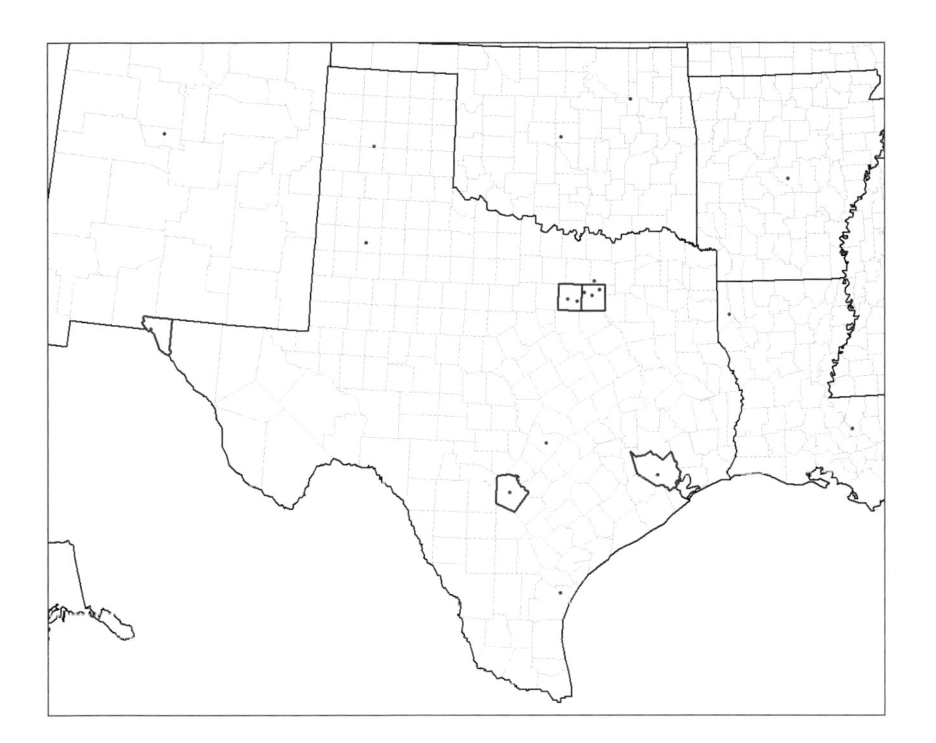

Show only selected records

1 **Open the Breast Cancer Deaths by County attribute table and click the "Show selected records" button.** This shows the records for only the features selected in the map.

Breast Cancer Deaths by County

OBJECTID *	Shape *	ID_	STATE_NAME	NAME2_	CWFBF00_04	RWF00_04	RBF00_04	LENGTH
2581	Polygon	4820	Texas	HARRIS	1887	25.6386	37.5864	211.336
2537	Polygon	4811	Texas	DALLAS	1239	23.7234	39.9342	120.393
2495	Polygon	4802	Texas	BEXAR	846	23.8372	37.1172	148.618
2700	Polygon	4843	Texas	TARRANT	820	24.5762	35.926	120.059
2551	Polygon	4814	Texas	EL PASO	410	26.3233	24.0889	147.14

1 (5 out of 3055 Selected)

2 **Click the "Show all records" button to show all records again.**

3 **Close the attribute table.**

Save the map document

1 **On the Menu bar, click File > Save As.**

2 **Save your map document as** Tutorial2-7YourName.mxd **to your Chapter2 folder in MyExercises.** Do not close ArcMap.

T 2-7

Tutorial 2-8
Creating a new layer of a subset of features

Sometimes just a subset of features is needed in a map layer. For example, in this tutorial, you will create a layer that has the counties you just selected.

1 **Right-click the Breast Cancer Deaths by County layer and click Selection > Create Layer From Selected Features.** This adds a new layer to the table of contents that contains just the five counties in Texas that had the highest number of breast cancer deaths.

2 **Rename the new layer** Top 5 Texas Counties, Female Breast Cancer Deaths 2000-2004 **and change the color fill to Mars Red.**

3 **Drag the new layer below Major U.S. Cities and clear the selected features.** The resulting map clearly shows the Texas counties that had the highest number of female breast cancer deaths between 2000 and 2004.

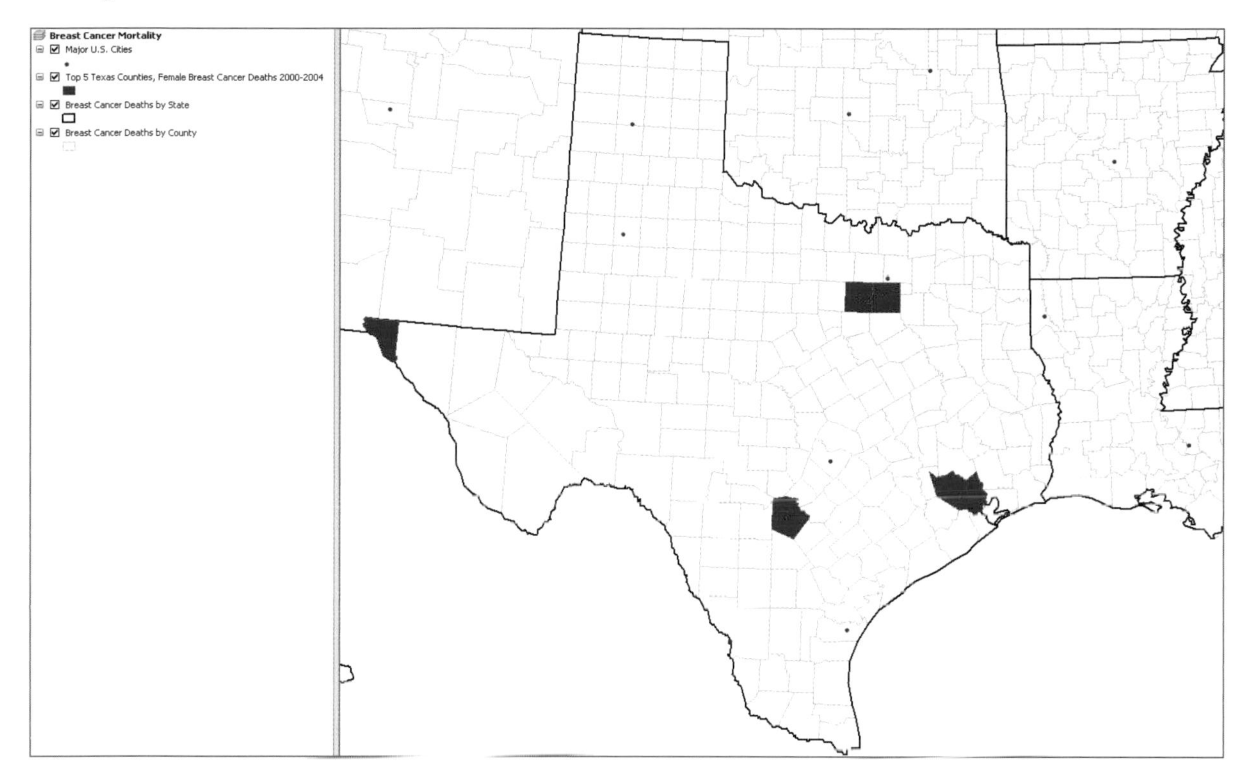

Save the map document

1 **On the Menu bar, click File > Save As.**

2 **Save your map document as** Tutorial2-8YourName.mxd **to your Chapter2 folder in MyExercises.** Do not close ArcMap.

Tutorial 2-9
Creating a point map based on a definition query

Sometimes just a subset of features is needed in a map layer. Suppose you have a layer that contains all the cities in the United States, but you want to display only the cities in Texas that have a population over 600,000. To do this, you can create a definition query to filter out all the cities that have population values outside the desired range but keep those that are in Texas in the desired range.

Create a definition query

1 **Click Selection > Select By Attributes.**

2 **In the Select By Attributes dialog box, click the Layer arrow and select Major U.S. Cities.**

3 **In the Select By Attributes dialog box, double-click "ST".**

4 **Click = for the logical operator.**

5 **Click Get Unique Values.** The resulting list has all the unique values in the ST attribute.

6 **In the Unique Values list, double-click 'TX'.**

7 **Click And for the logical operator AND.**

8 **Double-click "POP2007".**

9 **Click > for the logical operator.**

10 Press the SPACEBAR and type 600000. The completed query,

```
ST = 'TX' AND POP2007 > 600000,
```

yields a layer that contains only the cities in Texas that have a population over 600,000. If the query has an error, edit it in the lower panel of the Select By Attributes dialog box, or click Clear and repeat steps 2–9.

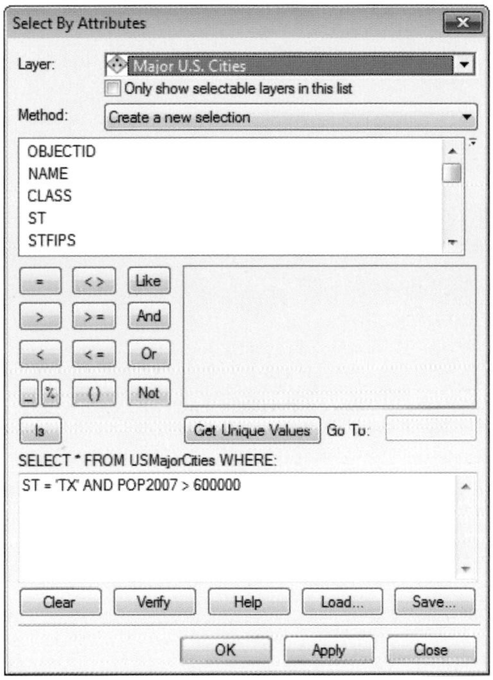

11 Click Apply > OK.

Create a layer from selected features

1 Right-click the Major U.S. Cities layer and click Selection > Create Layer From Selected Features. A new layer of just the selected cities in Texas is added to the table of contents.

2 Clear the selected features.

Rename and create a new symbol for the new layer

The symbol should be changed to differentiate it from the other layer that shows all the major US cities.

1 Right-click the "Major U.S. Cities selection" layer and click Properties.

2 Click the General tab and change the name of the layer to Major Texas Cities.

3 **Click the Symbology tab and click the Symbol button.**

4 **Change the symbol to a solid black circle and set the size to** 8. **Click OK twice.**

5 **Turn the Major U.S. Cities layer off to show only the major cities in Texas.** Although the years for population and breast cancer deaths are different, the map shows the proximity of deaths to the more highly populated cities in the state.

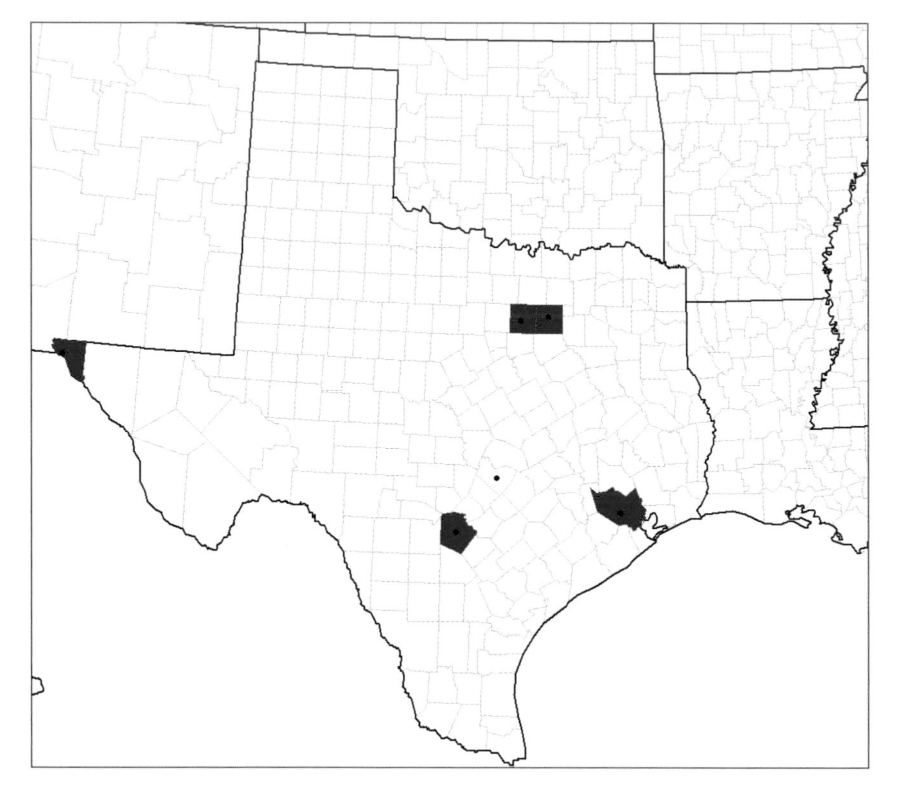

Save the map document

1 **On the Menu bar, click File > Save As.**

2 **Save your map document as** Tutorial2-9YourName.mxd **to your Chapter2 folder in MyExercises.** Do not close ArcMap.

Tutorial 2-10

Labeling major cities in Texas

Sometimes labels are needed to inform the map reader about features they are seeing on a map, such as the major cities in Texas. Because GIS features are connected to attribute data in tables, you can easily label map features using any data found in the feature's attribute table.

Set label properties and features

1 Right-click the Major Texas Cities layer and click Properties.

2 Click the Labels tab and select the "Label features in this layer" check box.

3 Click the Label Field arrow, and if necessary, select NAME from the list of available fields.

4 Click Symbol > Edit Symbol and then click the Mask tab.

5 Under Style, select Halo.

6 Click Symbol and choose a bright-yellow fill color.

7 Click OK three times.

8 Change the font to bold and the size to 10.

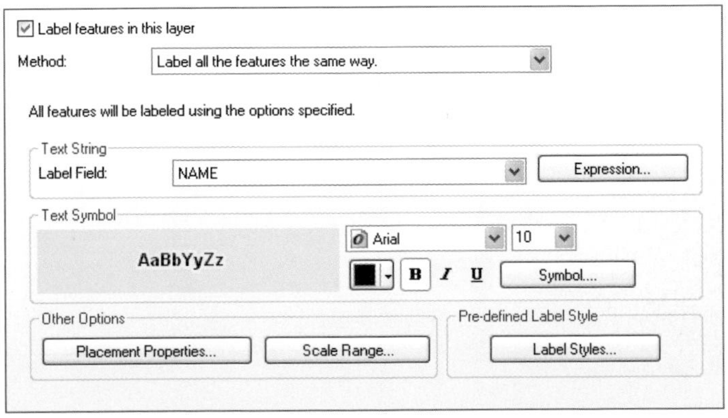

9 Click OK. ArcMap labels the most populated cities in Texas.

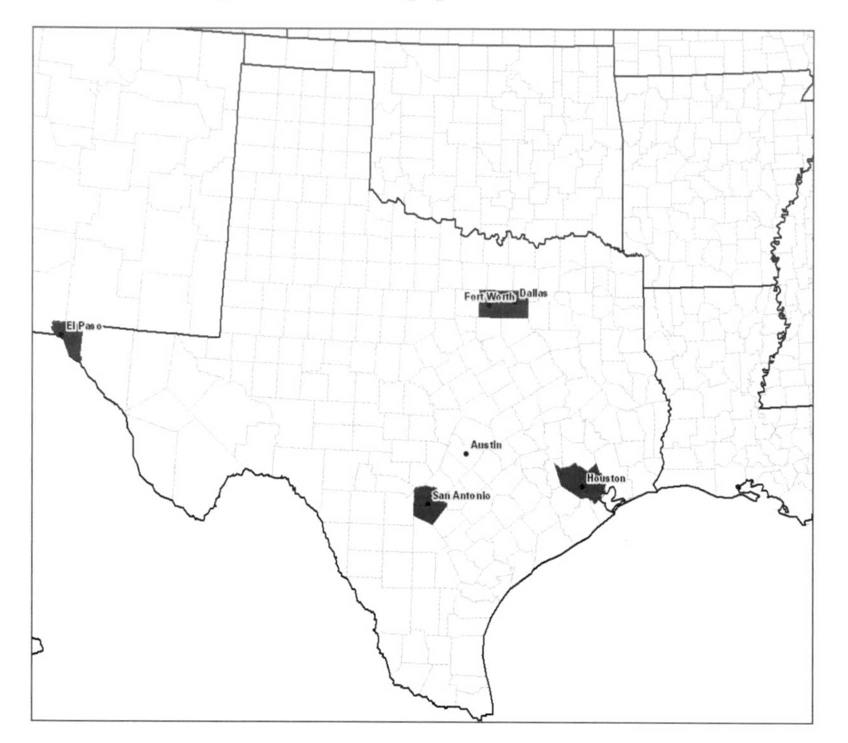

Remove labels

1 Right-click the Major Texas Cities layer and click Label Features. ArcMap turns the labels off.

2 Repeat step 1 to turn the labels back on.

Convert labels to annotation

Use labels to quickly generate maps that show text associated with a map feature. If you want to move individual labels, you'll need to convert labels to annotation text. In this exercise, you will convert the labels of Texas cities to annotation so that you can move them around on the map.

1 Right-click the Major Texas Cities layer and click Convert Labels to Annotation.

2 Under Store Annotation, select the "In the map" option. If you had features selected, you could choose "Selected features" under Create Annotation For to convert labels for those features only.

3 Click Convert. (See facing page.)

Convert Labels to Annotation

Store Annotation
In a database · In the map

Reference Scale
1:4,888,817

Create Annotation For
All features · Features in current extent · Selected features

Feature Layer	Annotation Group
Major Texas Cities	MajorTexasCities Anno

Destination: Annotation group stored in the map document

Convert unplaced labels to unplaced annotation

Convert · Cancel

Move labels

1 **On the Menu bar, click Customize > Toolbars > Draw.** The Draw toolbar is useful for moving labels, adding single labels, or adding text and other graphic elements.

2 **On the Draw toolbar, click the Select Elements tool.**

3 **Click the labels for Dallas, Fort Worth, and San Antonio, and using your own judgment, move the labels to a better position.**

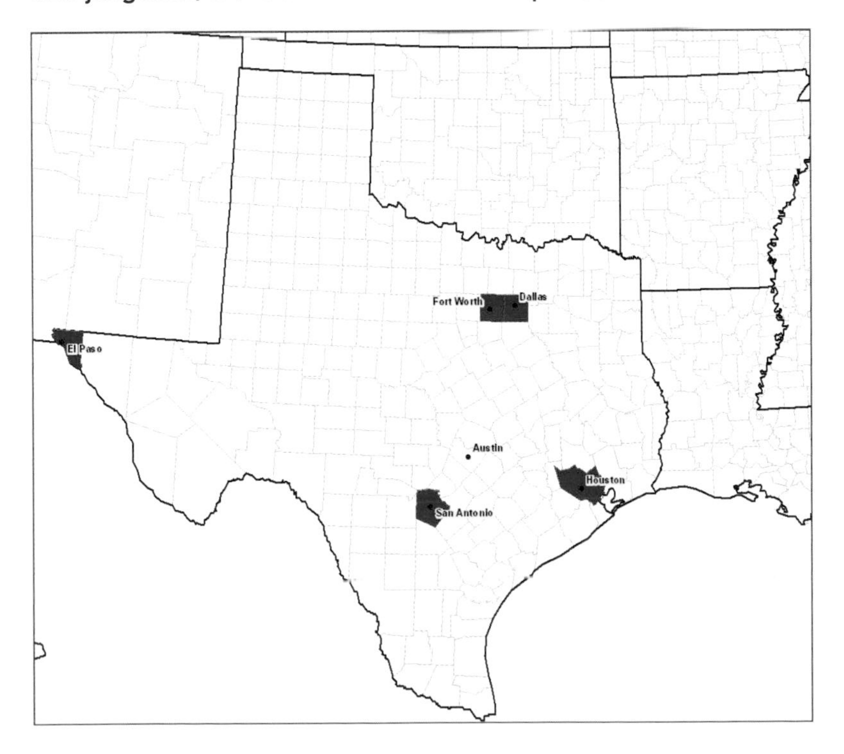

4 On the Menu bar, click Customize > Toolbars > Draw to close the Draw toolbar.

YOUR TURN

Use Advanced Sorting to create two new layers of the selected features for the top five Texas counties for white and black female mortality rates for 2000–2004 (RWF00_04 and RBF00_04). To start, for black female mortality rates, right-click State Name and Advanced Sorting, and sort first by RBF00_04 and then by County. Create a new layer from these selected features. Use a Mars Red fill color and 10% Simple hatch at a 45-degree angle. Repeat for white female mortality rates (RWF00_04) using the same fill color and hatch but at an angle of 135 degrees.

Hint: *To make a hatch 135 degrees, in the Symbol Selector dialog box, choose 10% Simple hatch as the pattern. Then click Edit Symbol, and in the Symbol Property Editor, choose a 135-degree angle.*

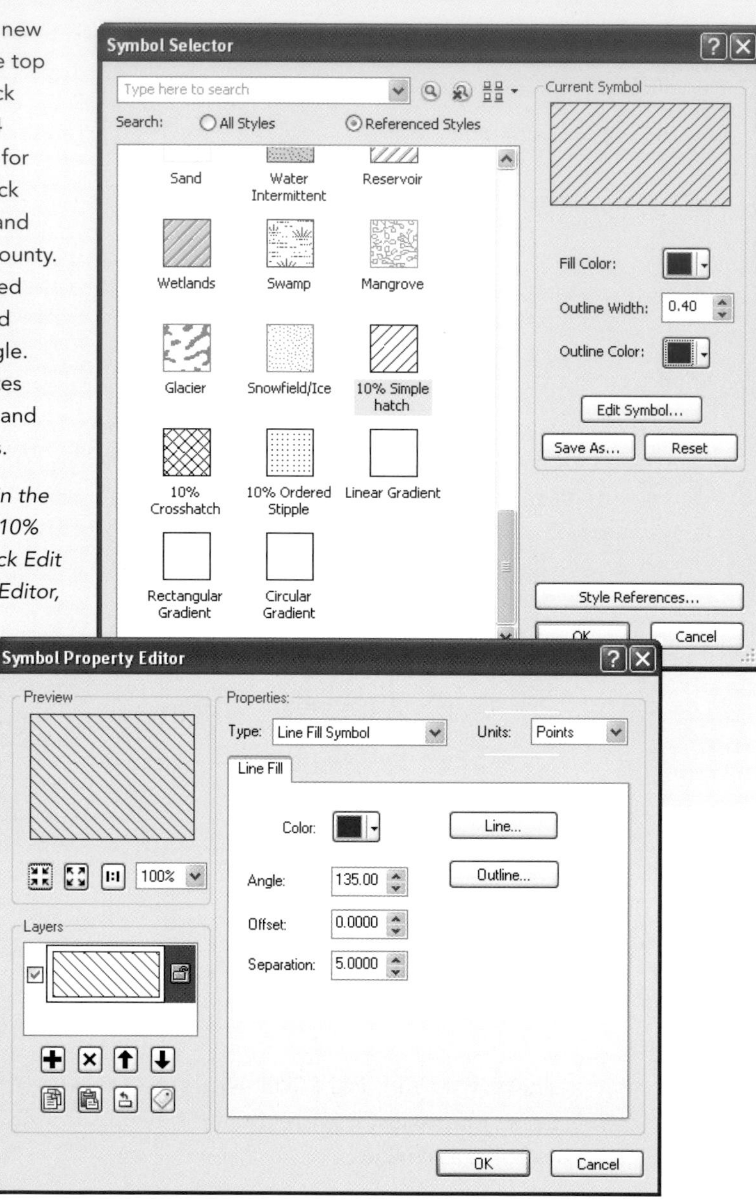

T 2-10

YOUR TURN continued

Notice that one Texas county (Crane) has a high mortality rate for both white and black females.

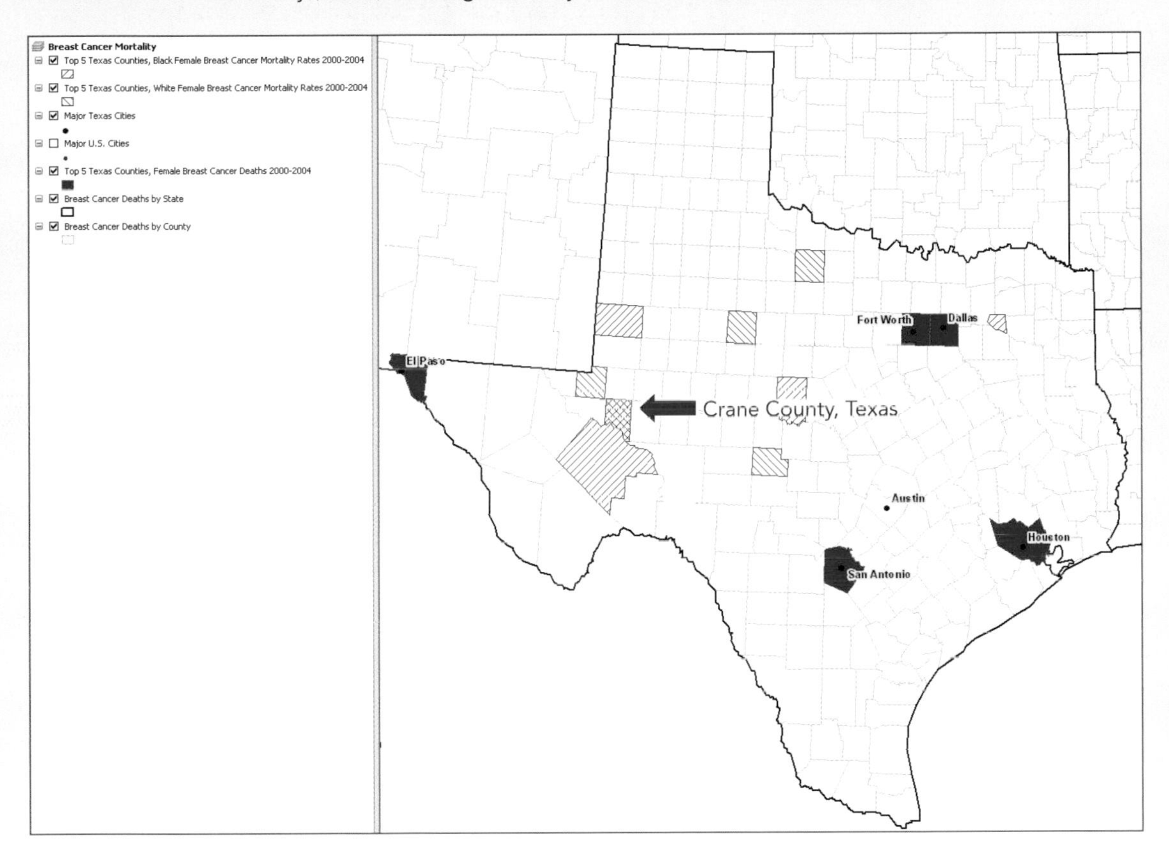

Save the project and exit ArcMap

1 **On the Menu bar, click File > Save As.**

2 **Save your map document as** Tutorial2-10YourName.mxd **to your Chapter2 folder in MyExercises.** This saves the current table and map information, including selected records and labels.

3 **Click File > Exit.** This closes ArcMap.

Summary

You now have a good start on making ArcMap work for you.

You have seen how a map document is composed of one or more map layers, which are added as needed and symbolized for the purpose at hand. You can symbolize map layers by changing symbol colors, outlines, shapes, and so forth. You can also add labels or annotation to identify map features.

You can change the portion or extent of the map layers you are viewing by zooming and panning the map. Spatial information is available at different map scales. Some information, such as cancer mortality rates by state in the United States, can be seen by zooming far out to the full extent of the map. Additional information is available at a finer scale by zooming to a state and viewing breast cancer mortality by county, with cities providing context. Zooming and panning are essential interactive tools for understanding both general and detailed information at different scales. Sometimes you will find a close-up view of features that you will want to revisit. In that case, you can create a spatial bookmark that allows you to quickly go back to that view.

Each point, line, and polygon map layer is linked to a feature attribute table that lists all the available attributes. You saw that each feature has its own data record, and if you select a feature on the map, ArcMap automatically selects its record. The opposite is true as well: If you select a table record, ArcMap selects the feature on the map. You can use the Identify, Select Features, Find, and Label tools to interact with the features on your map.

Of course, you are working with map documents for a reason—to find patterns regarding health, diseases, and related topics and convey this information to others. The essential information comes from how the features are spatially arranged in the map layers and from the health data records behind these features, which can be found in the attribute tables. For example, you sorted breast cancer mortality rates for counties by state in the county attribute table, selected the top five counties in the state, and then viewed the spatial arrangement of the selected counties on the map, using cities for additional spatial context. These are unique and useful capabilities made possible by GIS.

Assignment 2-1
Examine male lung cancer mortality rates by state

The National Cancer Institute (NCI) has a variety of websites to access cancer statistics and build interactive maps. Its Cancer Mortality Maps website provides interactive maps, graphs, text, tables, and figures showing geographic patterns and time trends of cancer death rates for more than 40 cancers from 1950 to 1994. GIS maps and data can also be found at http://gis.cancer.gov/research and surveillance.cancer.gov. These are excellent sites for building maps using predefined variables provided by NCI. If you want to create more-detailed or customized maps, you'll need to use a desktop GIS application.

In this assignment, use ArcMap to build maps showing lung cancer mortality for white and black males in the United States. Use a GIS attribute table to determine the states that had the highest mortality rates, and then display them in a map and in a Word document report.

Start with this data

- *\EsriPress\GISTHealth\Data\NCI.gdb\LungState:* a polygon feature class of lung cancer statistics by state and a data dictionary attribute table as follows:

Attribute	Definition
RWM00_04	Mortality rate per 100,000, white males, 2000–2004
RBM00_04	Mortality rate per 100,000, black males, 2000–2004

Create lung cancer mortality maps for US states

Create a map document called **Assignment2-1YourName.mxd** and save it to your Chapter2 folder in MyAssignments, using relative paths. Add the LungState layer modified as a Hollow fill with a medium-gray outline, size 1.0. Label every state by its abbreviation, using a yellow halo mask.

Get statistics and export maps

Using the layer attribute table, select the five states that had the highest lung cancer mortality rates for black males from 2000 to 2004. Create a new layer of only these selected features and rename it to reflect the new selection. Symbolize it as a dark-green 10% Simple hatch (45 degrees) and an outline width of 2.0. Using the selected records from the attribute table, create a table in a Microsoft Word document that shows the state names and black male mortality rates (sorted highest to lowest) for the top five selected states only.

Repeat these steps for white male lung cancer mortality rates for the top five states using a dark-blue 10% Simple hatch (135 degrees) and an outline width of 2.0. Using the selected records from the attribute table, create a table in a Microsoft Word document that shows the state names and white male mortality rates (sorted highest to lowest) for the top five selected states only.

Export the map as a JPEG file called **Assignment2-1YourName.jpg** and save it to your Chapter2 folder in MyAssignments.

Save your map document as **Assignment2-1YourName.mxd** to your Chapter2 folder in MyAssignments.

Create a Word document

Create a Microsoft Word document called **Assignment2-1YourName.docx** and save it to your Chapter2 folder in MyAssignments.

Include the following:

- Title
- Your name
- A few bullets mentioning any patterns that you observe from each of the following three exhibits:
  - Exhibit 1: table for black male lung cancer mortality rates, including a caption at the top
  - Exhibit 2: table for white male lung cancer mortality rates, including a caption at the top
  - Exhibit 3: map image inserted with a caption explaining black and white male mortality rates

WHAT TO TURN IN

If your work is to be graded, turn in the following files:

- ***ArcMap document:*** \EsriPress\GISTHealth\MyAssignments\Chapter2\Assignment2-1YourName.mxd
- ***Image file:*** \EsriPress\GISTHealth\MyAssignments\Chapter2\Assignment2-1YourName.jpg
- ***Microsoft Word document:*** \EsriPress\GISTHealth\MyAssignments\Chapter2\Assignment2-1YourName.docx

If instructed to do so, instead of individual files, turn in a compressed file, **Assignment2-1YourName.zip**, that includes all the preceding files. Do not include path information in the compressed file.

Assignment 2-2
Examine male lung cancer mortality rates by county

Detailed maps for US states show interesting patterns. One state, Kentucky, has relatively high lung cancer mortality rates for both black and white males. In this assignment, create a detailed map for a state health official in Kentucky that shows the Kentucky counties that had a mortality rate over 150 for black and white males between 2000 and 2004.

Start with this data

- *\EsriPress\GISTHealth\Data\NCI.gdb\LungState:* polygon features of lung cancer data by US state
- *\EsriPress\GISTHealth\Data\NCI.gdb\LungCounty:* polygon features of lung cancer data by county and a data dictionary attribute table as follows:

Attribute	Definition
RWM00_04	Mortality rate per 100,000 white males, 2000–2004
RBM00_04	Mortality rate per 100,000 black males, 2000–2004
CWMBM00_04	Count of white and black male lung cancer deaths, 2000–2004

- *\EsriPress\GISTHealth\Data\UnitedStates.gdb\USMajorCities:* point features of US cities including census demographics

Create detailed cancer mortality maps for Kentucky counties

Create a new blank map document called **Assignment2-2YourName.mxd** and save it to your Chapter2 folder in MyAssignments, using relative paths. Add the layers for states, counties, and major cities. Symbolize States using a Hollow fill, black outline, size 2.0; Counties using a Hollow fill, medium-gray outline; and Major Cities using a black circle, size 8. Label cities with the city name using a halo label. Zoom to Kentucky and save your zoomed-in view as a spatial bookmark called **Kentucky** so you can easily return to it.

Select Kentucky counties that had black male lung cancer mortality rates over 150 (2000–2004) and create a new layer of these selected counties. Rename the layer accordingly and choose a color and fill that you think is effective. Export this map as a JPEG file called **Assignment2-2AYourName.jpg** and save it to your Chapter2 folder in MyAssignments.

Repeat this selection process and create a new map layer of the Kentucky counties that had white male mortality rates over 150 (2000–2004). Export this map as a JPEG file called **Assignment2-2BYourName.jpg** and save it to your Chapter2 folder in MyAssignments.

Create a third selected layer of the five counties that had the highest number (count) of both white and black males (2000–2004). Export this map as a JPEG file called **Assignment2-2CYourName.jpg** and save it to your Chapter2 folder in MyAssignments.

Export a map as a JPEG file called **Assignment2-2DYourName.jpg** that has all the map layers turned on and save it to your Chapter2 folder in MyAssignments.

Save your map document as **Assignment2-2YourName.mxd** to your Chapter2 folder in MyAssignments.

Create a PowerPoint presentation

Create a Microsoft PowerPoint presentation called **Assignment2-2YourName.pptx** and save it to your Chapter2 folder in MyAssignments. Include the following:

- Title slide, including your name
- A slide showing Kentucky counties that had black male mortality rates over 150 from 2000 to 2004 with the map image inserted, including a caption at the top
- A slide showing Kentucky counties that had white male mortality rates over 150 from 2000 to 2004 with the map image inserted, including a caption at the top
- A slide showing Kentucky counties that had the highest count of black and white male lung cancer deaths between 2000 and 2004 with the map image inserted, including a caption at the top
- A slide showing all map layers with the map image inserted, including a caption at the top
- A summary slide that includes observations: List the two counties whose black and white male mortality rates were both over 150

WHAT TO TURN IN

If your work is to be graded, turn in the following files:

- ***ArcMap document:*** \EsriPress\GISTHealth\MyAssignments\Chapter2\Assignment2-2YourName.mxd
- ***Microsoft PowerPoint document:*** \EsriPress\GISTHealth\MyAssignments\Chapter2\Assignment2-2YourName.pptx

Note: *The interim JPEG files are not required for submission.*

If instructed to do so, instead of individual files, turn in a compressed file, **Assignment2-2YourName.zip**, that includes all the preceding files. Do not include path information in the compressed file.

Chapter 3

Designing maps for a health study

Objectives

- Investigate spatial patterns of uninsured and poor populations
- Design and build numeric scales for mapping attributes
- Symbolize numeric scales for polygons using color ramps
- Symbolize numeric scales for points using size-graduated point markers
- Map the relationship between two variables
- Build professional map layouts for presentations and reports
- Export map layouts as image files
- Create multiple output pages

Health-care scenario

Suppose that you have the ability to direct state funds to help finance health-care costs for uninsured populations in Texas. Probably most of the uninsured are poor, so you'll want to investigate the correlation between uninsured populations and poverty indicators, including unemployment and minority status. You also want to locate the target populations on a map to see where the funds should be concentrated.

Solution approach

Much of what needs to be done involves using cartographic (map design) principles to convey information about the underlying attributes of graphic features. So, this section provides concepts and guidelines for that purpose.

The graphic elements that can be used to symbolize maps include fill color and patterns for polygons; outline width, pattern, and color for lines—including outlines for polygons and point markers; and shape, size, and color for point markers. In general, maps cannot display continuous variation in numeric attributes because the human eye cannot readily interpret small changes in graphic elements. Instead, an approach that is analogous to making bar charts to symbolize continuous variables in data tables can be used to depict large changes in graphic elements.

An example is a choropleth map that uses solid fill color for polygons based on a relatively small number of intervals covering the range of an attribute. The right-side boundary of an interval is called a break value and is included in the interval, but the left side is not. For example, you will use 20 and under, 21–25, 26–30, and 31–35 for the percentage of uninsured persons per county in Texas, with break values of 20, 25, 30, and 35. The interval 21–25, for example, contains polygons that have a percentage of uninsured greater than 21 and less than or equal to 25.

Except for the 0–20 interval, these are equal-width intervals with each one covering a range of 5 percentage points. To make things easier to interpret, the break values were set to multiples of 5. Taken as a whole, these intervals include, or span, the complete range of attributes stored for this variable. ArcMap has several other options for designing intervals. A helpful one for analysts uses quantiles that break up attribute values into equal-size groups. For example, for four intervals, quantiles are the same as the more familiar quartiles, where each interval has 25% of the observations. Another useful option is to manually choose whatever break values you want. Many phenomena have long-tail distributions to the right, with many low values and relatively few but far-ranging high values. (A long-tailed probability distribution is one that assigns relatively high probabilities to regions far from the mean or median.) In this case, using a manual numeric scale with interval widths that double is often valuable—for example, 0–5, 5–15, 15–35, and 35–75, with interval widths of 5, 10, 20, and 40.

The choice of colors for intervals is based on color value, which is the amount of black added to a color. A monochromatic color scale uses a single color, with light to medium to dark shades of the same color. Usually, the darker the color, the higher the interval of values—this makes it easy to interpret a map at a glance. Also, if you make a black-and-white copy of a map that has a monochromatic scale, the map retains valid visual information by its shades of gray. ArcMap software generates monochromatic and multicolor color scales called color ramps. A design tip for using monochromatic color ramps is to include more light shades and fewer dark shades because the human eye is better at discriminating light shades.

The approach to symbolizing points depends more on variations in the shape and size of point markers than on color. A point is a mathematical object that has no area, but to see a point on a map, you have to plot a point marker that does have area. Perhaps the most effective way to show variation in a numerical attribute of a point feature is to vary the size of a fixed-shape point marker—that is, use size-graduated point markers. For example, you might use five intervals and five circular point markers with increasing radii for increasing intervals. Often, it is sufficient to use the same color for all sizes of a point marker of an attribute, but you can also add a monochromatic color ramp to the fill color of a point marker. Another design tip is to exaggerate the size intervals by increasing the differences in radii between successive point markers by more than the proportional increases in interval values.

These are the principles you will apply to studying the spatial pattern and correlation of uninsured and poor populations. The trick to plotting both populations on the same map is to use a county based choropleth map for one variable and size-graduated point markers located at the centroid (center point) of counties for the other variable. ArcMap automatically creates the polygon centroids for this purpose.

It is often the case that you will need to present your findings and write them up in a report or provide them as hard copies to be used for decision making. This calls for professional-quality, unique stand-alone maps, which goes beyond the interactive map views ArcMap software presents on a computer screen. As you may have guessed, ArcMap has the capacity to easily produce these professional-quality maps in the form of map layouts that can be printed as hard-copy maps. Map layouts have all the features that are necessary for use outside ArcMap: a title, map, neatline, legend, scale bar, and so forth. A neatline places a border around the map, and the legend explains symbols and numeric scales used on the map. Scale is a graphic representation of distance using a straight line that has a few distances marked off. ArcMap can also automate map outputs through Data Driven Pages, explored in tutorial 3-8.

Tutorial 3-1

Creating a choropleth map for the uninsured population in Texas

Your first task is to build a choropleth map for the percentage of uninsured by county in Texas. As is the case for all symbolization in ArcMap, this process is highly automated so you will need to make only a few selections to render the entire map layer rather than having to paint each graphic feature individually.

Open a map document

1 **Start ArcMap and open Tutorial3-1.mxd.** A new, empty map is displayed.

Next, you will add layers to the map and symbolize them.

Add a layer and change its name

1 **On the Standard toolbar, click Add Data.**

2 **Browse through the Data folder to UnitedStates.gdb, click TXCounties, and click Add.**

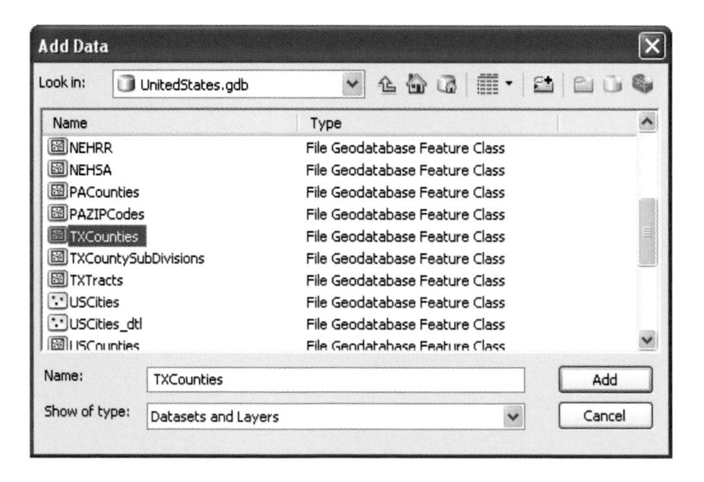

ArcMap adds Texas counties and picks an arbitrary fill color for the polygons. You will change the color later in this tutorial.

3 **In the table of contents, right-click the TXCounties layer and click Properties.**

4 **In the Layer Properties dialog box, click the General tab.**

5 **Type** % Population Uninsured **as the new layer name.**

6 **Click OK.**

Select an attribute to display the uninsured population

The Symbology tab in the Layer Properties dialog box allows you to use unique colors to symbolize your data using intervals that cover the range of a numeric attribute. There are several classification schemes to choose from. ArcGIS for Desktop Help describes all these classification methods. Generally, it is best to use a monochromatic color scale—that is, one color in increasingly darker shades progressing from small- to large-value intervals, or vice versa. ArcMap has many prebuilt progressions of color, called color ramps, that are monochromatic. In this exercise, you will classify data for the percentage of uninsured population in Texas counties.

1 **Right-click the % Population Uninsured layer and click Properties.**

2 **Click the Symbology tab.**

3 **In the Show panel, click Quantities > Graduated colors.**

T 3-1

4 Under Fields, click the Value arrow, scroll to the bottom of the list, and click PCT_UNINS. Only numeric fields appear in the Value list.

Layer Properties

General | Source | Selection | Display | Symbology | Fields | Definition Query | Labels | Joins & Relates | Time | HTML Popup

Show:
Features
Categories
Quantities
Graduated colors
Graduated symbols
Proportional symbols
Dot density
Charts
Multiple Attributes

Draw quantities using color to show values. Numeric field Import...

Fields
Value: PCT_UNINS
Normalization: none

Classification
Natural Breaks (Jenks)
Classes: 5 Classify...

Color Ramp:

Symbol	Range	Label
	14.700000 - 19.500000	14.700000 - 19.500000
	19.500001 - 21.900000	19.500001 - 21.900000
	21.900001 - 24.600000	21.900001 - 24.600000
	24.600001 - 28.400000	24.600001 - 28.400000
	28.400001 - 35.000000	28.400001 - 35.000000

Show class ranges using feature values
Advanced

OK Cancel Apply

5 Click OK. The result is five classifications of uninsured total population ranging from lowest to highest values with darker colors representing higher values. ArcMap picks an arbitrary color ramp and a method of creating intervals, called natural breaks, for the polygons. You will learn how to change the colors and classification methods later.

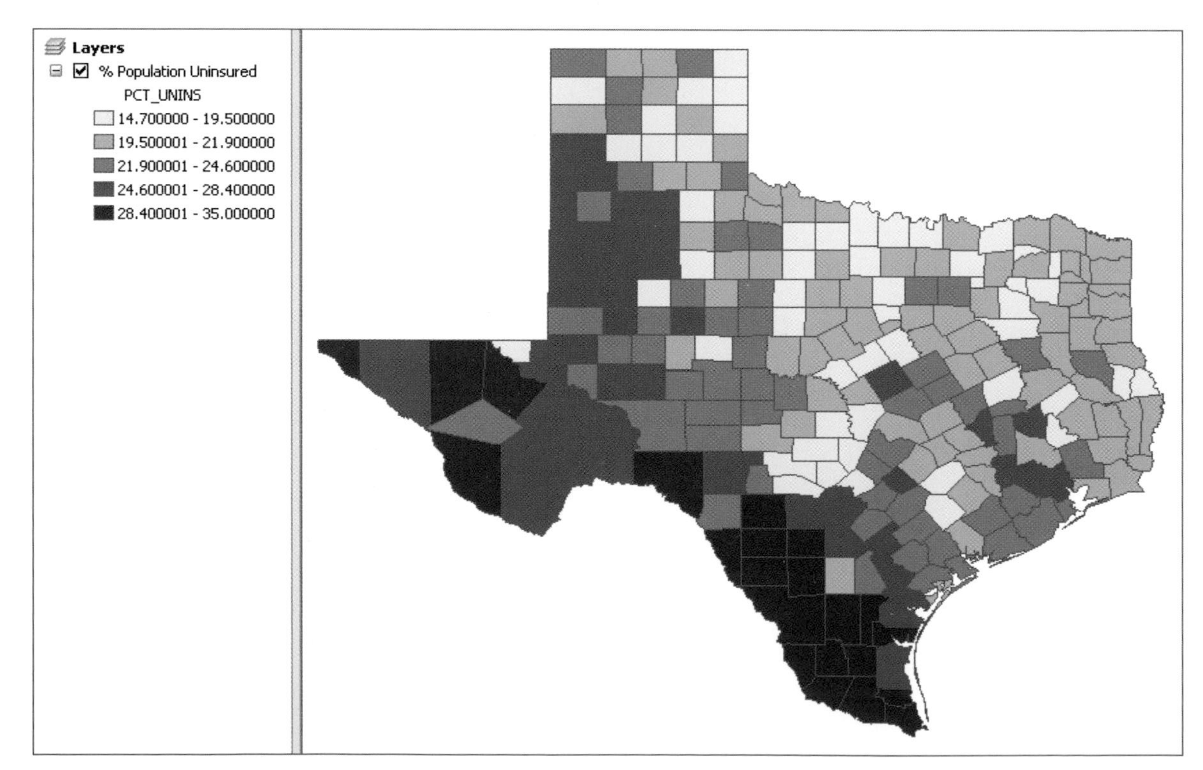

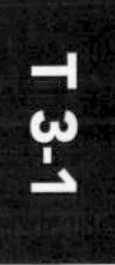

Create custom classifications

One of the powerful features of desktop GIS is the ability to create your own custom classifications and to choose or modify color ramps. In this exercise, you will create your own custom legend for the percentage of population that is uninsured.

1 **Right-click the % Population Uninsured layer, click Properties, and click the Symbology tab.**

2 **Under Classification, click the Classes arrow and change the number of classes to 4.**

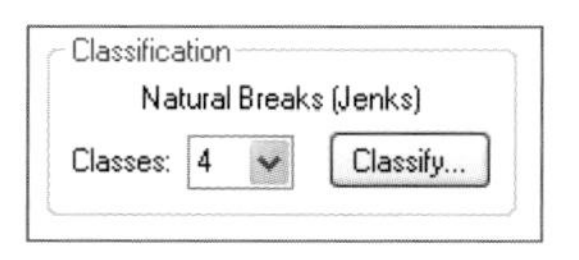

3 **Under Classification, click the Classify button.** The Classification dialog box shows the current classification method, classification statistics, a histogram of the data, and a list of the current classification break values.

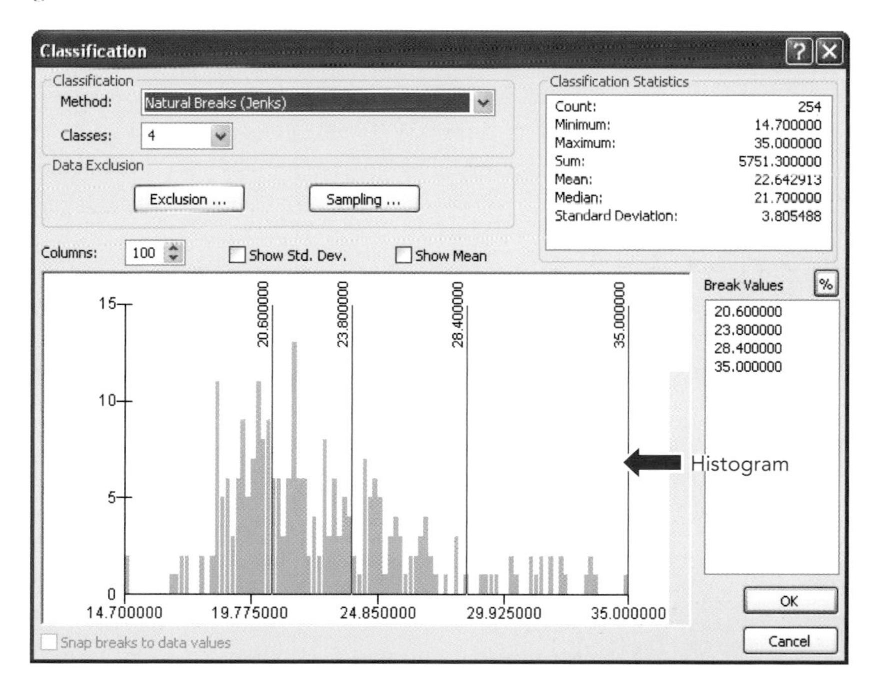

The next task is to break up the range of uninsured population into intervals, as you would do if you were creating a bar chart for this data.

Manually change classification values for the percentage of uninsured

1. **Under Classification, click the Method arrow and click Manual.**
2. **In the Break Values list, click the first value, 20.600000, to highlight it.**
   Notice that the blue line in the graph corresponding to that value turns red.
3. **Type** 20 **and press ENTER to move to the next break value.**
4. **Repeat steps 2 and 3 to create the following break values:** 25, 30, 35.
5. **Click OK.**

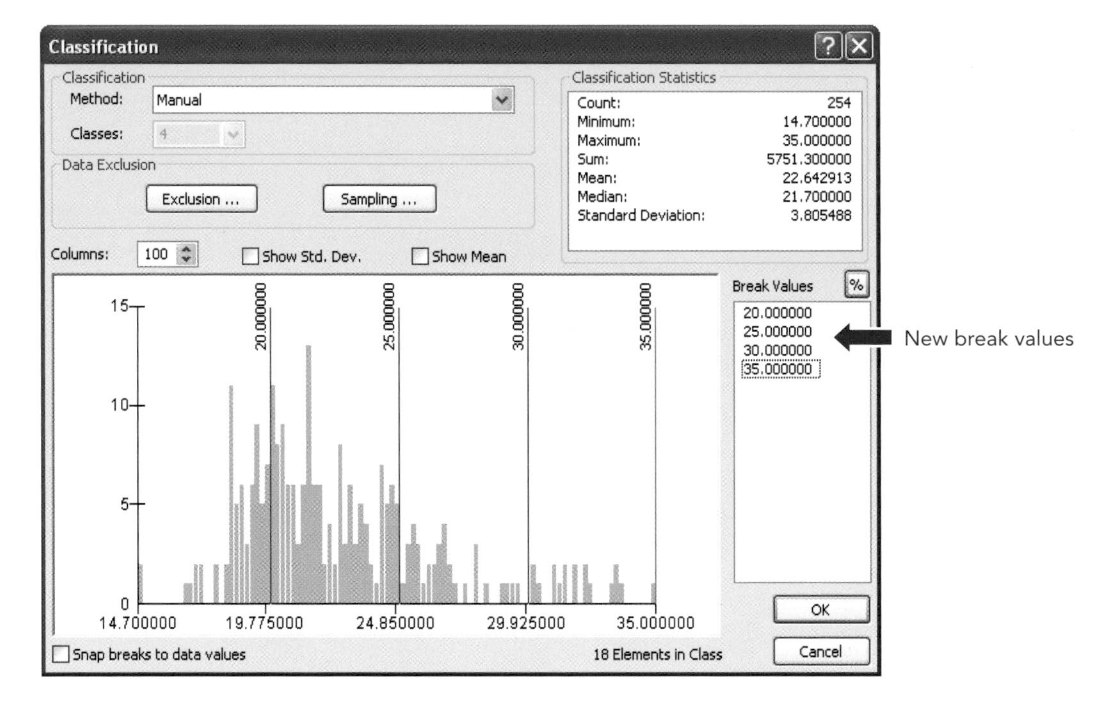

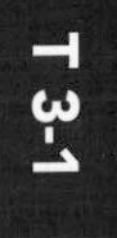

Change labels

1 In the Layer Properties dialog box, click the Symbology tab, click the Label column heading, and then click Format Labels.

2 In the Category list, select Percentage and click the Numeric Options button.

3 Set the "Number of decimal places" to 0 and click OK three times.

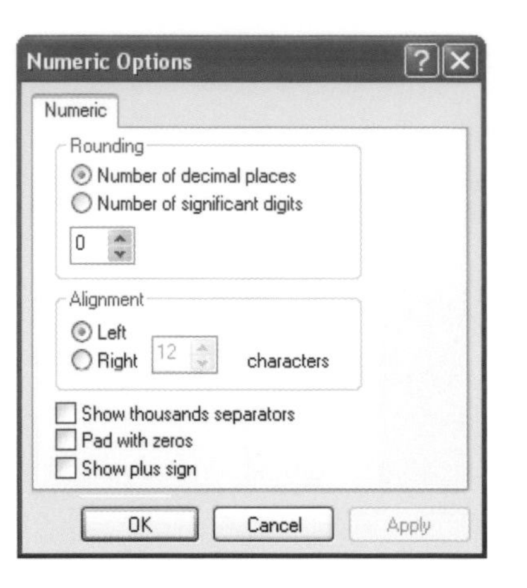

The changes to the Layers legend—fixed intervals of width 5, no decimal places, and the use of percent signs (%)—make the map easier for lay audiences to interpret.

Layers
% Population Uninsured
PCT_UNINS
15% - 20%
21% - 25%
26% - 30%
31% - 35%

Build a custom color ramp

Generally, it is best to have more classes in light colors and fewer classes in dark colors, because the human eye can differentiate lighter colors more easily than darker colors. In this exercise, you will build a custom color ramp that has lighter colors.

1 Right-click the % Population Uninsured layer, click Properties, and click the Symbology tab.

2 Click the Color Ramp arrow, scroll to the top, and click the fourth color ramp from the top (shades of blue).

3 Right-click the Color Ramp box and click Properties.

Color Ramp:
✔ Graphic View
Properties...
Save to style...

Symbol	Range	Label
	14.700000 - 20.000000	
	20.000001 - 25.000000	21% - 25%
	25.000001 - 30.000000	26% - 30%
	30.000001 - 35.000000	31% - 35%

4 Click the Color 1 color box and select Arctic White.

5 Click the Color 2 color box and select Dark Navy.

Colors

Color 1:

Color 2:

6 Click OK twice. The % Population Uninsured map now has a new custom color ramp, ranging from white to dark blue. You can also double-click each color box in the Symbology tab of a map layer's Layer Properties dialog box to change the classification colors individually.

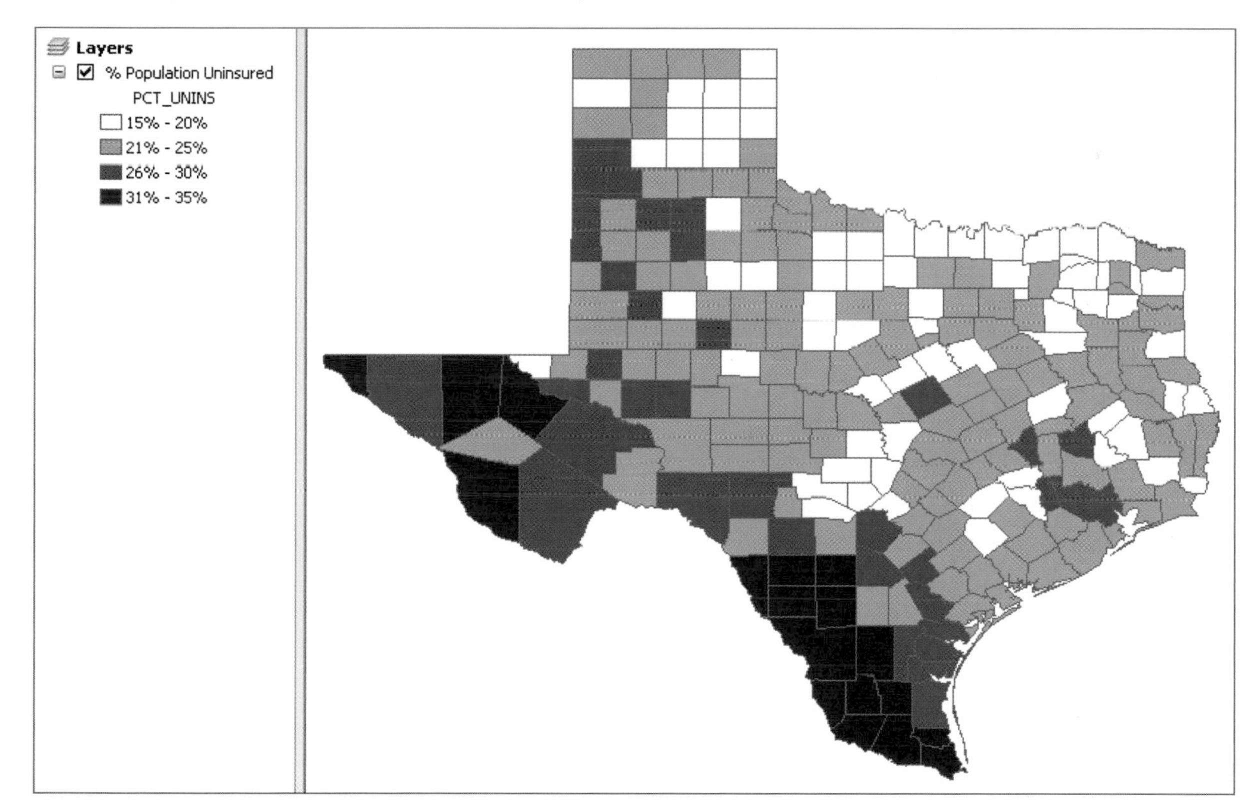

Save the Texas uninsured population choropleth map

1 On the Menu bar, click File > Save As.

2 Save your map document as Tutorial3-1YourName.mxd **to your Chapter3 folder in MyExercises.** Do not close ArcMap.

Tutorial 3-2
Creating a point map for the percentage of unemployed in Texas

In this tutorial, you will add unemployment data as points to your uninsured choropleth map so you can look for a correlation between the unemployment rate and the number of people who don't have health insurance. To show variations in unemployment, you will break up that variable's range into intervals similar to those for the insured, but this time you will use the point marker size instead of a color ramp to differentiate the intervals—the larger the point marker size, the larger the interval value.

Symbolize unemployment data as graduated point markers

1. **If it is not already open, open the map document you created in tutorial 3-1—Tutorial3-1YourName.mxd saved to your Chapter3 folder.**

2. **On the Standard toolbar, click Add Data and add the layer TXCounties from the United States geodatabase in the Data folder.**

3. **In the table of contents, double-click the TXCounties layer.** This is a shortcut to opening the Layer Properties dialog box.

4. **Click the General tab and change the name of the layer to** % Population Unemployed**.**

5. **Click the Symbology tab, and in the Show panel, click Quantities > Graduated symbols.**

6. **Under Fields, change Value to PCT_UNEMP.**

7. **Change the Template symbol to a red circle, Symbol Size to a range of** 2 **to** 24**, and Background fill and Outline to no color.** (See facing page.)

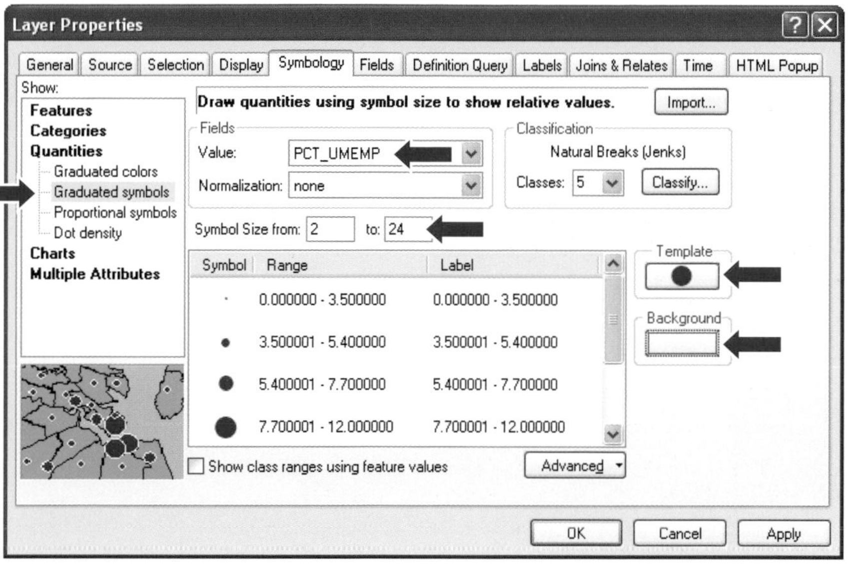

8 Click OK.

Modify point classifications

The default classifications for the points need to be modified so that an even comparison can be made to the uninsured population.

1 **Double-click the % Population Unemployed layer, click the Symbology tab, and click the Classify button.**

2 **In the Method list, click Equal Interval.**

The resulting interval break values are not whole numbers. To make the numeric scale easier to interpret, you will manually adjust the break values to even intervals of a width of 4.

3 **Change the break values to** 4, 8, 12, 16, 20.9 **and click OK.**

4 **Click the text of each line in the label and change the labels to** under 4%, 4.1% - 8%, 8.1% - 12%, 12.1% - 16%, 16.1% - 20.9%. Notice that labels can be a combination of text and numeric values.

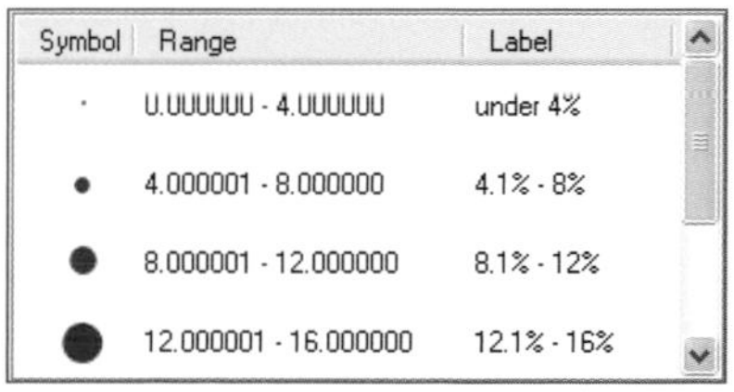

Symbol	Range	Label
·	U.UUUUUU - 4.UUUUUU	under 4%
•	4.000001 - 8.000000	4.1% - 8%
●	8.000001 - 12.000000	8.1% - 12%
●	12.000001 - 16.000000	12.1% - 16%

5 **Click OK.** The resulting map shows the counties layer twice: once as a choropleth map that has graduated colors and once as a point map that has graduated point markers. You can see the direct positive correlation between the unemployed and uninsured populations.

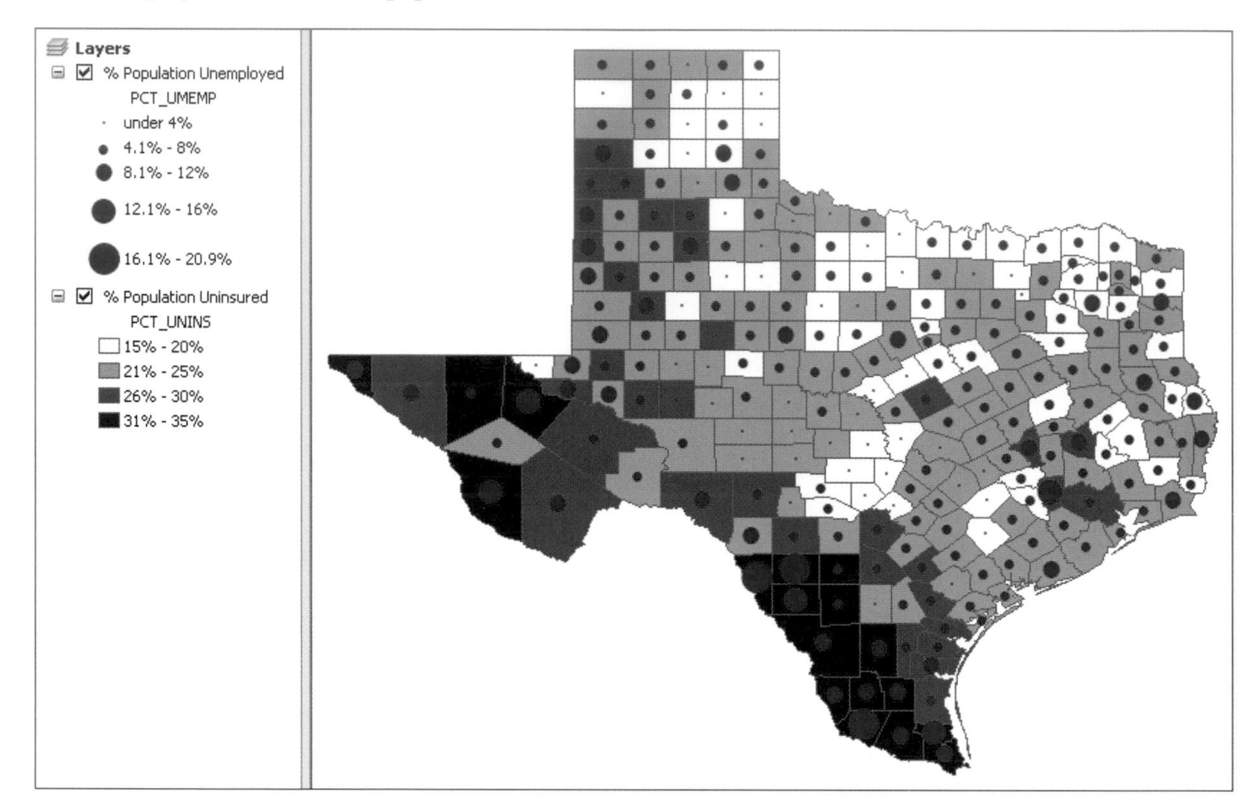

Save the graduated point marker and choropleth map

1 **On the Menu bar, click File > Save As.**

2 **Save your map document as** Tutorial3-2YourName.mxd **to your Chapter3 folder in MyExercises.** Do not close ArcMap.

Tutorial 3-3

Making a scatterplot comparing uninsured with unemployed populations

Scatterplots display pairs of attributes and may reveal a relationship between the values plotted. In this tutorial, you will create a scatterplot showing the positive correlation between uninsured and unemployed populations.

Create a scatterplot

1 On the Menu bar, click View > Graphs > Create Graph.

2 In the Create Graph Wizard, in the "Graph type" list, click Scatter Plot.

3 In the "Y field" list, scroll down and click PCT_UNINS.

4 In the "X field (optional)" list, scroll down and click PCT_UNEMP.

5 Click to clear the "Add to legend" check box.

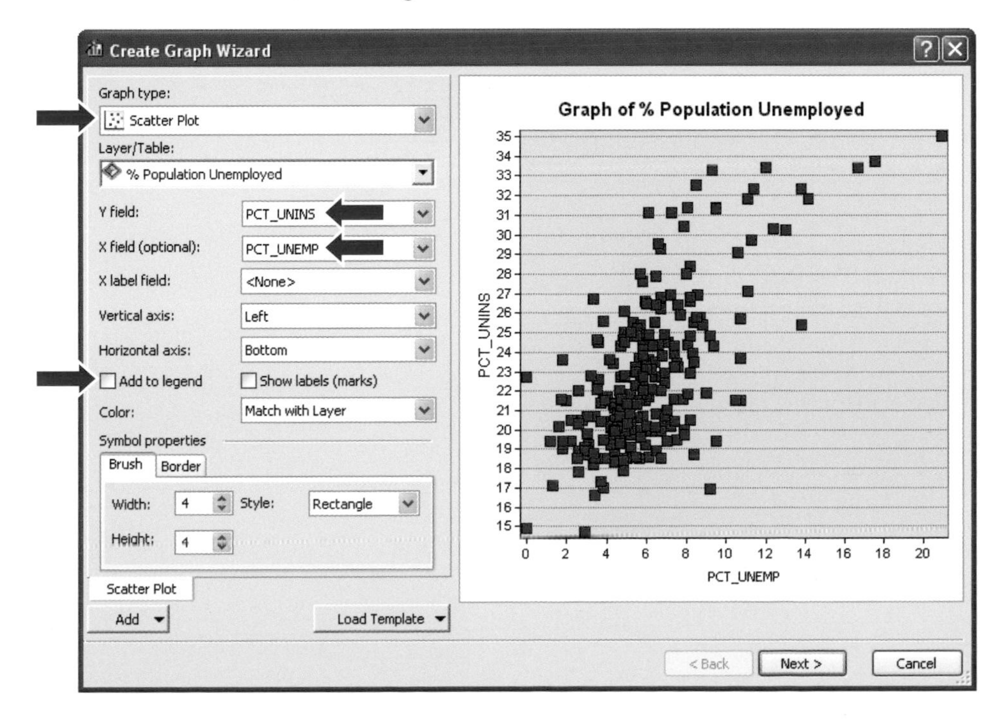

6 **Click Next.**

7 **In the Title box, type** Relationship of Uninsured and Unemployed Populations.

8 **Click to clear the "Graph legend" check box.**

9 **In the Axis properties panel, click the Left tab, and for Title, type** Percentage Uninsured.

10 **Click the Bottom tab, and for Title, type** Percentage Unemployed.

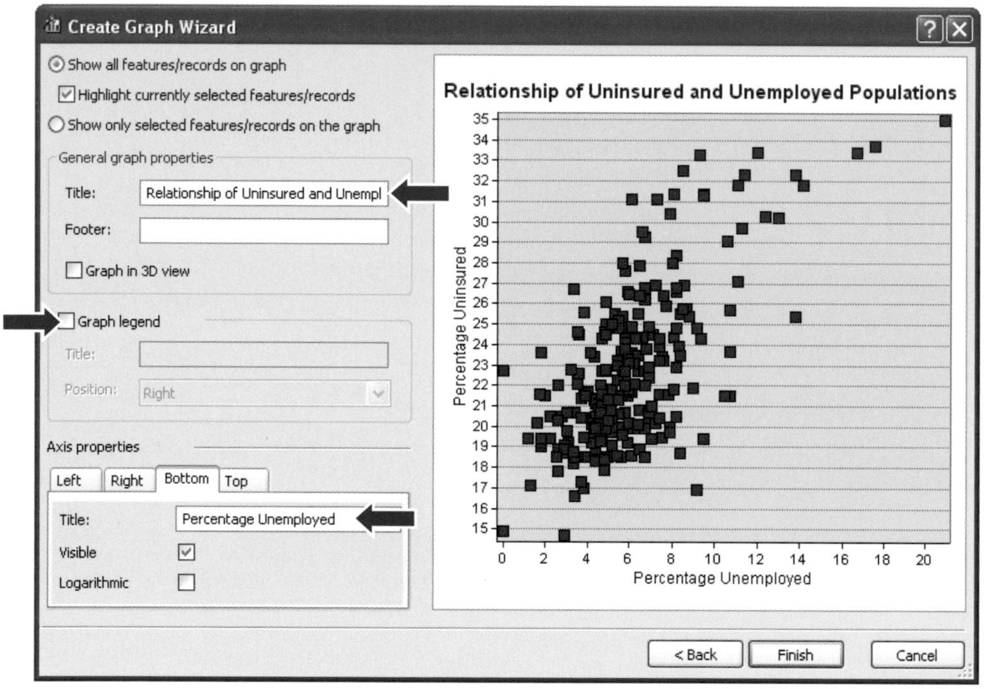

11 Click Finish. The result is a scatterplot that helps to summarize and support the results of the correlation between the unemployed and uninsured populations. Right-clicking anywhere on the graph opens a context menu that allows you to make revisions to your graph by clicking Advanced Properties or Properties. For example, you can add the graph to the layout of your current map or export it to a variety of graphic formats.

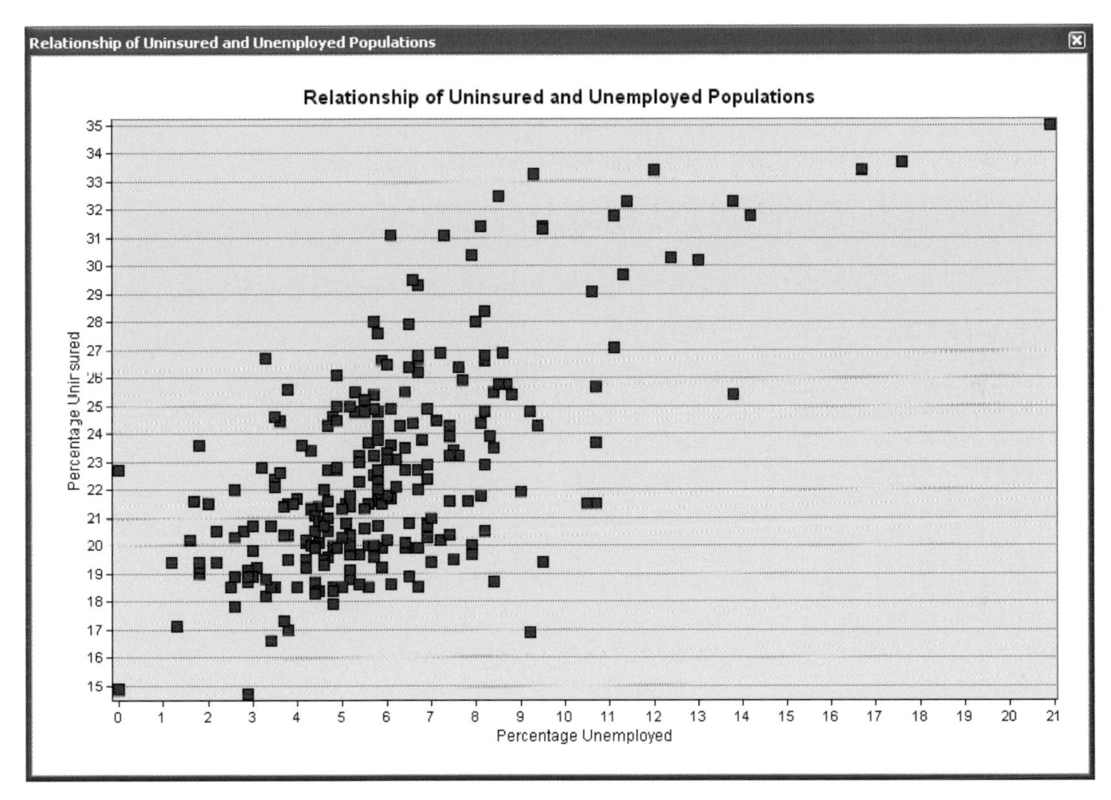

YOUR TURN

Search ArcGIS for Desktop Help to learn more about the types of graphs you can create.

Save the map and scatterplot

1 **On the Menu bar, click File > Save As.**

2 **Save your map document as** Tutorial3-3YourName.mxd **to your Chapter3 folder in MyExercises.** Do not close ArcMap.

Tutorial 3-4
Working with layer files

ArcMap has features that allow you to save and reuse your symbology, including classification schemes, colors of choropleth maps, and graduated point markers. To do this, you can save layer symbology to a layer (.lyr) file. Layer files allow you to use the same layer symbology across several maps.

Create a layer file

1 Close the scatterplot window.

2 In the table of contents, right-click % Population Unemployed and click Save As Layer File.

3 Browse through MyExercises to your Chapter3 folder.

4 Type Unemployed.lyr **for Name and click Save.**

YOUR TURN

Save the % Population Uninsured layer to a file called **Uninsured.lyr**, also saved to your Chapter3 folder in MyExercises. You will use this layer file in an upcoming task.

Create a group layer and add saved layers

You can also group several layers into a group layer, whose layers can be turned on and off by one click of the mouse, allowing for better organization of the layers in your map.

1 On the Menu bar, click File > New.

2 In the New Document dialog box, click Blank Map and click OK.

3 In the table of contents, right-click Layers and click New Group Layer.

4 Right-click the resulting New Group Layer and click Properties.

5 In the Group Layer Properties dialog box, click the General tab.

6 For Layer Name, type Texas Unemployed/Uninsured Comparison**.**

Group Layer Properties
General | Group | Display
Layer Name: Texas Unemployed/Uninsured Comparison ☑ Visible
Description:
Credits:
Scale Range
You can specify the range of scales at which this layer will be shown:
◉ Show layer at all scales
○ Don't show layer when zoomed:
Out beyond: <None> (minimum scale)
In beyond: <None> (maximum scale)
OK | Cancel | Apply

7 Click the Group tab and click the Add button.

8 Browse through MyExercises to your Chapter3 folder.

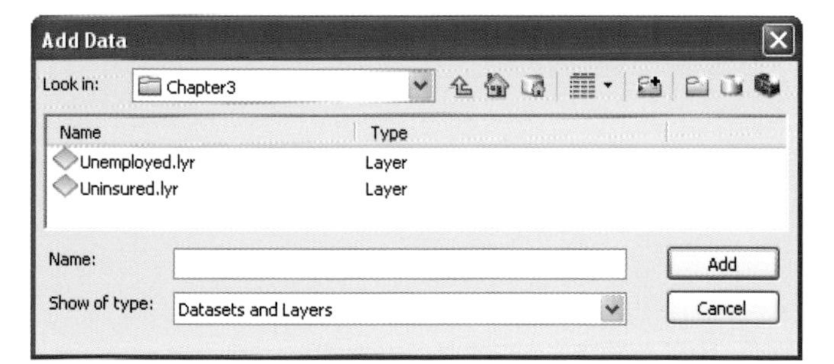

9 Select the layer names by holding down SHIFT and clicking Unemployed.lyr and Uninsured.lyr. Click Add and then OK. The resulting map document displays the already symbolized Texas polygon and point features comparing unemployed with uninsured in a group layer.

10 Collapse the tree structure of the existing layers in the table of contents by clicking the leftmost boxes for % Population Uninsured and % Population Unemployed, which have a minus sign (-). You can reverse this process by clicking the plus sign (+), which indicates that they can be expanded.

Layers
- Texas Unemployed/Uninsured Comparison
  - % Population Uninsured
  - % Population Unemployed

YOUR TURN

Turn the existing group layer off and create a new group layer called **Texas Uninsured/Hispanic Population Comparison**. Add the Uninsured.lyr file that you saved. Add the TXCounties layer again, this time showing the number of Hispanic people in Texas (field HISPANIC) as graduated point markers. Use the following cut points: **10,000, 30,000, 90,000, 270,000, 1,119,751**. Label as you see fit. Save this layer as **HispanicPopulation.lyr** to your Chapter3 folder in MyExercises. You will use this layer file in an upcoming task.

Save the new Texas health study comparison map

1 **On the Menu bar, click File > Save As.**

2 **Save your map document as** Tutorial3-4YourName.mxd **to your Chapter3 folder in MyExercises.** Do not close ArcMap.

Tutorial 3-5
Creating print layouts for a health-care study

In many cases, you will want to produce a paper copy or file copy of a map for distribution or use in a report or presentation. You will want to have a stand-alone map that has a title, map, legend, and possibly other components. ArcMap has a layout view for this purpose and several prebuilt templates for producing different kinds of layouts.

Choose a prebuilt layout template

For a quick map layout, you can use one of the provided templates.

1 **On the Menu bar, click File > Open, browse through your Maps folder if necessary, and open Tutorial3-5.mxd.** A new, empty map appears.

2 **Click View > Layout View.**

3 **Click Customize > Toolbars > Layout (if it is not already selected).**

4 **On the Layout toolbar, click the Change Layout button, scroll to the right, and click the Traditional Layouts tab. Click LetterLandscape.mxd.**

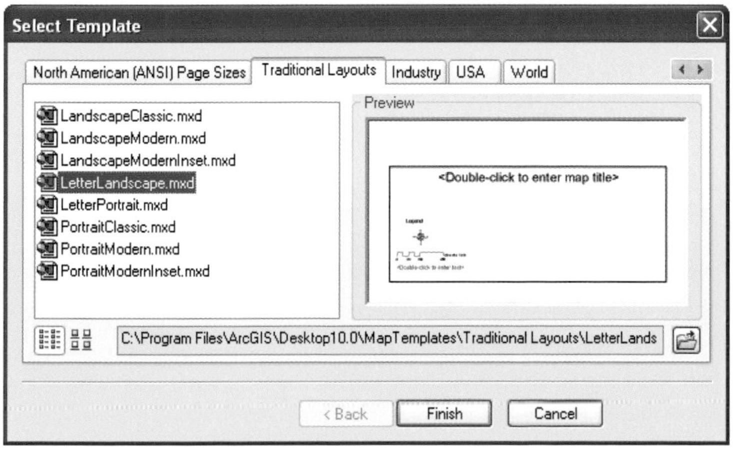

5 Click Finish.

A prebuilt map layout appears. Next, you simply need to add layers to the template.

YOUR TURN

Click Change Layout again and explore the other prebuilt layout templates. Notice the templates for industry standards as well as USA and World maps. Click Cancel when you are finished browsing.

Add layers to the map layout

1. **On the Standard toolbar, click Add Data.**
2. **Browse through MyExercises to your Chapter3 folder and add the Uninsured and Unemployed layers.**
3. **In the map data frame, double-click the title and change it to** Texas Uninsured and Unemployed Comparison. You may need to change the font size to fit the text on the map.
4. **Click the map scale to select it, and then right-click it and click Delete. Delete the north arrow the same way.** The map scale and north arrow are not needed for this map.
5. **Double-click the legend. In the Legend Properties dialog box, click the General tab and delete the word "Legend."**
6. **In the Map Layers, add % Population Unemployed and % Population Uninsured to Legend Items if they are not already there.**
7. **Click OK.**
8. **On the Tools toolbar, click the Fixed Zoom Out button.**
9. **Double-click the "Double-click to enter text" box in the lower-left portion of the template and type** Source: Data obtained from U.S. Census Bureau, 2000 and 2005. **Click OK, and then move the text to the right edge of the layout.** You should always include the data source of your map layers and attribute tables, including the date the data was collected. The resulting map layout is suitable for many uses.

10 On the Tools toolbar, use the Select Elements button to move the legend to the lower-left corner of the map layout, and then resize the legend to make it fit.

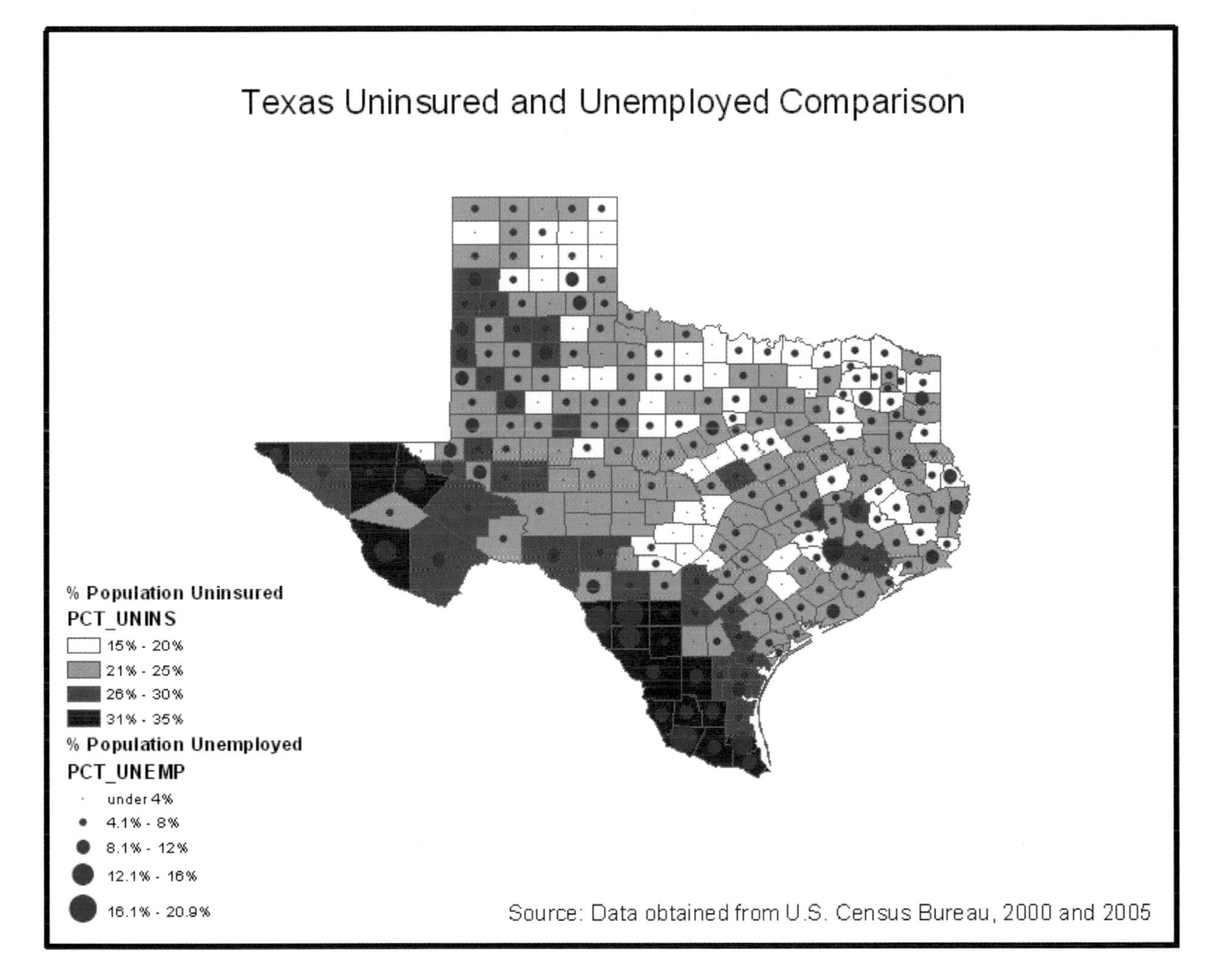

Save the map and layout

1 On the Menu bar, click File > Save As.

2 Save your map document as Tutorial3-5YourName.mxd to your Chapter3 folder in MyExercises. Do not close ArcMap.

Tutorial 3-6

Creating custom map layouts for multiple maps

It is often effective to place two or more maps in the same layout to facilitate comparisons. Choose the same classification break values when comparing similar maps. For example, if you want to compare uninsured minority populations, such as blacks and Hispanics, use the same break values for both populations.

To create multiple maps, you'll need to create multiple data frames. A data frame is a fundamental element in a map. When you create a map, it contains a default data frame to which you add layer files. This data frame is listed in the table of contents.

Build a custom layout grid

1 On the Standard toolbar, click the New button and click Blank Map. Click OK.

2 On the Menu bar, click View > Layout View.

3 Right-click the outer border of the layout and click Page and Print Setup.

4 Under Paper, change the size to Legal and select the Landscape option.

5 Under Map Page Size, select the Use Printer Paper Settings check box. Click OK. ▶

6 At the top of the map document, click the horizontal ruler at the 0.5 in., 5.5 in., 6.0 in., 11.0 in., and 13.5 in. marks.

7 At the left side of the map document, click the vertical ruler at the 1.5 in. and 7.0 in. marks.

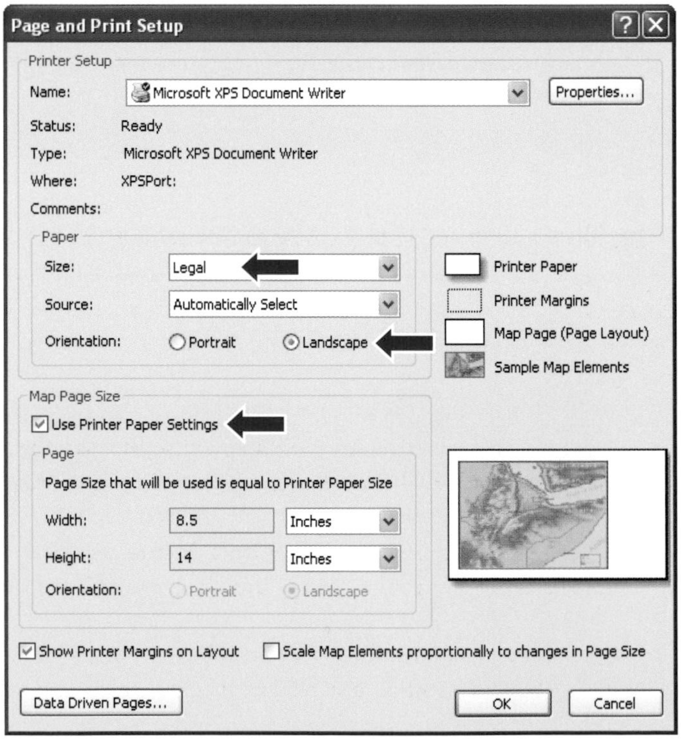

8 Use the Select Elements tool and drag the Layers data frame so that its upper-left corner snaps to the intersection of the 0.5 in. horizontal guide and the 7.0 in. vertical guide.

9 Drag the lower-right corner of the data frame to snap it to the intersection of the 5.5 in. horizontal guide and the 1.5 in. vertical guide. The layout should look like the figure.

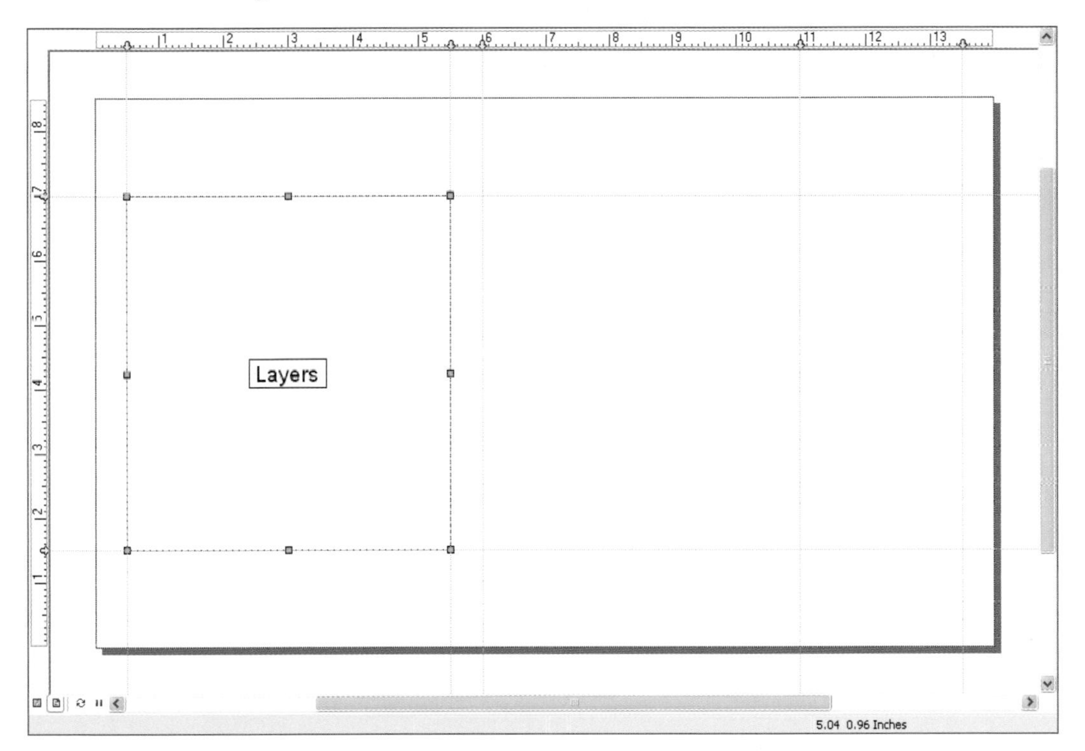

Add layers and create multiple data frames

In the first data frame, you will add Uninsured and Hispanic populations. In the second data frame, you will add Uninsured and black populations. You may need to use the zoom buttons on the Layout toolbar to be able to better see the legend items.

1 On the Standard toolbar, click Add Data, browse through MyExercises to your Chapter3 folder, and add Uninsured.lyr and HispanicPopulation.lyr.

2 On the Menu bar, click Insert > Data Frame and drag or modify the new data frame to fit in the guides beside the original frame.

3 On the Standard toolbar, click Add Data, browse through MyExercises to your Chapter3 folder, and add Uninsured.lyr.

4 With the new data frame still active, click Add Data again and add TXCounties from the United States geodatabase in the Data folder.
The resulting layer in the new data frame is a single color and needs to be classified.

When you have more than one data frame in a map, you need to be aware of which data frame is active. Many of the ArcMap tools and commands work in only the active data frame. The active data frame is the frame that is highlighted with the blue boxes on the layout page. Its name also appears in bold in the table of contents. You can click another data frame to make it active or right-click the data frame in the table of contents and click Activate.

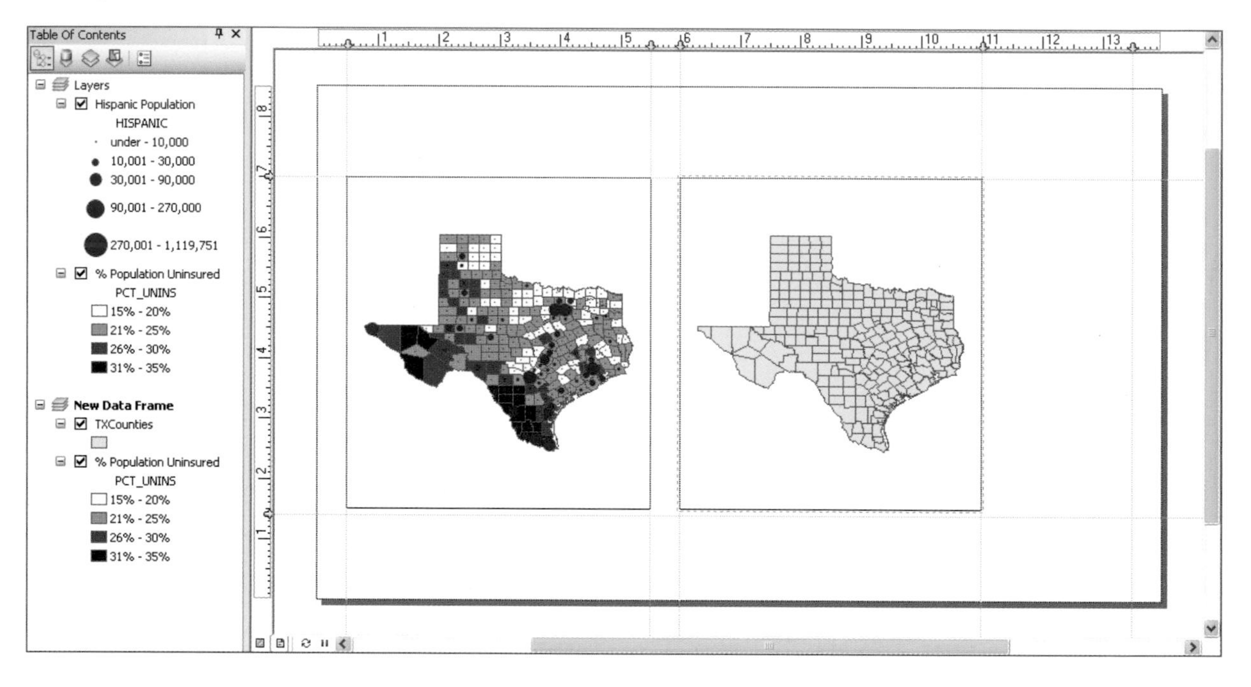

Classify data

1 In the table of contents, double-click the TXCounties layer, click the Symbology tab, and click the Import button.

2 In the Import Symbology dialog box, click the Browse button to locate an existing layer file.

3 Browse through MyExercises to your Chapter3 folder, click the HispanicPopulation.lyr file, and click Add. Click OK.

4 In the Import Symbology Matching Dialog box, click the Value Field arrow, click BLACK, and click OK. ▶

Import Symbology Matching Dialog

Select field(s) from the current layer to match to the field(s) used in the imported symbology definition:

Value Field

HISPANIC

BLACK

Normalization Field

OK Cancel

5 In the Layer Properties dialog box, click OK.

The data frame shows the black population of Texas using the same classification as the Hispanic population. Both maps show the same % Population Uninsured map layer.

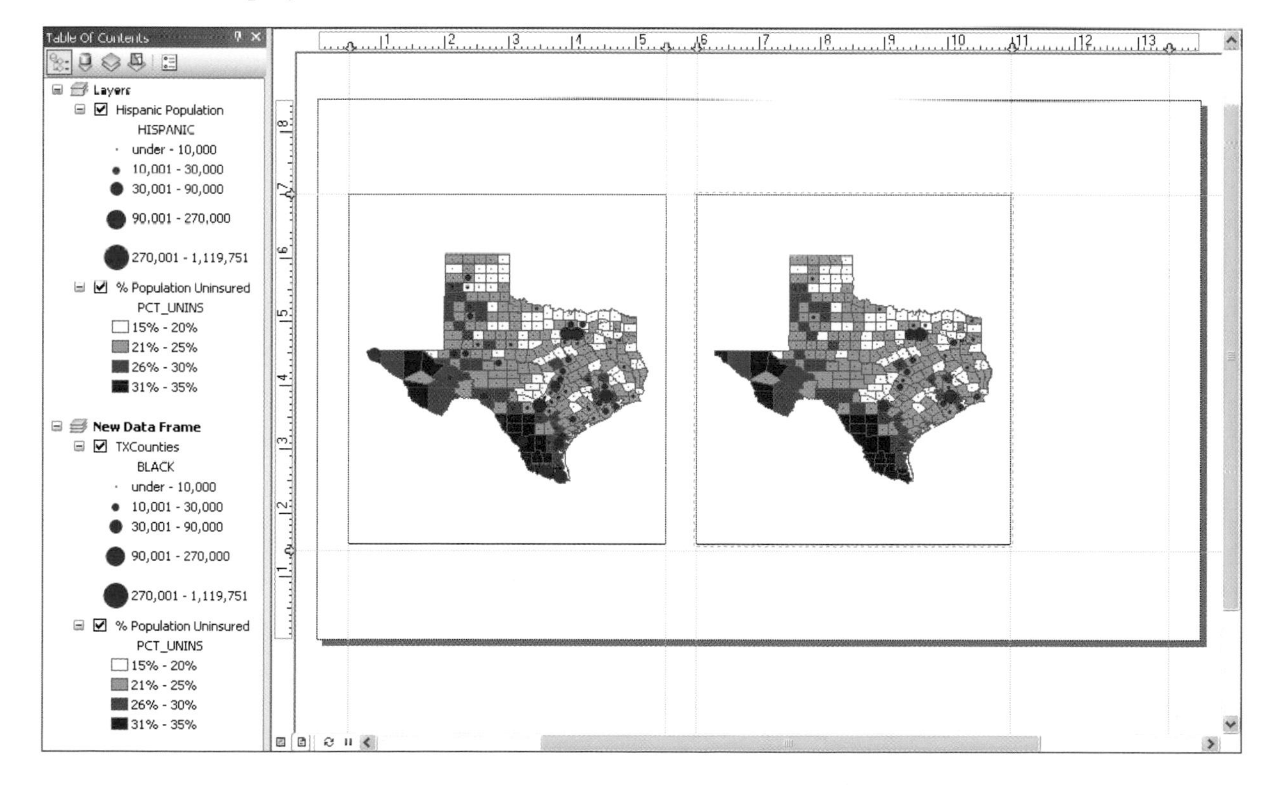

YOUR TURN

Rename the newly added TXCounties layer to **Black Population**.

Rename data frames

Similar to layers, you can rename a data frame and change its properties.

1 **In the table of contents, right-click the original data frame (currently named Layers) and click Properties.**

2 **Click the General tab, and for Name, type** Texas Hispanic Population Compared to Uninsured. **Click OK.**

3 **Rename the other data frame** Texas Black Population Compared to Uninsured. The new data frame names appear in the table of contents. ▶

Texas Hispanic Population Compared to Uninsured
Hispanic Population
under 10,000
10,001 - 30,000
30,001 - 90,000
90,001 - 270,000
270,001 - 1,119,751
% Population Uninsured
15% - 20%
21% - 25%
26% - 30%
31% - 35%

Texas Black Population Compared to Uninsured
Black Population
under 10,000
10,001 - 30,000
30,001 - 90,000
90,001 - 270,000
270,001 - 1,119,751
% Population Uninsured
15% - 20%
21% - 25%
26% - 30%
31% - 35%

Delete field names in the table of contents

Sometimes, field names are not very descriptive, and you will want to delete or rename them in the table of contents. The changes automatically update the layout's legend. Each field name appears directly under the layer name.

1 **In the table of contents, single-click the first instance of PCT_UNINS, pause, and click again so the text is highlighted.**

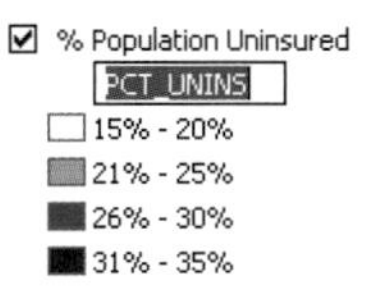

2 **Press DELETE and click anywhere in the table of contents.** The field name disappears from the table of contents.

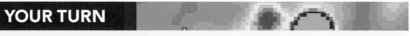

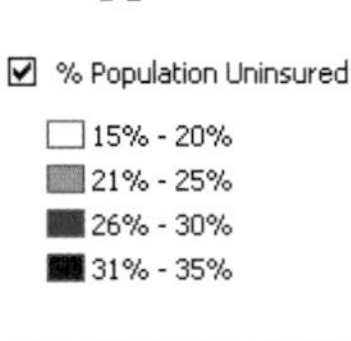

Delete the remaining field names in the table of contents.

T 3-6

Add map titles and text

You need to add an overall title to your map, as well as titles for both data frames. The overall title should be in larger type.

1 **On the Menu bar, click Insert > Title, and in the title box, type** Texas Minority Population Compared to Uninsured.

2 **Change the symbol font to bold, size** 28, **and move the title to the appropriate location in the layout.**

3 **Click Insert > Title. Right-click the title, click Properties, and type** Hispanic Population and Uninsured.

4 **Change the symbol font size to** 18 **and place the title just above the corresponding data frame in the layout.**

YOUR TURN

Create a title for the **Black Population and Uninsured** data frame and add text for the data source: **U.S. Census Bureau, Population (2000) and Uninsured (2005).**

Add and modify a legend

If you want precise control over the legend elements created by ArcMap, you can convert a legend to graphics and edit individual legend elements. *Note: The legend created by ArcMap is dynamic and automatically reflects any changes you make to symbolization; however, a legend converted to graphics is static and does not reflect subsequent changes to symbolization.* Once a legend is converted to graphics, it cannot be converted back to a dynamic legend, so you may want to make converting your legend to graphics the final step. In this exercise, you will convert your legend to graphics to modify the legend elements. You can also delete the field names in the legend if you didn't already delete them in the table of contents. If deleting field names isn't necessary, you can use the Legend Properties dialog box to modify your legend.

1 **Make Texas Hispanic Population Compared to Uninsured the active data frame.**

2 **Click Insert > Legend, click Next four times, and then click Finish.**

3 **Move the legend to the lower-right corner of the page and resize it to fit the available space.**

4 **Right-click the legend and click Convert To Graphics.**

5 **Right-click the legend again and click Ungroup.** This allows you to edit individual parts of the legend.

6 **Double-click the word Legend and change it to** Total Number of People. **Click OK.**

7 **Select and move this title and the graduated point markers of the legend to make space between this grouping and the uninsured classes.**

8 **Right-click the title Total Number of People and click Copy.**

9 **Right-click anywhere in the layout and click Paste.**

10 **Move the title above the uninsured legend and rename it** % Population Uninsured.

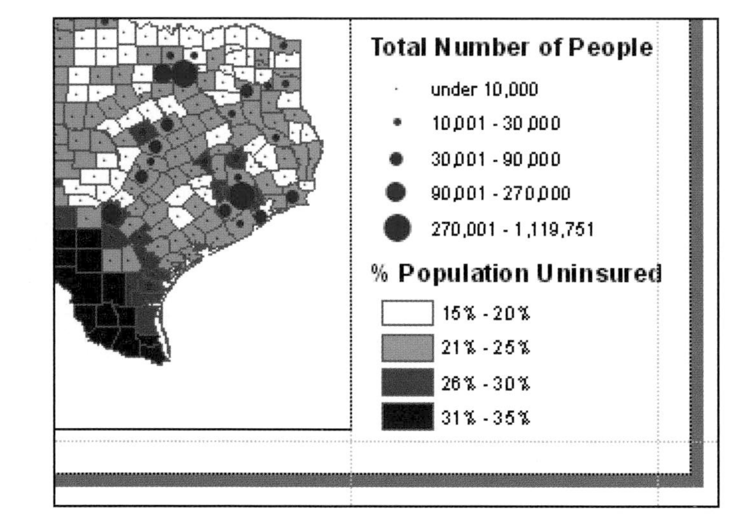

Unify map scales

The map scales for both data frames need to be set exactly the same. Otherwise, one map may be slightly larger than the other, which will bias the map reader toward that map.

1 **Click in the Hispanic Population data frame to make it active.**

2 **On the Standard toolbar, click in the Map Scale box to the right of the Add Data button.**

3 **Type the scale** 1:13,000,000. **Then press ENTER.**

YOUR TURN

Set the scale for the Black Population data frame to **1:13,000,000**, so it matches the first data frame scale.

Congratulations! You have just created a sophisticated map layout that compares two maps. Other map elements that might be interesting to add include a neatline (border around the map), map author (your name and the date the map was created), bar charts, graphs, photographs, and other graphics.

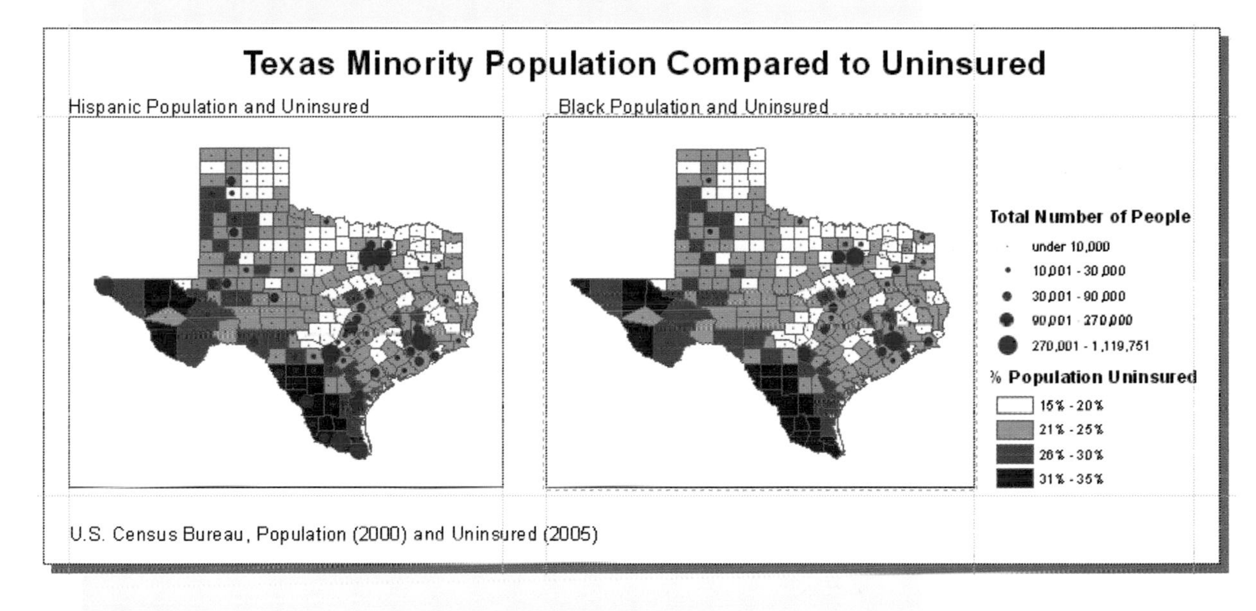

Save the map and multiple-data-frame layout

1 **On the Menu bar, click File > Save As.**

2 **Save your map document as** Tutorial3-6YourName.mxd **to your Chapter3 folder in MyExercises.** Do not close ArcMap.

Tutorial 3-7
Exporting maps

You will often need to share your maps with others or to use maps and other software for presentations or publication. You can export ArcMap maps to many image formats, or simply copy and paste map elements into other applications such as a Microsoft Word document, Microsoft PowerPoint presentation, or web page.

Export a map to an image file

1. **In the map layout, go to the Menu bar and click File > Export Map.**

2. **Browse through MyExercises to your Chapter3 folder.**

3. **Click the "Save as type" arrow and click TIFF.** Other common image types include raster formats, JPEG, bitmap, PNG, and GIF. Other export types include Adobe PDF software and the vector formats AI (Adobe Illustrator), SVG (scalable vector graphics), and EPS (encapsulated PostScript).

4. **For File Name, type** Tutorial3-7YourName.tif. **Click Save.** ▶

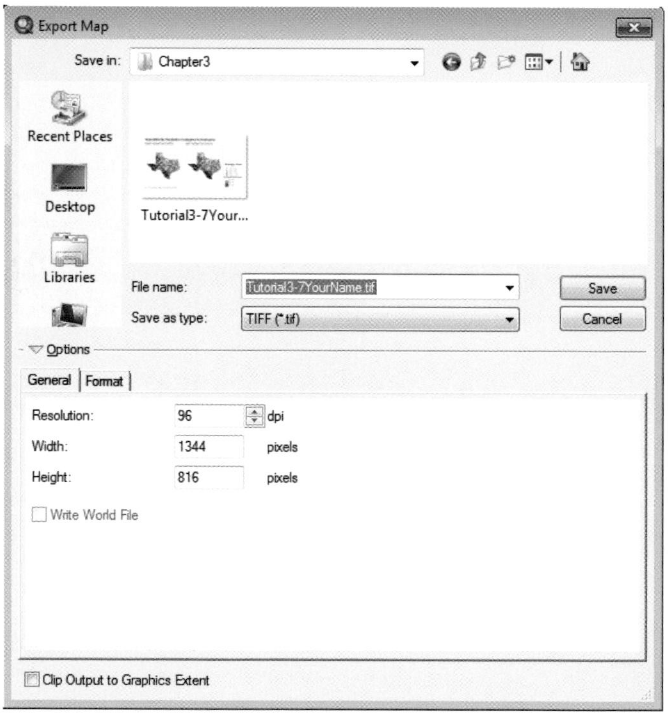

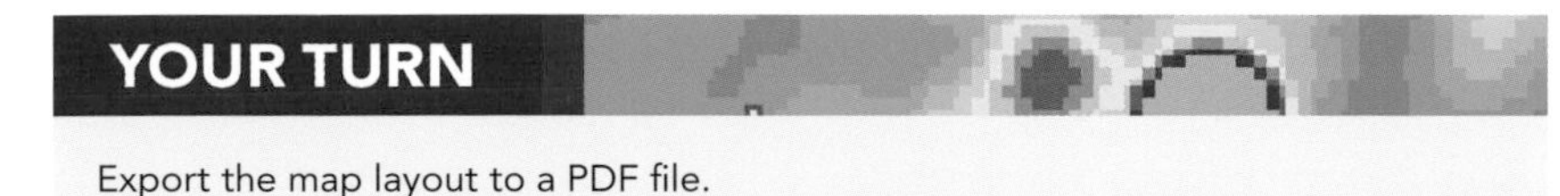

Export the map layout to a PDF file.

Copy and paste map images

You will often use maps in Microsoft PowerPoint presentations or in Word documents, and it may be better to copy the map components individually. That way, you can edit parts of the map in PowerPoint or Word.

1 **In the map layout, click Select Elements and select one of the two data frames.** Blue boxes appear around the data frame selected. You can also select multiple elements by holding down SHIFT or CTRL while selecting.

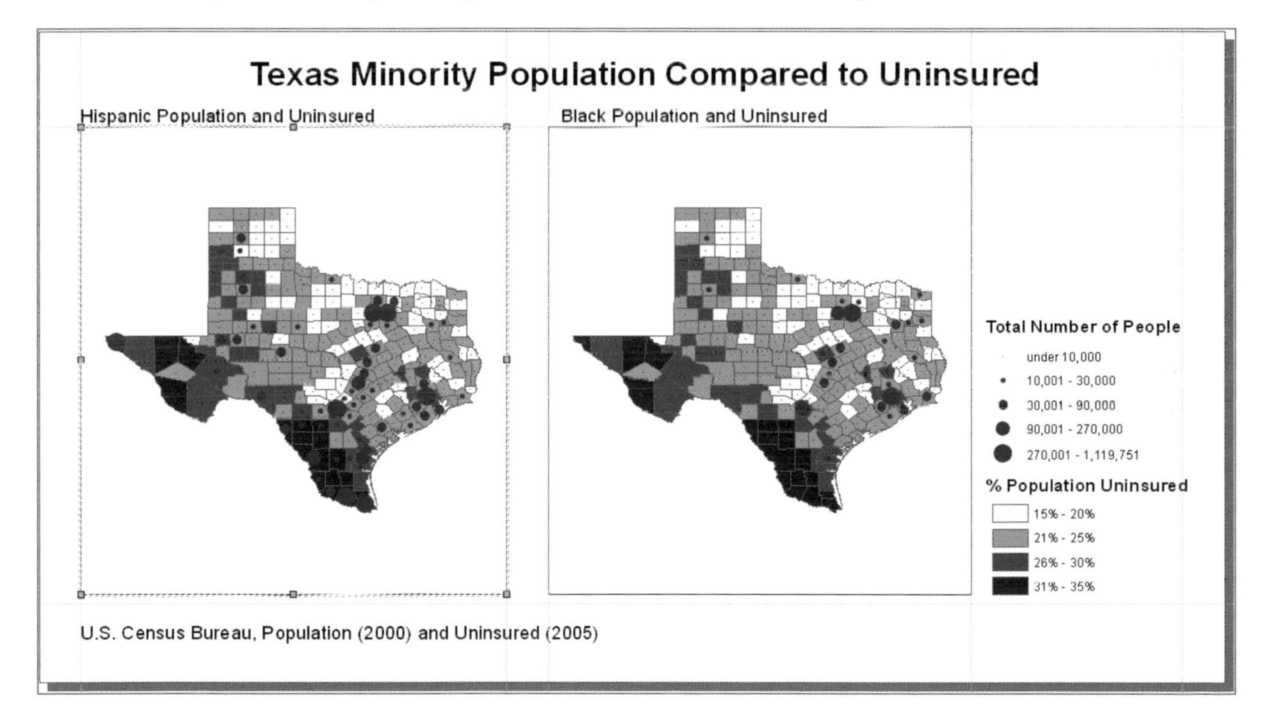

2 **Click Edit > Copy.** Alternatively, you can press CTRL+C.

3 **Start another application such as PowerPoint.**

4 Press CTRL+V. The map element is pasted into the application and you can edit it there.

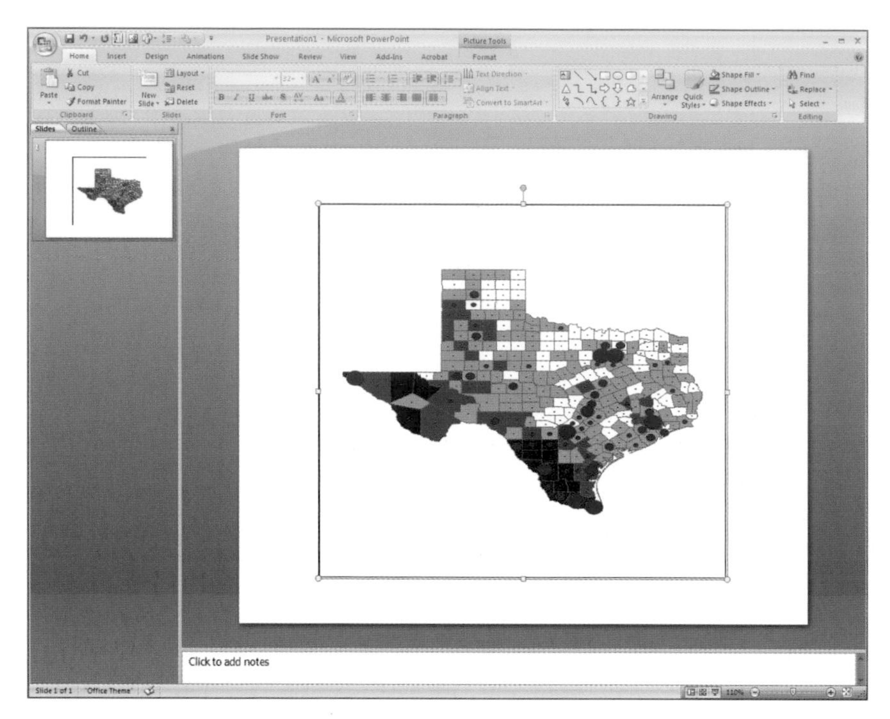

YOUR TURN

Copy and paste other map elements into Microsoft Word or another Windows application.

Save the map

1. **On the Menu bar, click File > Save As.**

2. **Save your map document as** Tutorial3-7YourName.mxd **to your Chapter3 folder in MyExercises.** Do not close ArcMap.

Tutorial 3-8
Creating multiple output pages

Sometimes it is desirable to produce many maps from a single layout, in which each map has a different extent—for example, each neighborhood within a municipality, each municipality within a county, or each state or province within a country. ArcMap Data Driven Pages serve this purpose. You have to define each extent in an index layer that includes the collection of extents as polygons, such as counties, states, or provinces. The output is a collection of images, or even a PDF. Suppose the health director of a state needs a PDF that includes a map for each major city in Texas that shows the number of Hispanic people who live there. Multiple output pages can be used to create these maps in a few simple steps.

Apply Data Driven Pages

1 **On the Menu bar, click File > Open, browse through the Maps folder if necessary, and open Tutorial3-8.mxd.** The map document opens zoomed in to the city of Austin, Texas, the state capital.

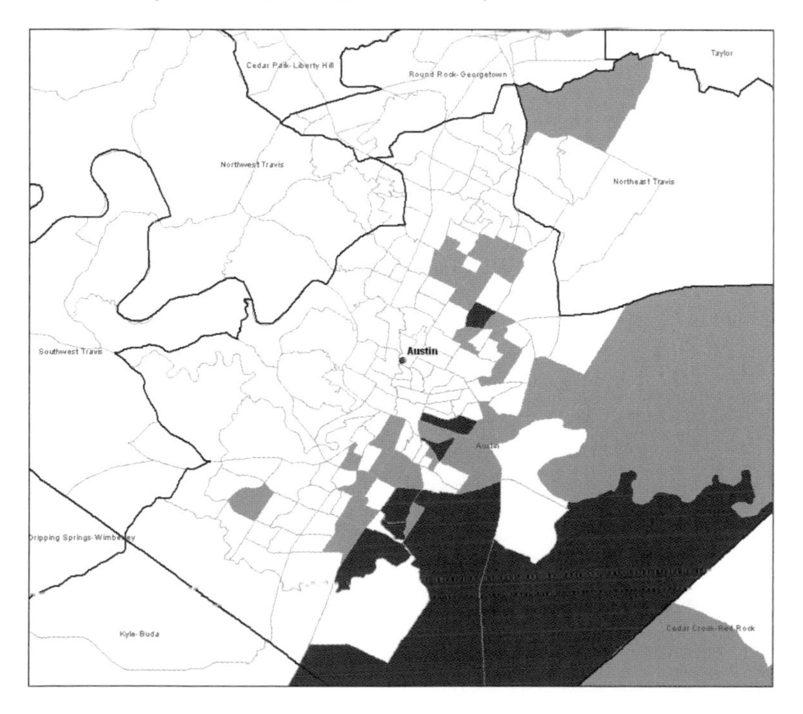

2 Click Customize > Toolbars > Data Driven Pages.

3 On the Data Driven Pages toolbar, click the Data Driven Page Setup button .

4 In the resulting dialog box, select the Enable Data Driven Pages check box, and for Layer (second drop-down list in the left panel), select Major Cities. Set both Name Field and Sort Field to NAME. Click OK. ▶

Setup Data Driven Pages

Definition | Extent

What are data driven pages?

An index layer is used to produce multiple output pages using a single layout. Each page shows the data at a different extent. The extents are defined by the features in the index layer.

☑ Enable Data Driven Pages

Index Layer
Data Frame: Texas Hispanic Population Study
Layer: Major Cities
Name Field: NAME
Sort Field: NAME
☑ Sort Ascending

Optional Fields
Rotation: none
Spatial Reference: none
Page Number: none
Starting Page Number: 1

OK | Cancel

5 On the Data Driven Pages toolbar, click the First Page button . The map extent switches to the first city by alphabet, Amarillo.

6 On the Data Driven Pages toolbar, click the Next Page button . The map extent switches to the next city by alphabet, Arlington.

7 Click the Previous Page button to return to Amarillo.

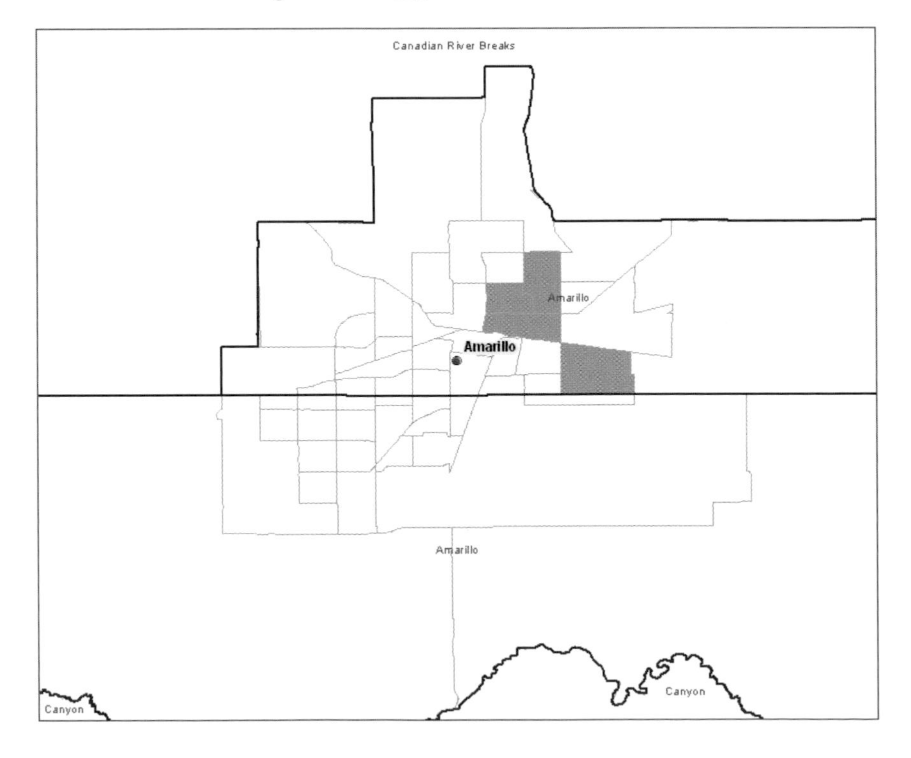

8 **Click View > Layout View.**

9 **Click Insert > Dynamic Text > Data Driven Page Name.** ArcMap places a small text box in the center of your map that has the city name Amarillo.

10 **Drag the inserted text box to the top at the center of the page, double-click it, click Change Symbol, and set Size to** 22 **and Style to B for bold. Click OK twice.**

YOUR TURN

In the layout, resize and relocate the map to your liking, enter a map scale of **1:225,000**, and insert a legend and a scale bar.

Output Data Driven Pages

1 **On the Menu bar, click File > Export Map.**

2 **Browse through MyExercises to your Chapter3 folder, change the "Save as type" box to PDF (*.pdf), change "File name" to** TexasCityHispanicStudy_A-D.pdf**, and click the Options button to expose the options.** This creates a PDF of the five major cities in Texas whose names begin with A, B, C, or D.

3 **Click the General tab and type** 300 **for dpi. Click the Pages tab, click the Page Range option, and type** 1-5 **in the Page Range text box. Click the General tab again and click Save.** ▶

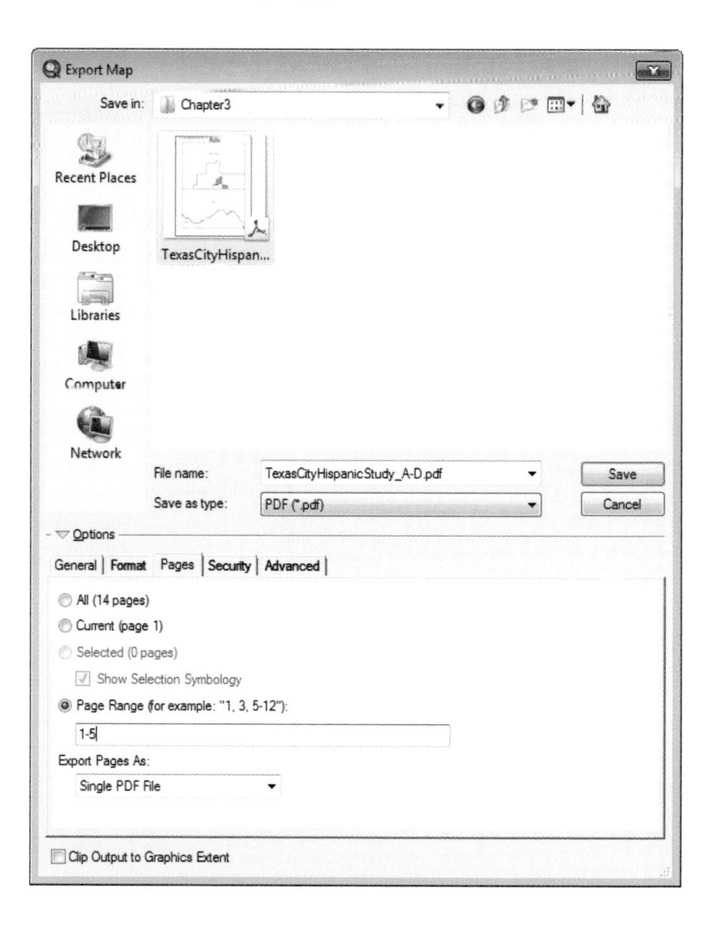

T 3-8

4 **Open a My Computer window, browse through MyExercises to your Chapter3 folder, double-click TexasCityHispanicStudy_A-D.pdf to open the file in Adobe Acrobat or an equivalent program, and view the resulting document.** The PDF has maps for Amarillo, Arlington, Austin, Corpus Christi, and Dallas.

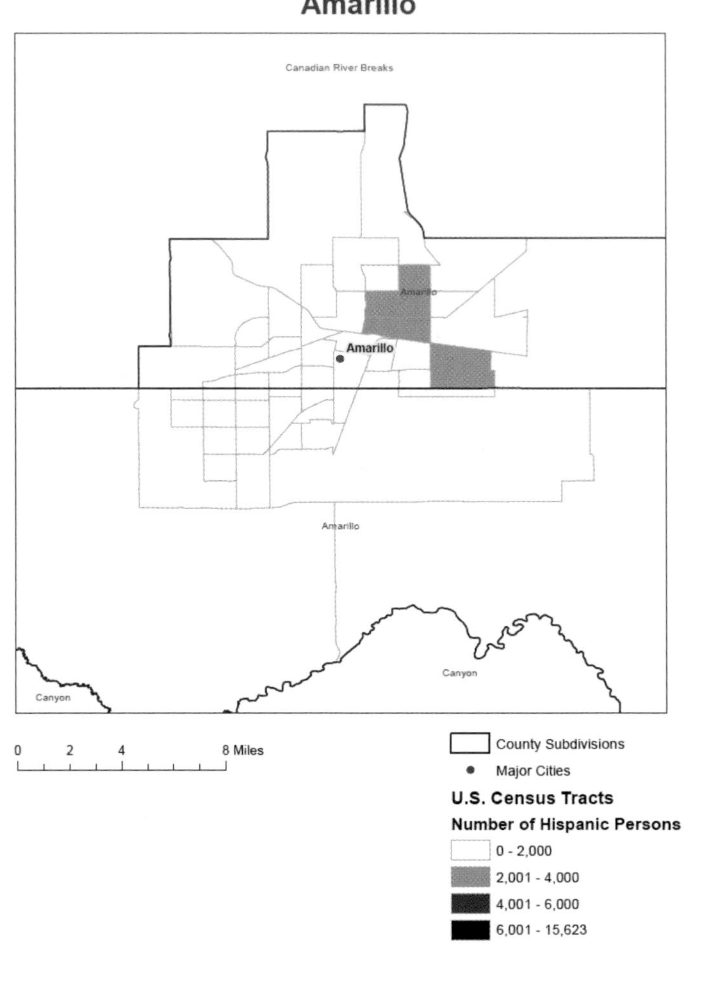

Create a PDF for the next five cities.

Save the map

1 **On the Menu bar, click File > Save As.**

2 **Save your map document as** Tutorial3-8YourName.mxd **to your Chapter3 folder in MyExercises.** Close ArcMap.

Summary

The mapping exercises in these tutorials revealed some interesting and perhaps useful patterns of uninsured populations in Texas. First, as expected, you saw a high correlation between being uninsured and being poor. The maps that you made, however, showed further that much of the poor and unemployed populations are along the border of Texas and Mexico. The location of Hispanic and black minority populations—often among the poor—seems less a factor in explaining locations of uninsured populations. Further research is needed to better understand this preliminary result.

In this chapter, you learned how to symbolize maps using numeric attributes of points and polygons. Unless you are working in the transportation field, you will rarely use lines, such as streets and rivers, for more than spatial context. Thus in analytic mapping, lines are generally shown in background colors. You learned about using numeric scales to design intervals to cover the range of an attribute. Equal-width intervals, quantiles, and increasing-width intervals are commonly used in mapping. Numeric intervals can be rendered by using monochromatic color ramps for polygons and size-graduated point markers for points.

The health-care maps you design in ArcMap are primarily used for reports and presentations. A well-designed map layout can become the best vehicle for communicating your findings to policy and decision makers. You can very easily use ArcMap to generate professional map layouts that include a map or maps, a title, a distance scale, a legend for interpreting symbols, and so forth. You can use your maps in reports and presentations by simply exporting your map layouts as image files and inserting them into Microsoft Word documents or PowerPoint presentations.

Besides teaching you how to build map layouts, this set of tutorials has also advanced your map design skills in the use of sophisticated maps to compare two variables—in this case, the percentage of uninsured per county versus the percentage of unemployed or minority populations. You learned how to create choropleth and graduated point marker maps, which can be viewed together in the same map composition. Moreover, you found that map layouts that have two map compositions side by side allow for comparison of three variables at the same time. You found a correlation between uninsured populations and poverty indicators, as expected, but the map also provided information on where and how densely clustered the health insurance problem is.

ArcMap is a flexible software package that allows extensive custom mapping. You created custom break points for choropleth and graduated point marker maps, which makes the maps easy to interpret because of the uniform scales used.

Now you are in a good position to create effective interactive maps in ArcGIS for exploring and researching important spatial patterns. Plus, you have the skills to convert finished maps into map products that others can understand and use.

Assignment 3-1

Compare uninsured with minority populations in California counties

State of California health officials suspect that in California counties, census variables like uninsured populations correlate with other census variables like minority populations, and thus have asked you to explore this phenomenon using GIS. They then want you to present your findings to a team of health policy analysts. Your task in this assignment is to make a map that compares this data and to produce a map layout and brief Microsoft PowerPoint presentation for the health officials to consider in making a decision.

Start with this data

- *\EsriPress\GISTHealth\Data\UnitedStates.gdb\CACounties:* polygon features of California counties using US Census data (2000 and 2005) and the following attribute fields:
  - *BLACK:* Total black population, year 2000
  - *HISPANIC:* Total Hispanic population, year 2000
  - *POP2000:* Total population, year 2000
  - *UINPCT:* Percentage of uninsured population per county, year 2005

Create a comparison map of census data

Create a map document called Assignment3-1YourName.mxd and save it to your Chapter3 folder in MyAssignments, using relative paths. Prepare your map as follows:

- 11 x 8½ in. landscape layout with three data frames of equal size and map scale, including the following:
  - One for the percentage of uninsured population
  - One for the percentage of black population
  - One for the percentage of Hispanic population
- Use logical classification breaks and colors.
- Rename all data frames and layers.
- Include a title and or subtitles, legend(s), data source, and text including map author (you).
- Do not label counties.

Export the layout as a JPEG called **Assignment3-1YourName.jpg** to your Chapter3 folder in MyAssignments.

Hint: *To show the population percentages, choose the race in the Value field (for example, Black) and Pop2000 in the Normalization field.*

Create a PowerPoint presentation

Create a Microsoft PowerPoint presentation called **Assignment3-1YourName.pptx** and save it to your Chapter3 folder in MyAssignments. Include the following:

- Title slide including your name
- Slide including observations about California counties and the uninsured and minority populations
- Inserted map layout image

WHAT TO TURN IN

If your work is to be graded, turn in the following files:

- ***ArcMap document:*** \EsriPress\GISTHealth\MyAssignments\Chapter3\Assignment3-1YourName.mxd
- ***Microsoft PowerPoint presentation:*** \EsriPress\GISTHealth\MyAssignments\Chapter3\Assignment3-1YourName.pptx

If instructed to do so, instead of individual files turn in a compressed file, **Assignment3-1YourName.zip**, that includes all the preceding files. Do not include path information in the compressed file.

Assignment 3-2
Compare Texas population density with housing statistics

In addition to displaying and analyzing GIS data at the state level, analysts can also create demographic maps for a smaller geographic area such as a county, city, or neighborhood. For example, basic population and housing data is available for US Census tracts, block groups, and blocks, which are subdivisions of counties. In 2005, displaced persons from Hurricane Katrina in New Orleans, Louisiana, moved to Houston, Texas, and many permanently relocated there. An interesting study would be to examine the population and housing statistics in cities in Harris County, Texas, where Houston is located. These GIS maps could help public officials prepare for or alleviate economic and health-related stress factors in these cities. In this assignment, you will create choropleth and point maps that compare population with vacant housing units in two Texas cities to determine housing opportunities.

Start with this data

- ***\EsriPress\GISTHealth\Data\UnitedStates.gdb\HarrisCountyTracts:*** polygon features of Harris County census tracts using the following US Census data:
  - ***POP04_SQMI:*** population density per square mile, year 2004
  - ***VACANT:*** Number of vacant housing units, year 2000
- ***\EsriPress\GISTHealth\Data\UnitedStates.gdb\HarrisCountyCities:*** point features of cities in Harris County, Texas

Create choropleth and point map layers

Create a map document called **Assignment3-2YourName.mxd** and save it to your Chapter3 folder in MyAssignments, using relative paths. Add the preceding layers and show the 2004 population as a choropleth map and vacant housing units as graduated point markers. Think carefully about your color, point size, and classification values. Add the Harris County cities using a halo label. Rename the data frame and map layers.

In an 8½ x 11 in. portrait map layout, show the data frame zoomed to the city of Pasadena at a scale of 1:150,000. Copy the data frame and zoom to the city of Baytown at the same scale. Include a title and subtitles, legend(s), a graphic scale bar in miles (see hint), north arrow, data source (including dates), and text including map author (you).

Export your map layout as a JPEG called **Assignment3-2YourName.jpg** and save it to your Chapter3 folder in MyAssignments.

> ***Hint:*** *Before inserting the graphic scale, right-click the data frame and click Properties. Click the General tab, and for Display Units, select Miles.*

WHAT TO TURN IN

If your work is to be graded, turn in the following files:

- ***ArcMap document:*** \EsriPress\GISTHealth\MyAssignments\Chapter3\Assignment3-2YourName.mxd
- ***Image file:*** \EsriPress\GISTHealth\MyAssignments\Chapter3\Assignment3-2YourName.jpg

If instructed to do so, instead of individual files turn in a compressed file, **Assignment3-2YourName.zip**, that includes all the preceding files. Do not include path information in the compressed file.

Assignment 3-3

Compare percentage in poverty with percentage unemployed

Comparison maps in a layout such as the one created in assignment 3-2 are very useful, but automated maps created from Data Driven Pages are often needed when comparing many areas that do not fit nicely into a single map layout. In this assignment, you will create multiple maps in one PDF comparing the percentage of population in poverty with the percentage of unemployed in Harris County, Texas.

Start with this data

- *\EsriPress\GISTHealth\Data\UnitedStates.gdb\HarrisCountyTracts:* polygon features of Harris County census tracts using the following US Census data:
  - *PCTPOV:* percentage of population in poverty, year 1999
  - *PCTUNEMP:* percentage of population unemployed, year 2000
- *\EsriPress\GISTHealth\Data\UnitedStates.gdb\HarrisCountyCities:* point features of cities in Harris County, Texas

Create Data Driven Pages

Create a map document called **Assignment3-3YourName.mxd** and save it to your Chapter3 folder in MyAssignments, using relative paths. Add the preceding layers and show the percentage of population in poverty as a choropleth map and the percentage of unemployed as graduated point markers. Think carefully about your color, point size, and classification values. Add the Harris County cities using a halo label. Rename the data frame and map layers.

Create a Data Driven Page using Harris County cities and the NAME field. Include the map layout title and data-driven dynamic text, scaled to 1:150,000, a legend, a graphic scale bar in miles, a north arrow, a data source and date(s), and text including map author (you).

Hints

- *Before inserting the graphic scale, right-click the data frame and click Properties. Click the General tab and select Miles for Display Units.*
- *Export your map layout including the first 10 Data Driven Pages as a PDF called* **Assignment3-3YourName.pdf** *and save to your Chapter3 folder in MyAssignments.*

WHAT TO TURN IN

If your work is to be graded, turn in the following files:

- ***ArcMap document:*** \EsriPress\GISTHealth\MyAssignments\Chapter3\Assignment3-3YourName.mxd
- ***Adobe PDF:*** \EsriPress\GISTHealth\MyAssignments\Chapter3\Assignment3-3YourName.pdf

If instructed to do so, instead of individual files turn in a compressed file, **Assignment3-3YourName.zip**, that includes all the preceding files. Do not include path information in the compressed file.

Chapter 4

Projecting, downloading, and using spatial data

Objectives

- Project world maps for health data analysis using different projections
- Prepare incidence and prevalence maps
- Download international data for health analysis
- Explore map projections for a single continent
- Import and project map layers for local analysis
- Download and import basemaps for local analysis

Health-care scenarios

This chapter has three health scenarios, covering map projections that are appropriate for health studies at the global, continental, country, and local levels. In addition, assorted GIS topics that occur at different geographic scales are also discussed.

In the first scenario, a public health official working for an international health organization wants to study a snapshot of HIV/AIDS data on a global scale. For example, the enormity of the HIV/AIDS problem is well known for sub-Saharan Africa. HIV/AIDS has created 13.2 million orphans in that part of the world, and the Joint United Nations Program on HIV/AIDS reports that in 2010 there were more than 42 million orphans there—that is, the same number of children living in the United States east of the Mississippi River. The public health official would like to have a map that clearly identifies other heavily affected parts of the world.

The second scenario focuses on a detailed HIV study for a single country in sub-Saharan Africa. You will download data for this study from HIV Spatial Data Repository, a website sponsored by the US government's PEPFAR (President's Emergency Plan for AIDS Relief) initiative and by ICF Marco, which collects national and subnational HIV prevalence data. PEPFAR was launched in 2003 to support partner nations around the world in response to HIV/AIDS and is the largest commitment by any nation in history to combat a single disease internationally. The second scenario also includes a brief return to the US map for male lung cancer mortality by county, seen in tutorials 1-3 and 1-4. Data for this study was downloaded from the National Cancer Institute website. This map is used solely to demonstrate various map projections for the continental United States.

The third scenario is at the municipal and neighborhood levels. The client is a task force of universities, schools, and health-care organizations working on reducing childhood obesity in Pittsburgh, Pennsylvania. Members of the task force want a map of parks and other areas used for outdoor activities around public schools to be used in designing school physical fitness programs. At this level, it is useful to include aerial-image basemaps, which you will download from the US Geological Survey website.

Solution approaches

This section provides information on map projections and designs for different geographic scales. There are many map projections at different scales, and you will learn about the capacity of ArcGIS to apply these different projections. In addition, the design of thematic maps varies based on scale, so there is a section on this topic as well. Finally, you will download or work with map layers in a variety of spatial data formats, so this section reviews some of the major formats.

Map projections for different geographic scales

The smaller the map scale—or the more of the world included on a map—the more types of distortion there are in a projected flat map. Various combinations of area, shape, direction, and distance are always distorted in maps of the world, hemispheres, continents, and large countries. As the map scale increases to the municipal, provincial, or state level, distortion decreases because a plane becomes a good approximation of the earth's surface for small areas. Nevertheless, mapmakers need to choose which projection to use for maps at all scales. For example, a good projection for a map at the world scale is the Robinson projection; a good projection for the continental United States and the display of disease incidence is the Albers Equal Area Conic projection, and good projections for substate areas of the United States are the state plane and universal transverse Mercator (UTM) projections—although there are many other good projections and considerations to be made in choosing between them (see ArcGIS for Desktop Help for more information about choosing projections).

Working with projections in ArcGIS

A major topic of this chapter is how ArcMap and ArcCatalog handle map projections. A map document can have one or more data frames in the table of contents. The GIS user can switch between data frames in data view or layout view to display separate maps for any of the data frames in the map document. Each data frame has its own collection of map layers along with a map projection.

A data frame can have multiple map layers, each with a different projection, as long as each map layer has a spatial reference—that is, data that records the map layer's projection and coordinate system. ArcMap can reproject map layers to the data frame projection on the fly so that they can be accurately displayed. A GIS analyst can change a data frame projection, and ArcMap will reproject all the data frame's map layers to the new common projection whenever the map document is opened.

Many spatial data formats, including those used in a geodatabase and in a shapefile, have spatial references. For example, a shapefile can have a projection file, and a geodatabase can have a feature class that stores spatial references in a table. If you have a map layer that does not have a spatial reference but you know its projection and coordinate system, you can use ArcCatalog to add the spatial reference to the map layer. Some GIS functions that you will learn about in a later chapter require that all layers have a projection.

An alternative for choropleth maps

One important side issue regarding small-scale maps is the display of count data by area in a choropleth map. Perceived meaning in a choropleth map comes from two signals: color value (or the darkness of a shade of color), which carries the primary information, and polygon size, which is a secondary but possibly false signal. The viewer's perception may be overly influenced by large polygons that have high color value, although small polygons that have high color value may be just as important, or even more important. For example, if a large and a small polygon have roughly the same large number of cases, they will both have the same high color value, even if the smaller polygon has more cases per square mile. If contagion is a factor in contracting a disease, the smaller polygon may be more important than the larger one. In addition to this inherent factor of size in choropleth maps, small-scale maps can have potentially large and systematic errors in polygon areas.

One remedy for small-scale maps is to use size-graduated point markers located at polygon centroids to symbolize variables such as disease incidence instead of using a choropleth map. Point marker size is then the only variable, eliminating confusion and distortion. For medium-scale maps (for example, of the continental United States), good equal-area projections are available that remove projection-induced errors in area, making choropleth maps a good choice. Figure 1.1 in chapter 1 uses this kind of projection. This choropleth map shows county boundaries, which are numerous and relatively small so that area does not carry much information and color value sends a clear signal. In this case, graduated point markers are too numerous to see and interpret, unless the viewer zooms to a particular section of the country.

The prevalence of a communicable disease, represented by cases per 10,000 people, reveals the extent of the diffusion of the communicable disease throughout a population. By this measure, a small country that has high disease prevalence shows up prominently on a map, whereas a large country that has low prevalence but a high raw count of cases shows up less prominently—the opposite of a map that portrays just raw counts. Again, graduated point markers located at polygon centroids are preferable to a choropleth map in such cases.

Spatial data formats

Map layers, which can be acquired from a variety of places, come in a variety of spatial data formats—all of which can be imported, transformed, and used directly in ArcCatalog and ArcMap. Some commonly encountered vector data formats that you will use in this chapter include the following:

- *ArcInfo coverage:* an older data format for earlier GIS products that places each map layer in its own folder, which contains several files. Many organizations still keep their map layers in this format.
- *.e00 interchange file:* another older data format that places an ArcInfo coverage into a single file, instead of a folder of files, for ease of transfer.
- *Shapefile:* an older but still widely used data format that has three or more files per map layer, each with the same file name but different extensions (for example, .shp, .dbf, .shx).
- *Geodatabase:* the latest spatial data format commonly used, in which all map data is stored in relational database format. The file geodatabase is built into ArcGIS technology and uses an internal database engine. ArcSDE software uses enterprise-level database packages that employ ArcGIS. Databases from Oracle and Informix are also used for geodatabases.
- *CAD:* drawings made from computer-aided design (CAD) software applications. Many architectural and engineering firms create and use CAD files to create GIS layers. ArcMap can add CAD files in the following formats: native AutoCAD (DWG), Drawing Exchange Files (DXF), and MicroStation (DGN).
- *Event table:* a table of point features that includes attributes for x,y coordinates. Some organizations include coordinates for point data, making it easy to map the data using any GIS package. Global Positioning System (GPS) data is a source of event data—for example, the location of data collected from a mobile phone can be shown as a series of points over time. ArcMap can directly display event table data as points.

With this background in hand, it's time to work on the tutorials for this chapter.

World projections

In these tutorials, you will create maps that compare estimates of the cumulative number of AIDS cases with the prevalence of AIDS in countries around the world. You will explore various map projections to determine which works best for a world health study.

Tutorial 4-1
Exploring map projections for a world AIDS study

Open an existing map

You will begin by opening the map document Tutorial4-1.mxd, which has three data frames, each of which has the same two map layers already symbolized. When you open the map document, all three data frames are unprojected, using geographic latitude-longitude coordinates. You will set the first data frame to the Mercator projection, the second to the cylindrical equal-area projection, and the third to the Robinson projection.

1 **Start ArcMap and open Tutorial4-1.mxd.** The map opens with three data frames, each with no projection.

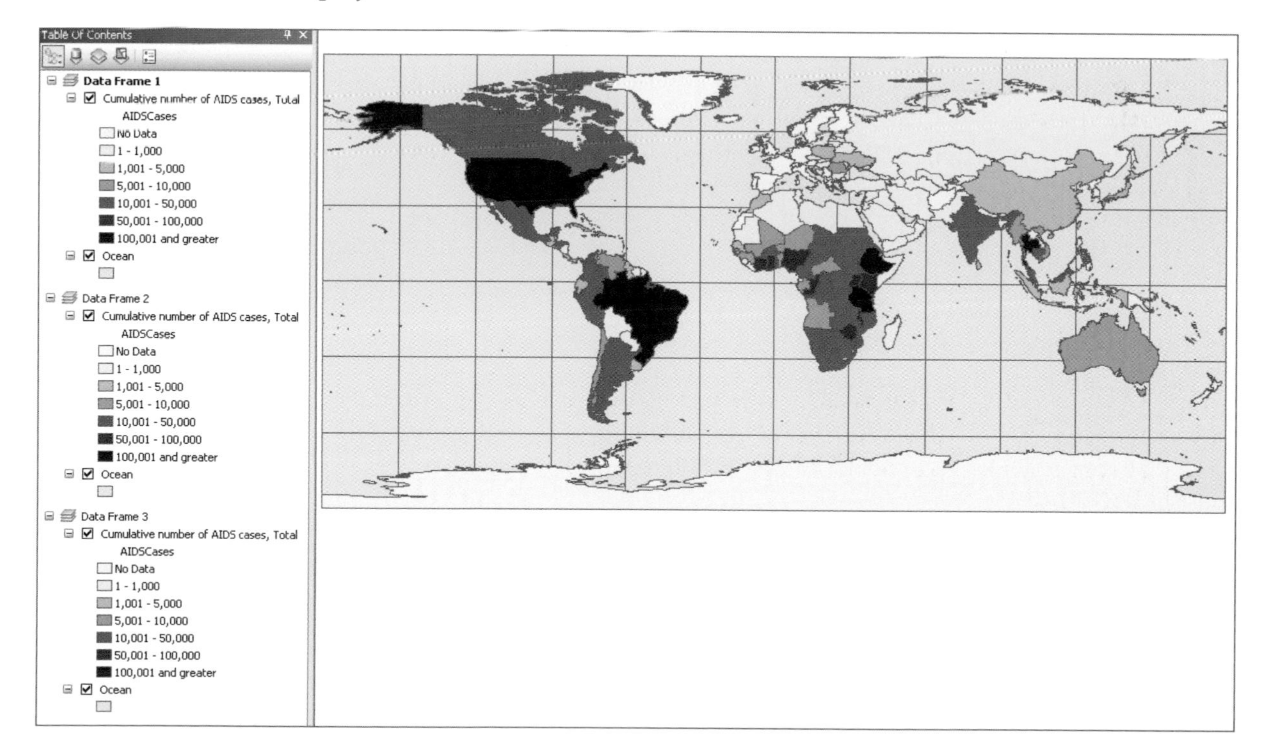

Change Data Frame 1 projection to Mercator

1. **In the table of contents, right-click Data Frame 1 and click Activate.** This step activates the map layers in Data Frame 1 for use in the map. Only one data frame can be active at a time. You will activate the other two data frames in turn.

2. **Move the pointer to the position shown in the figure.** Notice that the pointer is close to the (0,0) coordinate in the geographic coordinate system, as seen in the coordinates field at the bottom of the map document window.

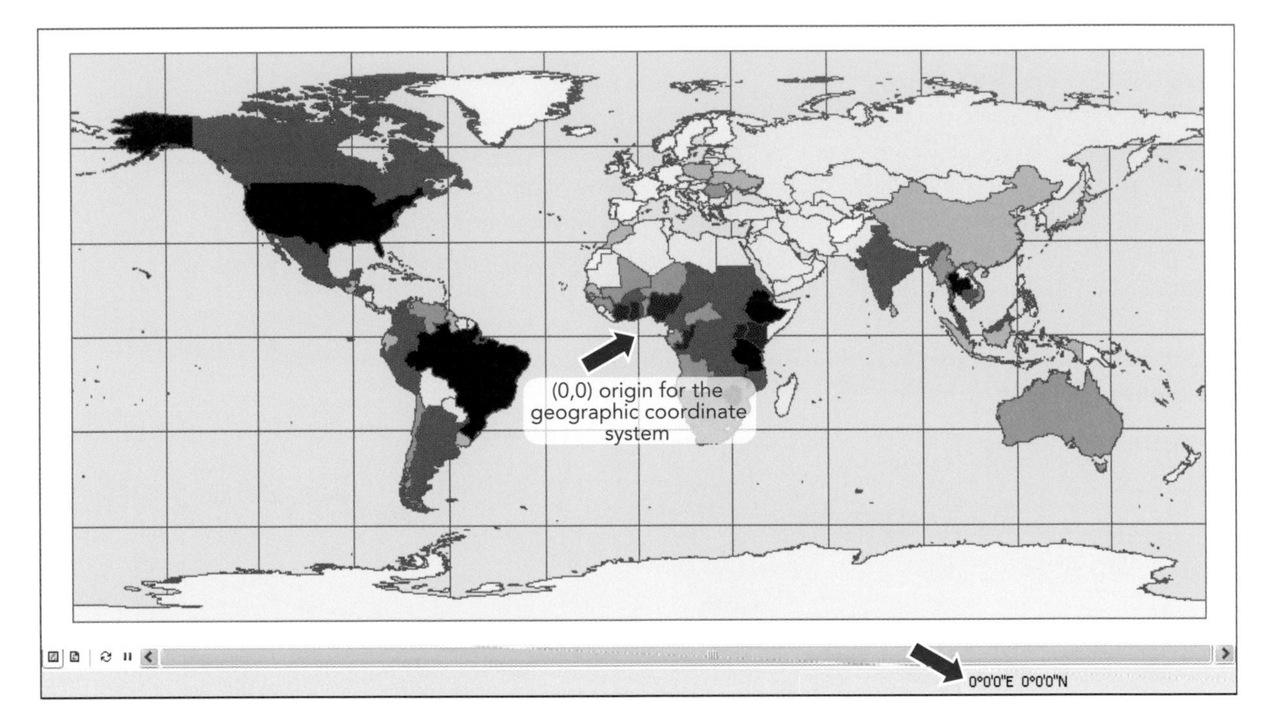

3. **Move the pointer around the map from the origin to the west, east, north, and south to see the range of values for the geographic coordinate system.**

4. **In the table of contents, right-click Data Frame 1, click Properties, and click the Coordinate System tab.**

5 In the top panel, click the plus sign (+) next to the Projected Coordinate System folder to expand its contents.

6 Inside the Projected Coordinate Systems folder expand the World folder.

7 Scroll down, click "Mercator (world)", and click OK.

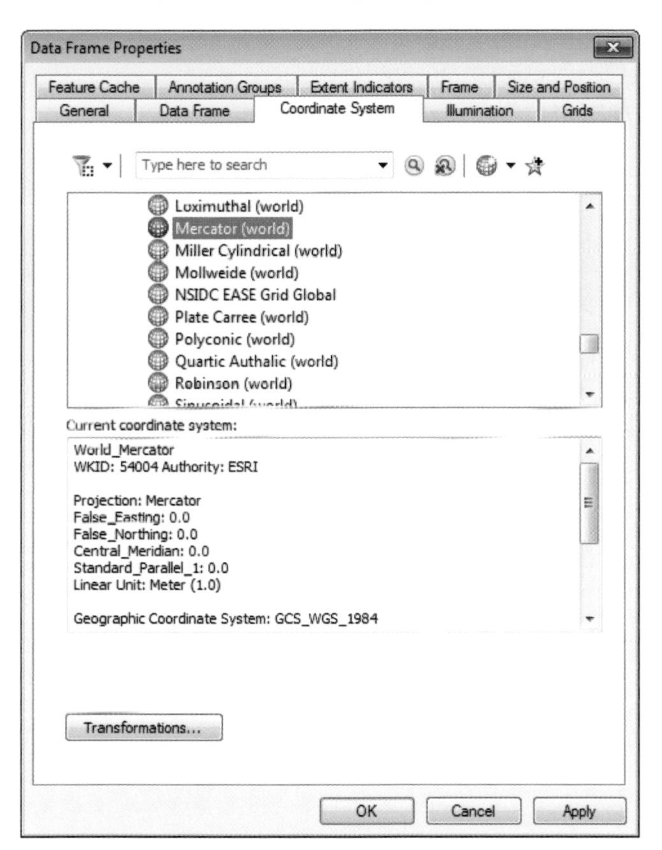

Rename the data frame

1 In the table of contents, click the Data Frame 1 title, wait a second or two, click it again, and type Mercator Projection to change the name of the data frame.

2 **On the Tools toolbar, zoom to the full extent.** The resulting map shows world AIDS cases using a Mercator projection. Notice how large Greenland and Antarctica are. These are enormous distortions.

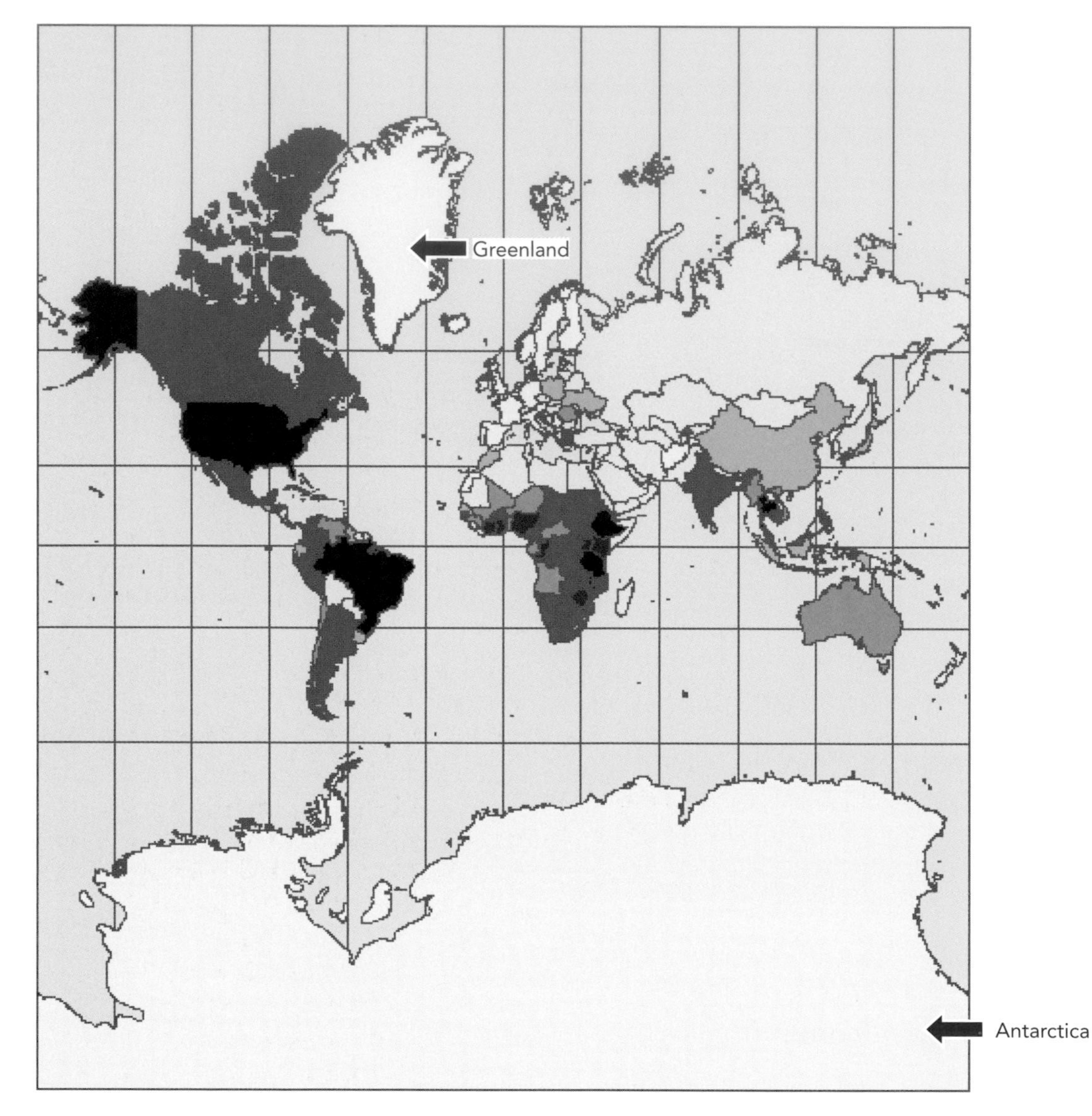

YOUR TURN

Repeat the preceding steps applying the "Cylindrical Equal Area (world)" projection to Data Frame 2 and the Robinson (world) projection to Data Frame 3. Recall that the Mercator is a conformal projection, preserving direction; the cylindrical equal-area projection preserves area; and the Robinson projection is a hybrid that minimizes the misrepresentation of shape, area, distance, and direction by allowing small amounts of distortion in each of these spatial properties.

Save the map document

1 **On the File menu, click Save As.**

2 **Save your map document as** Tutorial4-1YourName.mxd **to your Chapter4 folder in MyExercises.** Do not close ArcMap.

Tutorial 4-2
Symbolizing area maps using size-graduated point markers

Frequency data, such as the number of AIDS cases, is better shown by using graduated point markers for polygon centroids than using choropleth maps. In this tutorial, you will show the number of world AIDS cases using graduated point markers and the Robinson projection.

Start a new map document

1 **On the Menu bar, click File > New > My Templates > Blank Map, and click OK to begin a new map document.**

2 **In the table of contents, right-click the Layers data frame and click Properties.**

3 **Click the Coordinate System tab and click Projected Coordinate Systems > World, Robinson (world). Click OK.** At this point, no image will appear in the map window.

Each map layer you will add in the next step is a feature class that includes a projection (.prj) file. These files store the projection and coordinate information for a feature class.

The coordinates of the feature classes you will load are geographic (latitude and longitude). When you add the feature class, ArcMap reads the information in the projection file to determine its projection and coordinates, and then spatially adjusts the data to match the projection defined for the data frame, which you just defined as Robinson. The ability of ArcMap to read a projection file and automatically adjust spatial data according to the data frame projection is referred to as "on-the-fly projection."

On-the-fly projection is extremely useful when you are working with data layers stored in different projections and you need to correctly overlay these layers in the map. Keep in mind that on-the-fly projection is a temporary adjustment to the data that occurs only within the working map document—it does not permanently alter the coordinates of the layers.

4 On the Standard toolbar, click Add Data and add the Country and Ocean feature classes from the World geodatabase in the Data folder. The Ocean layer contains a graticule made up of lines of constant latitude and longitude at 30-degree intervals.

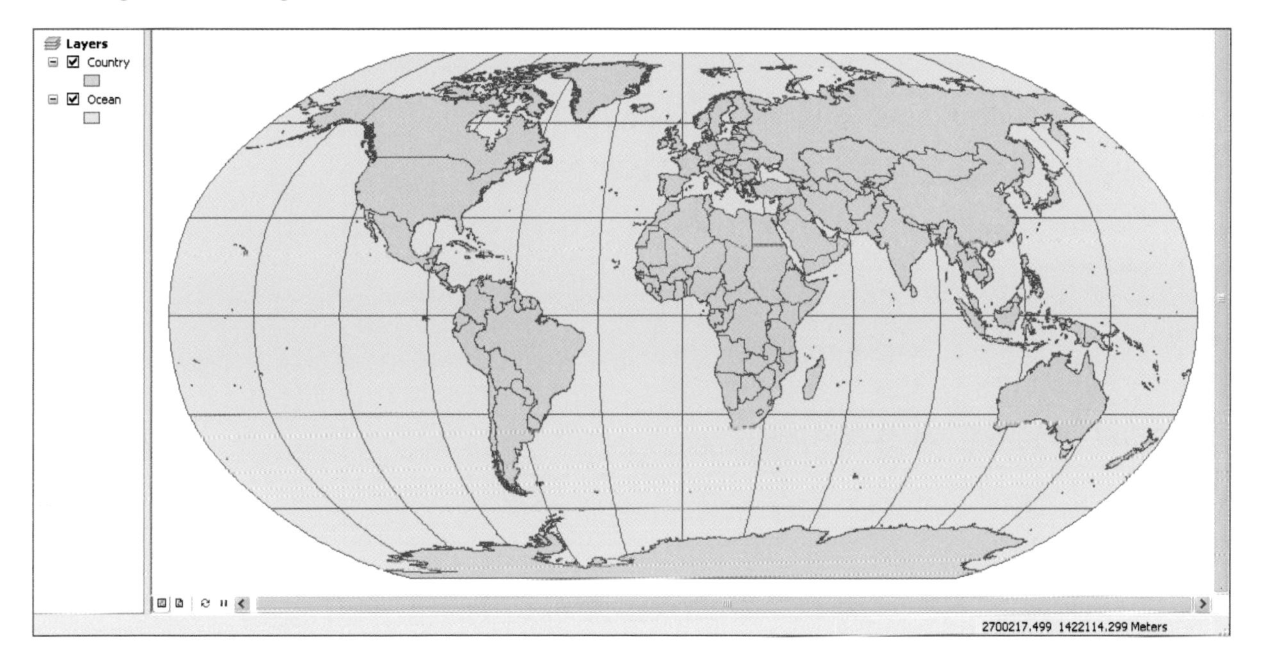

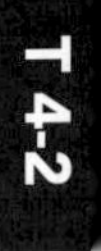

Symbolize layers

1 **In the table of contents, right-click the Country layer, click Properties, and click the Symbology tab.**

2 **In the Show panel, click Quantities > Graduated symbols.**

3 **Under Fields, click the Value arrow and click AIDSCases.**

4 **Click the Template button and change the symbol type to Circle 2 and a Mars Red fill color.**

5 **In the Symbology window, set the Symbol Size range to** 2 **to** 12.

6 **Click the Background button to set the background to Arctic White.**

7 Change the number of classes to 7 **and click the Classify button to define seven classes and manual break values of** 0, 1000, 5000, 10000, 50000, 100000, 900000. **Click OK.**

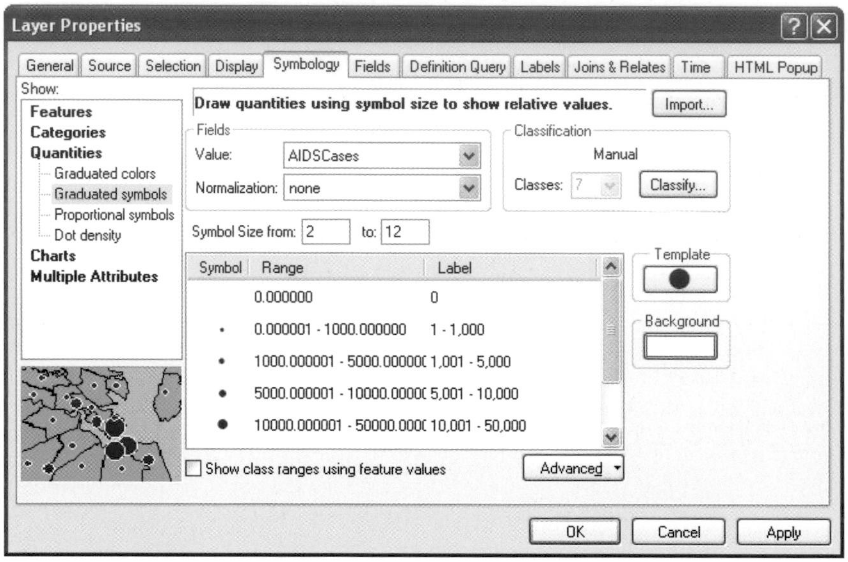

8 In the Symbol list, double-click the smallest red point marker symbol for the 0 class and change the point marker to Circle 1 and no fill color. This step makes the point marker for the 0 class invisible.

9 In the Symbol list, click the Label column heading, click Format Labels, change the number of decimal places to 0, **and select the "Show thousands separators" check box. Click OK twice.**

10 Symbolize the Ocean layer using a light-blue fill color and medium-gray outline.

11 In the table of contents, click each layer name, and then, in a second or two, click it again to activate the text pointer and type labels for Cumulative AIDS Cases **and** 30 Degree Graticule**, as shown in the figure.** Dark fill color in country polygons, as seen at the beginning of this chapter, makes for false perceptions. For example, the United States' AIDS problem was overblown and Eastern Europe's was understated. This map, however, clearly shows the volume of AIDS cases by country, with heavy concentrations in sub-Saharan Africa and a surprising number in Eastern Europe. Be aware that some countries, such as in Western Europe, have no AIDS data. These countries were reflected as polygons in the earlier choropleth map but not necessarily shown with graduated point markers. One solution could be to add text to the legend stating that there is no AIDS data for these countries.

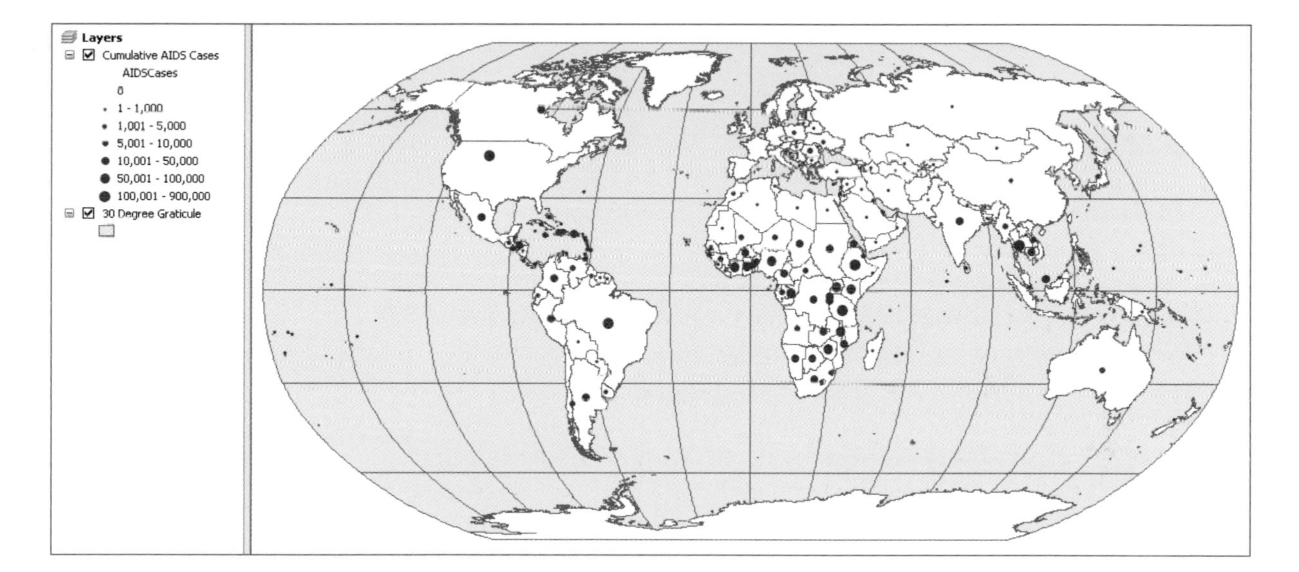

Save the map document

1 On the File menu, click Save As.

2 Save your map document as Tutorial4-2YourName.mxd **to your Chapter4 folder in MyExercises.** Do not close ArcMap.

Tutorial 4-3
Creating a prevalence map using point markers

Prevalence maps help to illustrate the progression of an infectious disease. In this tutorial, you will map AIDS prevalence (rate per 10,000 people) using graduated point markers and the Robinson projection. First, you will calculate the prevalence by creating a new field for the incidence rate.

Copy the Cumulative AIDS Cases layer

1 In the table of contents, right-click Cumulative AIDS Cases and click Copy.

2 On the Menu bar, click Edit > Paste and turn off the second copy of this layer in the table of contents by clicking to clear its check box.

Add and calculate a field

1 Right-click the first copy of Cumulative AIDS Cases and click Open Attribute Table.

2 In the attribute table of Cumulative AIDS Cases, click the Table Options button.

3 Click Add Field, and for Name, type AIDSRate; for Type, click Double; and then click OK.

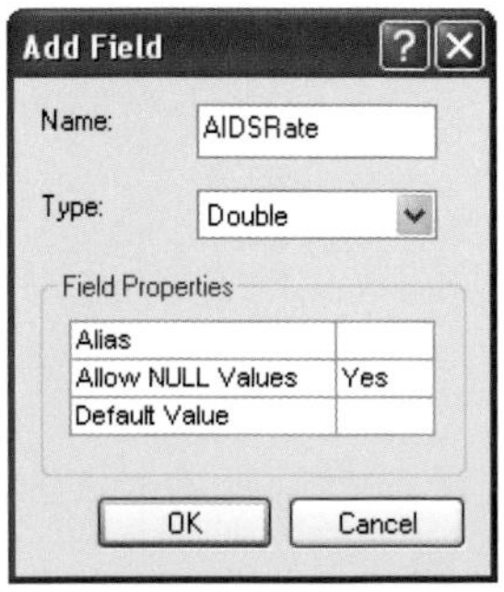

Add Field

Name: AIDSRate

Type: Double

Field Properties

Alias	
Allow NULL Values	Yes
Default Value	

OK Cancel

4 **Scroll to the right end of the attribute table, right-click the AIDSRate field name, and click Field Calculator. Click Yes to continue if you get a warning box about calculating outside an edit session.**

5 **In Field Calculator, scroll down the Fields list, double-click AIDSCases, and click the multiplication (*) button. Then type** 10000, **click the division (/) button, and double-click POP_CNTRY.**

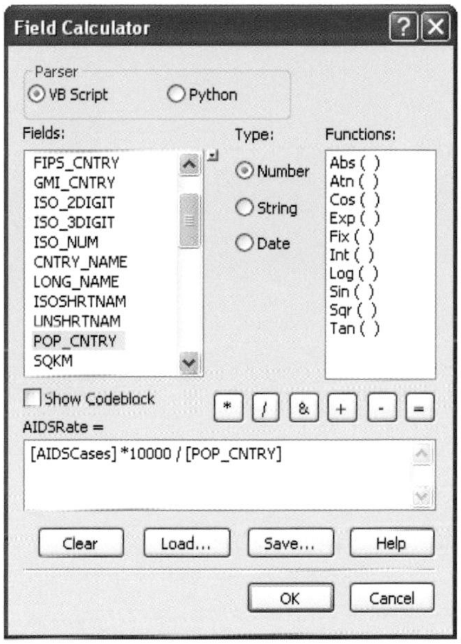

Field Calculator

Parser: VB Script / Python

Fields: FIPS_CNTRY, GMI_CNTRY, ISO_2DIGIT, ISO_3DIGIT, ISO_NUM, CNTRY_NAME, LONG_NAME, ISOSHRTNAM, UNSHRTNAM, POP_CNTRY, SQKM

Type: Number / String / Date

Functions: Abs ( ), Atn ( ), Cos ( ), Exp ( ), Fix ( ), Int ( ), Log ( ), Sin ( ), Sqr ( ), Tan ( )

Show Codeblock

AIDSRate =

[AIDSCases] *10000 / [POP_CNTRY]

Clear | Load... | Save... | Help | OK | Cancel

6 **Click OK.** The attribute table shows the prevalence of AIDS per 10,000 persons.

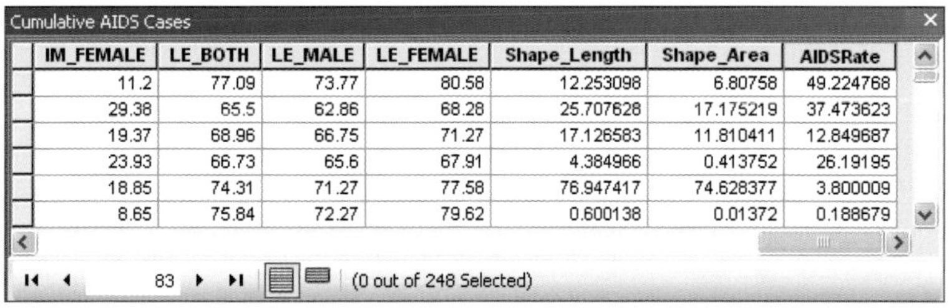

Cumulative AIDS Cases

IM_FEMALE	LE_BOTH	LE_MALE	LE_FEMALE	Shape_Length	Shape_Area	AIDSRate
11.2	77.09	73.77	80.58	12.253098	6.80758	49.224768
29.38	65.5	62.86	68.28	25.707628	17.175219	37.473623
19.37	68.96	66.75	71.27	17.126583	11.810411	12.849687
23.93	66.73	65.6	67.91	4.384966	0.413752	26.19195
18.85	74.31	71.27	77.58	76.947417	74.628377	3.800009
8.65	75.84	72.27	79.62	0.600138	0.01372	0.188679

83 (0 out of 248 Selected)

7 **Close the table when you are finished.**

YOUR TURN

Rename the top layer **AIDS Rate Per 10,000 Persons** and symbolize it using the newly calculated field AIDSRate to yield AIDS prevalence per 10,000 persons as shown in the figure. Compare the two portrayals of AIDS: incidence and prevalence. There are some notable differences. This map shows the alarming scope of AIDS in sub-Saharan countries and the Caribbean, de-emphasizing most of the rest of the world, compared with the previous map on incidence.

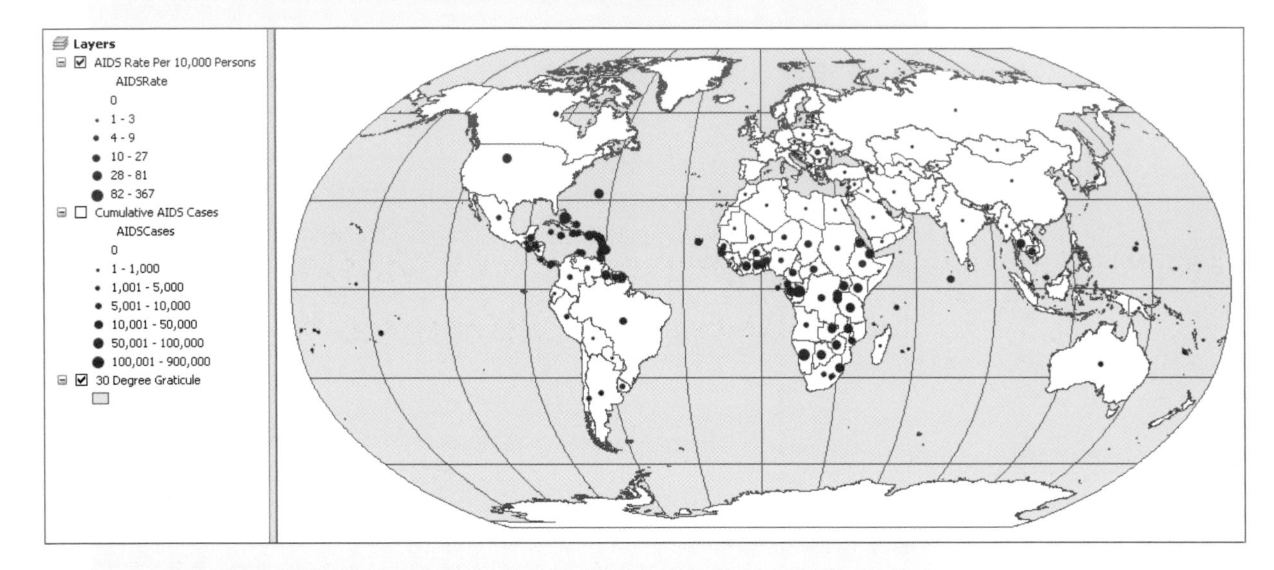

Save the map document

1 **On the File menu, click Save As.**

2 **Save your map document as** Tutorial4-3YourName.mxd **to your Chapter4 folder in MyExercises.** Do not close ArcMap.

Country-level data and continental projections

Often, more-detailed maps at a country level are needed to study a health condition. Map projections vary depending on the country of focus. Many health organizations provide health and GIS data to download from the Internet. In these tutorials, you will learn how to download data from the HIV Spatial Data Repository website, which is supported by PEPFAR. You will also learn about the best projections to use for the United States.

Tutorial 4-4
Downloading international HIV/AIDS data

In the following exercises, you will log on to the HIV Spatial Data Repository website and download subnational HIV prevalence data for Zambia, a country in Africa.

Download and extract HIV data for Zambia

1 **In a web browser, go to http://hivspatialdata.net/.**

2 **In the box "Attention ESRI GIS Tutorial for Health Users:", click "Download the Zambia DHS 2007 data for tutorial 4-4."** ▶

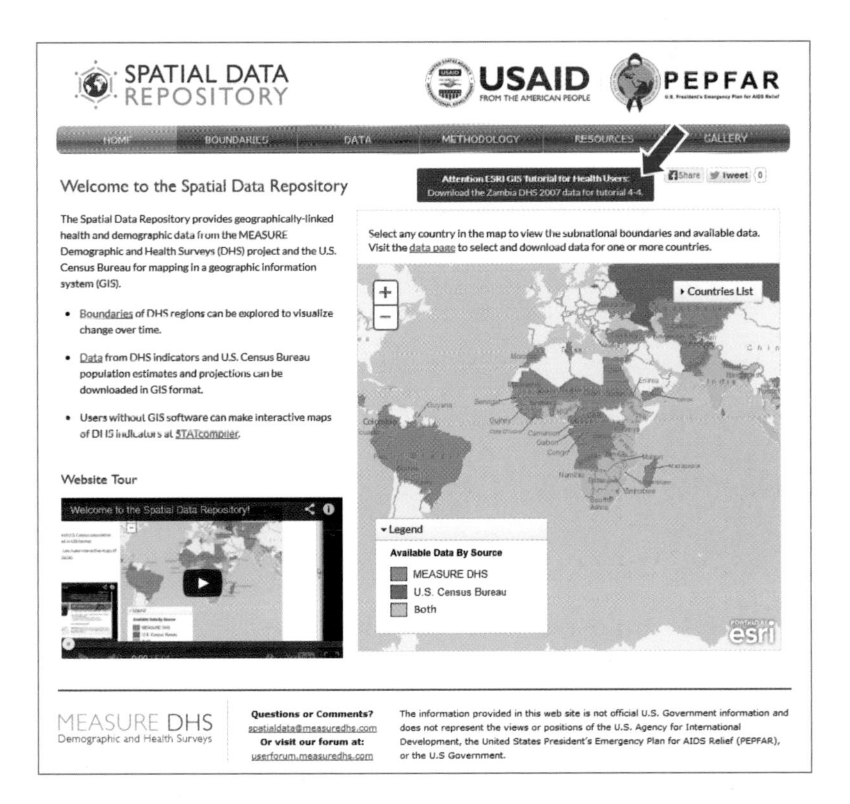

3 **Browse to** your Chapter 4 MyExercises folder, and save the compressed file ZM_DHS_07_GIS_Tutorial_for_Health.zip. Note that the FinishedExercises folder does not include this file and you must down-load it from the website.

4 In Windows Explorer, browse to your Chapter4 folder, double-click ZM_DHS_07_GIS_Tutorial_for_Health.ZIP, and extract all files to this location. The extracted files include the files needed for the shapefile (.dbf, .prj, .sbn, .sbx, .shp, .xml, and .shx), an image file (.gif) of Zambia's regions, and a Microsoft Excel spreadsheet (.xls) that has data and metadata. A README text file (readme.txt) that contains details describing these files is also included.

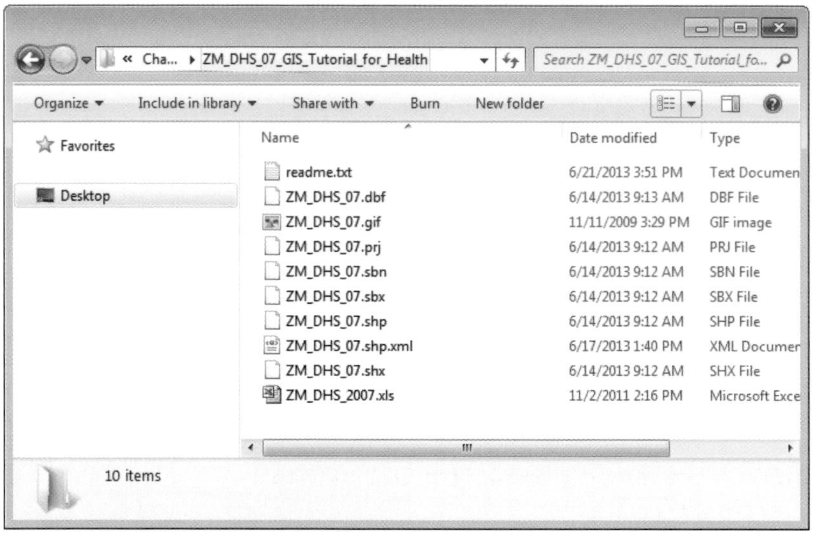

« Cha... ▸ ZM_DHS_07_GIS_Tutorial_for_Health

Organize ▾ Include in library ▾ Share with ▾ Burn New folder

Favorites

Desktop

Name	Date modified	Type
readme.txt	6/21/2013 3:51 PM	Text Documen
ZM_DHS_07.dbf	6/14/2013 9:13 AM	DBF File
ZM_DHS_07.gif	11/11/2009 3:29 PM	GIF image
ZM_DHS_07.prj	6/14/2013 9:12 AM	PRJ File
ZM_DHS_07.sbn	6/14/2013 9:12 AM	SBN File
ZM_DHS_07.sbx	6/14/2013 9:12 AM	SBX File
ZM_DHS_07.shp	6/14/2013 9:12 AM	SHP File
ZM_DHS_07.shp.xml	6/17/2013 1:40 PM	XML Documen
ZM_DHS_07.shx	6/14/2013 9:12 AM	SHX File
ZM_DHS_2007.xls	11/2/2011 2:16 PM	Microsoft Exce

10 items

YOUR TURN

Open readme.txt to see the description about the data. Open the .gif file to see the regions in Zambia. Close Windows Explorer when you are finished.

Explore metadata in Microsoft Excel

Some organizations provide metadata directly in GIS files and others provide it as text or spreadsheet documents. The metadata for Zambia DHS AIDS data is found in a Microsoft Excel spreadsheet.

1 Start Microsoft Excel and open the spreadsheet called ZM_DHS_07.xls, which was downloaded with the GIS layers to your Chapter4 folder in MyExercises.

2 Click the Indicator Key tab at the bottom of the spreadsheet. The Map_Code column corresponds directly to the ArcGIS attribute field.

	A	B	C	D
1	Map_Code	Indicator	Unit	Definition
2	SDR021_F	No Education among Women	Percentage (%)	Percentage of women age 15-49 who have no education
3	SDR021_M	No Education among Men	Percentage (%)	Percentage of men age 15-49 who have no education
4	SDR022_F	Secondary Education among Women	Percentage (%)	Percentage of Women age 15-49 who have secondary education or higher
5	SDR022_M	Secondary Education among Men	Percentage (%)	Percentage of Men age 15-49 who have secondary education or higher
6	SDR023_F	Primary Education among Women	Percentage (%)	Percentage of Women 15-49 who have completed primary or higher education
7	SDR023_M	Primary Education among Men	Percentage (%)	Percentage of Men 15-49 who have completed primary or higher education
8	SDR03_F	Media Exposure (Female 15-49)	Percentage (%)	Percentage of women age 15-49 who are exposed to at least one source of media (radio, television, newspaper or magazine) per week
9	SDR03_M	Media Exposure (Male 15-49)	Percentage (%)	Percentage of men age 15-49 who are exposed to at least one source of media (radio, television, newspaper or magazine) per week
10	V107	Birth registration (Children 0-4)	Percentage (%)	Percentage of children age 0 -4 whose births are reported as being registered

Regional Data | Indicator Key

T 4-4

Create a combined map comparing education and HIV prevalence

Zambia has the highest subnational percentage of HIV in Africa and the map you will create in this exercise will show details of the percentage of women age 15–49 (Map_Code SDR021_F) who have no education and the percentage of women age 15–49 who tested positive for HIV (Map_Code V150_F).

1 In a new map document, add the downloaded shapefile ZM_DHS_07.shp from your Chapter4 folder in MyExercises.

2 Right-click the ZM_DHS_07 layer, click Properties, and click the Symbology tab.

3 Change the settings to match those in the figure. The SDR021_F field is the percentage of women age 15–49 who have no education, as described in the Excel spreadsheet.

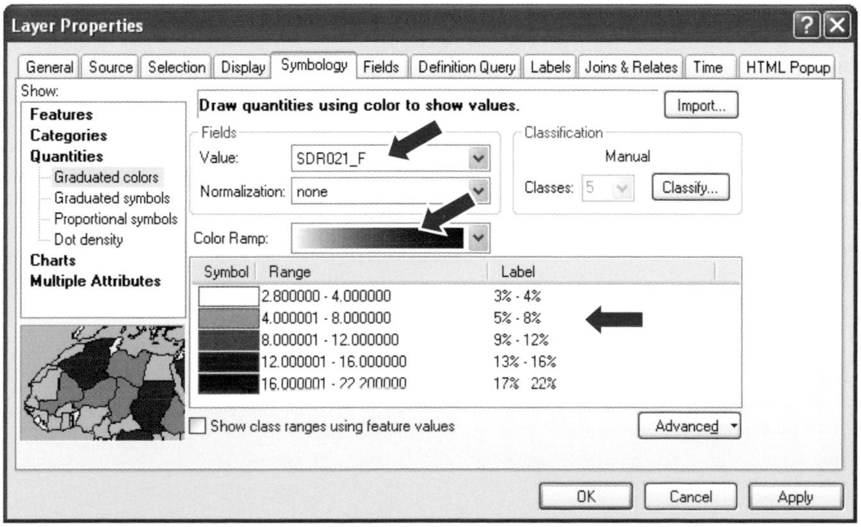
Layer Properties
General | Source | Selection | Display | Symbology | Fields | Definition Query | Labels | Joins & Relates | Time | HTML Popup
Show:
Features
Categories
Quantities
Graduated colors
Graduated symbols
Proportional symbols
Dot density
Charts
Multiple Attributes
Draw quantities using color to show values.
Import...
Fields
Value: SDR021_F
Normalization: none
Classification
Manual
Classes: 5
Classify...
Color Ramp:
Symbol | Range | Label
2.800000 - 4.000000 | 3% - 4%
4.000001 - 8.000000 | 5% - 8%
8.000001 - 12.000000 | 9% - 12%
12.000001 - 16.000000 | 13% - 16%
16.000001 - 22.200000 | 17% - 22%
Show class ranges using feature values
Advanced
OK
Cancel
Apply

4 **Rename the layer** % of women with no education **and remove the field name to match the legend in the figure.** ▶

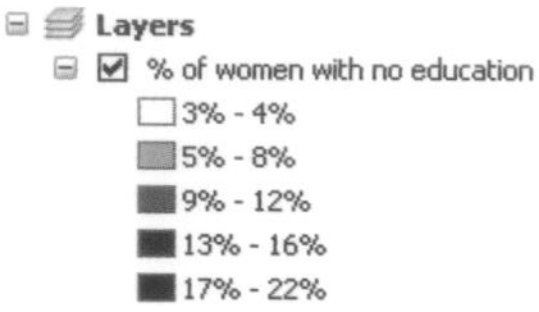

5 **Add the ZM_DHS_07 shapefile again, right-click the layer, click Properties, and click the Symbology tab.**

6 **Change the settings to match those in the figure.** The V150_F field is the percentage of women age 15–49 who tested positive for HIV.

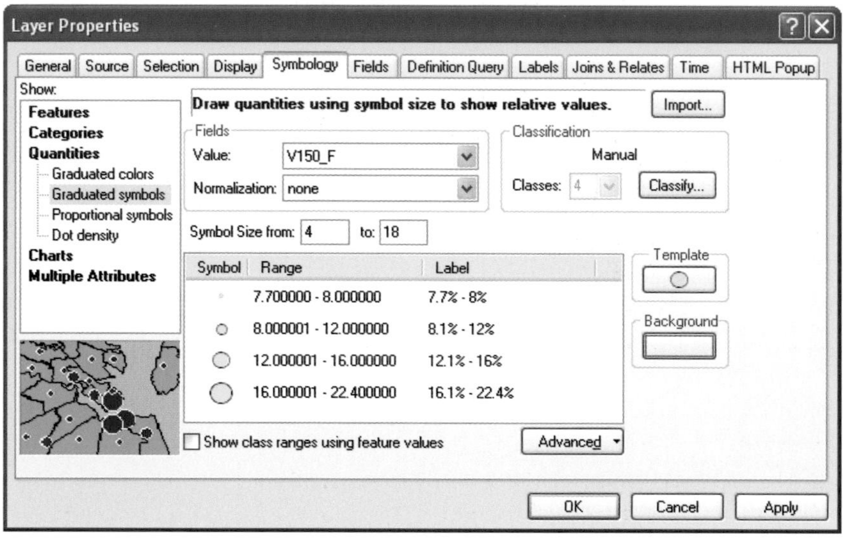

7 **Rename the layer** % of women who tested positive for HIV. ▶

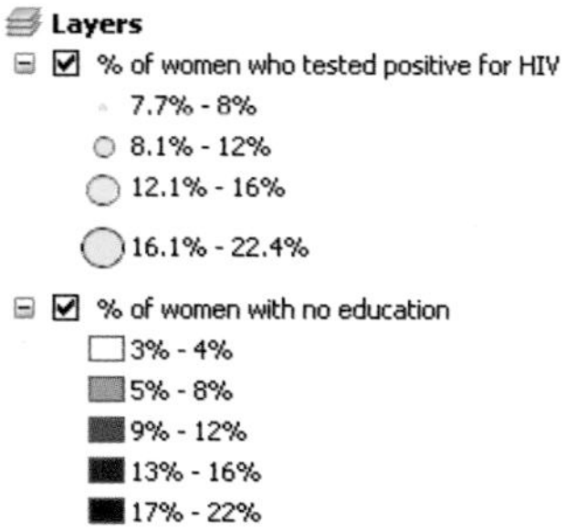

8 **Label the map using the REG_NAME field and a white halo. Convert the labels to annotation and move them so the graduated point markers are visible.**

9 Rename the data frame Zambia HIV study of women ages 15-49. Study the resulting map to see if there is a correlation between the percentage of females in a province who have no education and the prevalence of HIV in that province.

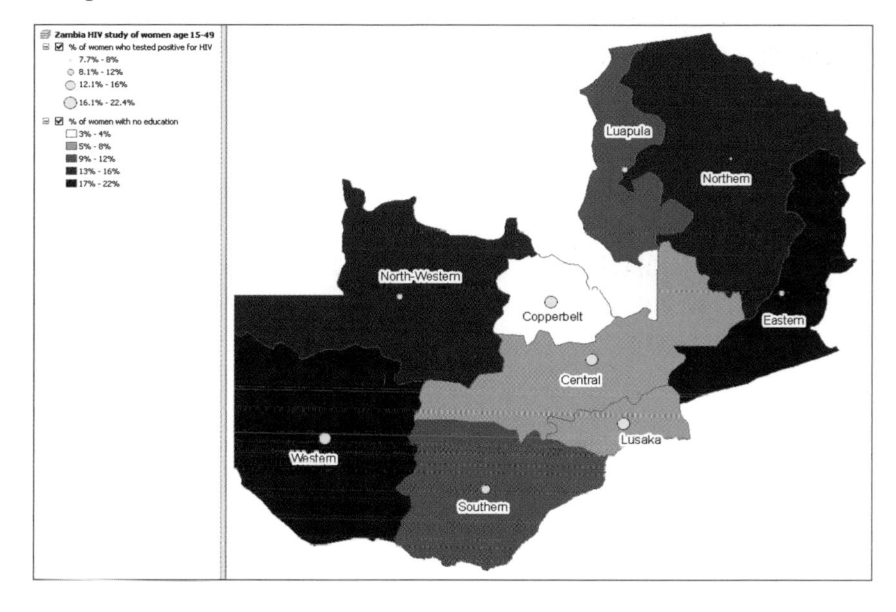

YOUR TURN

Create a map layout including the data source and date. Export the map as a JPEG image file called **Tutorial4-4YourName.jpg** to your Chapter4 folder in MyExercises.

Save the map document

1 On the File menu, click Save As.

2 Save your map document as Tutorial4-4YourName.mxd **to your Chapter4 folder in MyExercises.** Do not close ArcMap.

Tutorial 4-5
Exploring map projections for a US lung cancer study

In this tutorial, you will explore map projections for the 48 states of the contiguous United States. You already know how to change the projection of a data frame, so here you will open a finished map document in layout view and observe differences in the projections.

Study differences in the projections

1 **On the Menu bar, click File > Open, browse through the Maps folder, and open Tutorial4-5.mxd.** This is a map document in layout view that has four data frames for the contiguous 48 states, plus four selected cities. The spatial reference used for the geographic coordinates data frame is in the Data Frame Properties on the Coordinate System tab under Geographic Coordinate Systems > North American Datum (NAD) 1983. For the two US contiguous projections, see Projected Coordinate Systems > Continental North America.

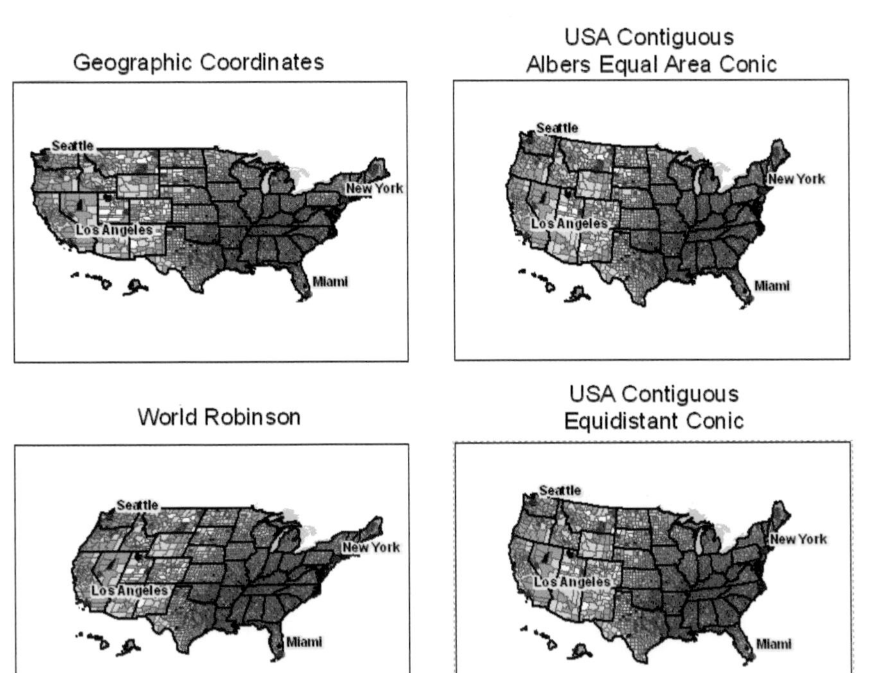

2 **In Layout View, click the data frame for Geographic Coordinates.** This step makes the data frame active. The geographic coordinates flatten the map in the north–south direction.

3 **Click View > Data View.**

4 **On the Tools toolbar, click the Measure button .** The Measure window opens and the Measure Line tool is activated. The current map units are meters, but miles are more familiar in the United States, so you will change the units to Miles.

5 **In the Measure window, click the Choose Units arrow.**

6 **Click Distance > Miles and leave the Measure window open.**

7 **Move the pointer to the city of Los Angeles and click it.**

8 **Move the pointer to New York and double-click it.** The distance shown in the dialog box should be about 2,461mi.

9 **Measure the distance between New York and Miami.** The distance should be about 1,086 mi. Both distances are as the crow flies.

YOUR TURN

Activate the other data frames and observe how the projections look. The Robinson projection, although very attractive for viewing the world as a whole, has undesirable distortions when viewing the United States by itself. Both the equal-area and equidistant projections are comparable in appearance and good choices for use. The equal-area conic projection was used in figure 1.1 in chapter 1 using the same data. Use the Measure tool to measure distances between the selected cities. The actual distance between Los Angeles and New York is 2,441 mi, showing that the Albers Equal Area Conic is the best projection to use if measurements are necessary.

Save the map document

1 **On the File menu, click Save As.**

2 **Save your map document as** Tutorial4-5YourName.mxd **to your Chapter4 folder in MyExercises.** Do not close ArcMap.

Local-level spatial data

In the next tutorials, you will create a map showing neighborhood "walkability" by adding layers from a variety of sources, in various data formats, and in various projected coordinate systems. You will carry out several steps involving data frame and map layer projections. You will start with several layers obtained from the Pittsburgh City Planning Department, all saved as NAD 1983 Pennsylvania South state plane coordinates. To these layers, you will add data from an ArcInfo interchange file, which you will import into an ArcInfo coverage and then transform into a shapefile. You will also add a CAD drawing from an engineering firm and an XY table of schools including latitude and longitude coordinates.

Tutorial 4-6
Adding and symbolizing existing map layers

In this exercise, you will add layers of varying levels of detail. You will see that the coordinate system of the data frame is automatically set by the first layer added to the map document. You will learn how to label multiple layers at once and how to adjust the layer transparency and scale range.

Add neighborhood layers

1 **On the Menu bar, Click File > New > My Templates > Blank Map, and click OK to begin a new map document.**

2 **On the Standard toolbar, click Add Data, browse through the Data folder to Pittsburgh.gdb, click Neighborhoods, and click Add.**

3 **In the table of contents, right-click the Layers data frame, click Properties, and click the Coordinate System tab.** You can see that the current coordinate system is NAD_1983_StatePlane_Pennsylvania_South_FIPS_3702_Feet. The data frame automatically inherits the projection of the first map layer added, if you have not explicitly already set the data frame projection. So, regardless of the projection of additional layers, ArcMap projects them on the fly to the state plane coordinates of Neighborhoods. This assumes that each map layer has a projection file that has the correct projection assigned.

4 **Click OK and symbolize the map using a Hollow symbol and an outline width of** 1.15. Check the coordinates in the lower-right corner of the map to see that they are in feet units, corresponding to state plane units.

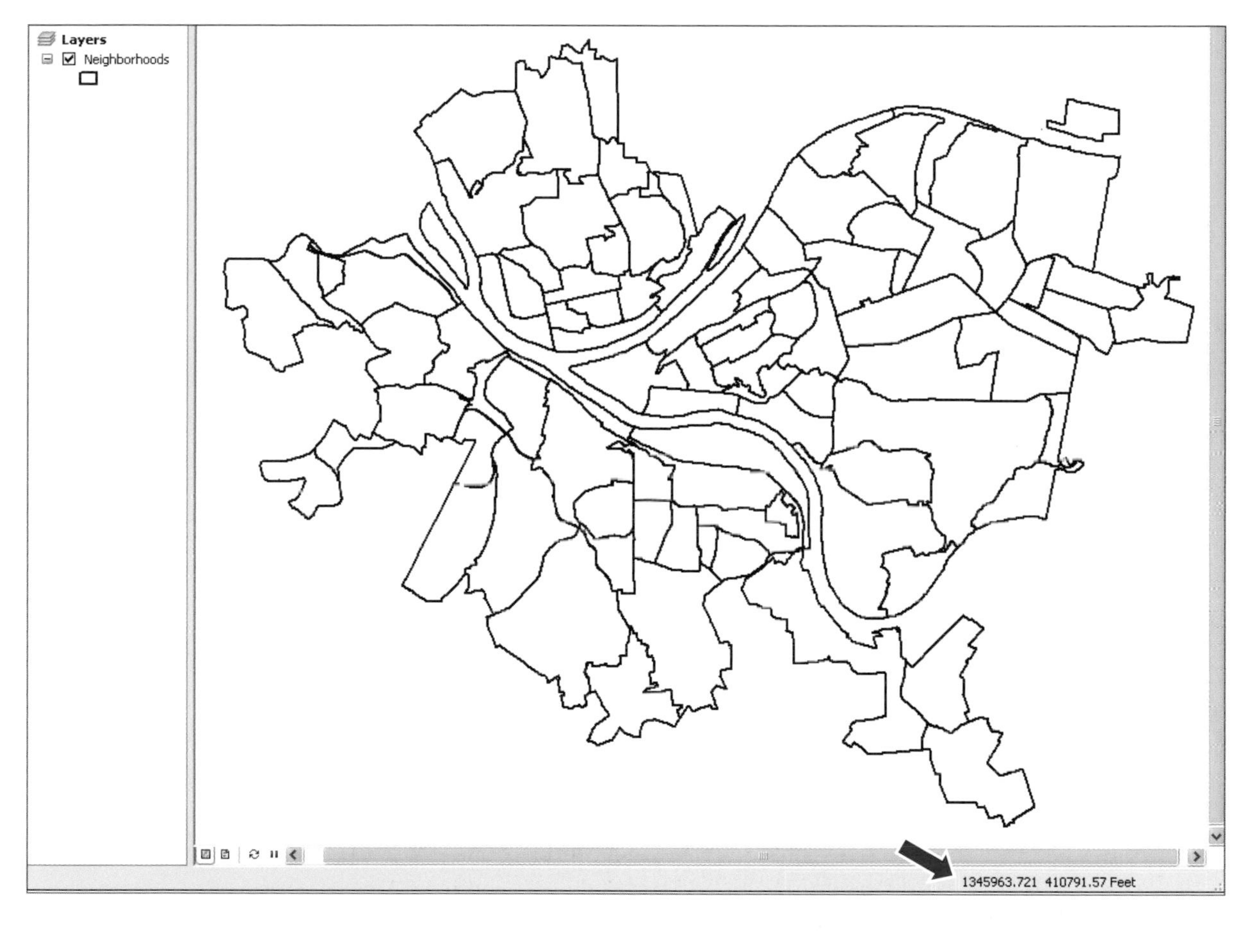

YOUR TURN

Add the following layers from Pittsburgh.gdb to the map document: Parks, Sidewalks, and Topo25ft. Symbolize these layers so that Sidewalks is a light-gray color, Parks is a medium-green color, and Topo25ft is a light-tan color. Move Neighborhoods to the top of the table of contents, followed by Parks, Sidewalks, and Topo25ft.

Label multiple layers

1 In the table of contents, right-click Layers and click Labeling > Label Manager.

2 In the Label Manager dialog box, select the check boxes for Neighborhoods, Parks, and Topo25ft.

3 Under Topo25ft, click Default, and for Label Field, click ELEV; for Text Symbol color, choose a medium brown. For Placement Properties Orientation, select Curved.

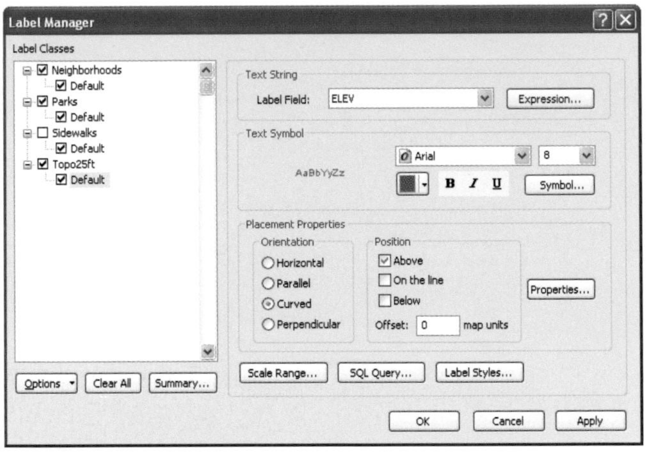

4 Under Neighborhoods, select Default; under Placement Properties, click the Properties button; then click the Placement tab and select the "Remove duplicate labels" option. Click OK twice.

The end result is a very jumbled and unusable map, which you will remedy in the next "Your Turn" exercise.

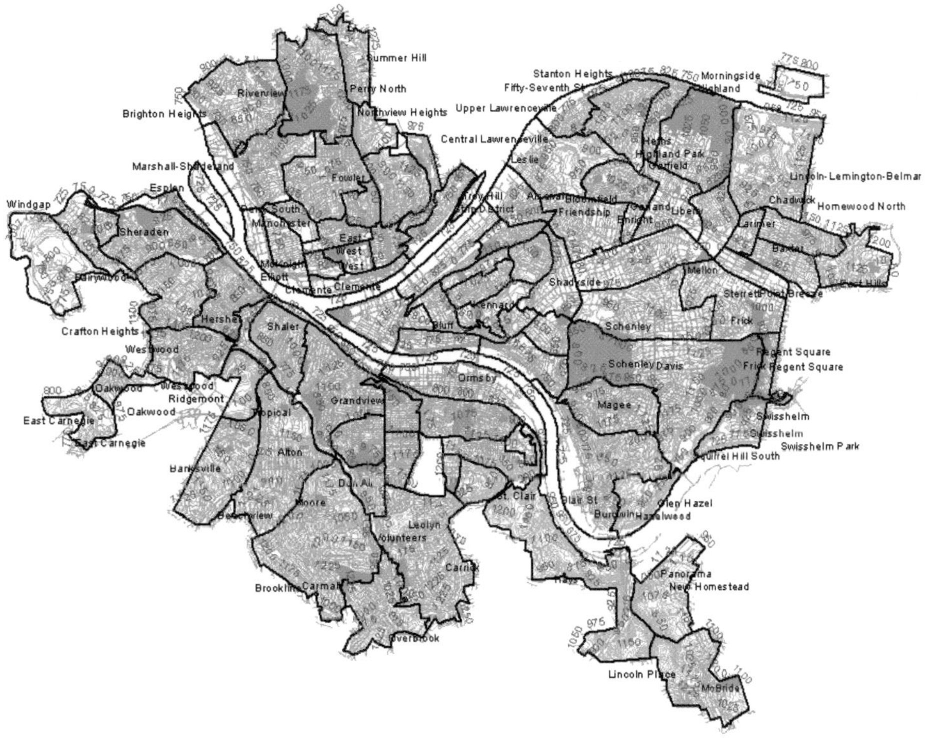

YOUR TURN

Add a white, size 1 halo to the Parks layer labels and set Label Manager to remove duplicate labels. Give Neighborhoods a blue, size 2 halo label.

Set parks as semitransparent

1 **Right-click any toolbar and click Effects.**

2 **Click the Layer arrow and click Parks.**

3 **Click the Adjust Transparency button .**

4 **Slide the transparency level to 50% and close the Effects toolbar.**

Set scale ranges

In this exercise, you will set layers to turn on when zoomed below a scale of 1:24,000, which is a common scale for viewing detailed features in a map. Alternatively, you could zoom to a scale that you find appropriate, read the scale from the Standard toolbar, and use it to set scale range properties.

1 **Right-click the Topo25ft layer and click Properties.**

2 **Click the General tab and select the "Don't show layer when zoomed" option.**

3 **Click the "Out beyond" arrow, click 1:24,000, and click OK.** The topography layer is no longer displayed at the current scale.

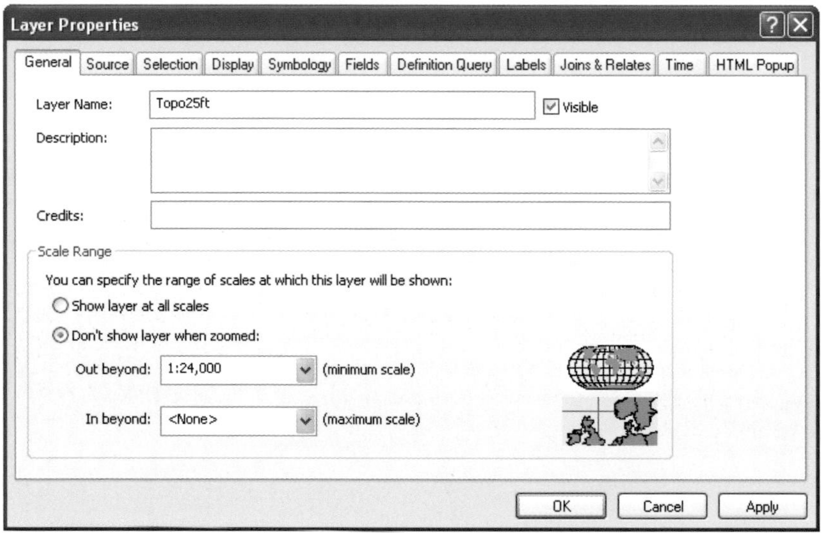

4 **Zoom in on the map until you are at or below a scale of 1:24,000.** You will see the topography layer appear when zoomed at or below a scale of 1:24,000.

5 Zoom out to the full extent of the map.

YOUR TURN

Change the scale to turn the sidewalks and parks off when zoomed beyond 1:24,000. Try out your map at exactly 1:24,000 by setting that scale in the scale field on the Standard toolbar and pressing ENTER.

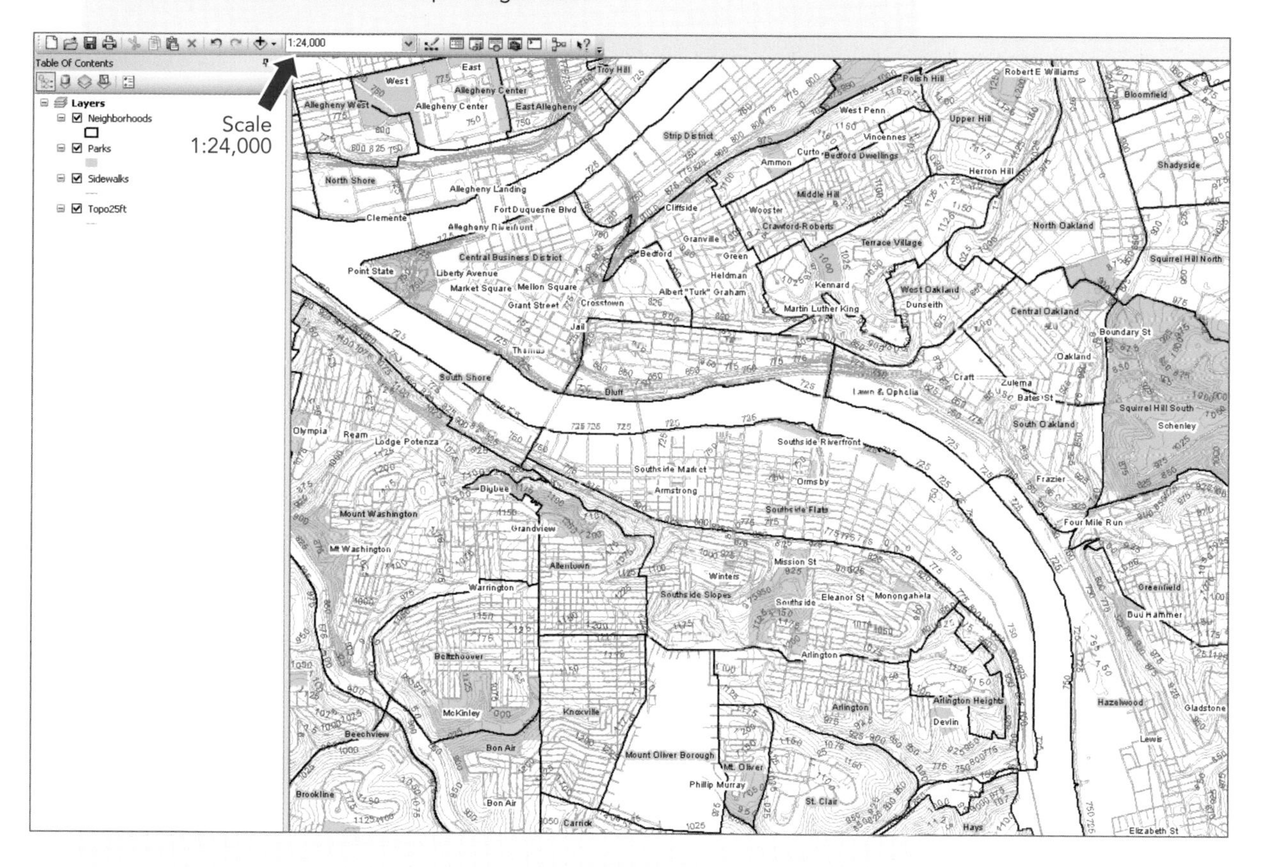

Save the map document

1 On the File menu, click Save As.

2 Save your map document as Tutorial4-6YourName.mxd **to your Chapter4 folder in MyExercises.** Do not close ArcMap.

Tutorial 4-7
Working with spatial-data formats

A file geodatabase is an integral part of working with spatial-data formats. A file geodatabase, which is merely a collection of files in a file folder, is flexible and simple to use. Nonetheless, you need a special utility program to build and maintain a file geodatabase—and that is ArcCatalog. Some of the functionality of ArcCatalog is also available in ArcMap in the Catalog window, which you will use in this tutorial. The Catalog window allows you to do some utility work in ArcMap without opening the separate application program, ArcCatalog. Because the file geodatabase is the preferred ArcMap format, you will first build it, and then import all remaining files into it.

Open the Catalog window

To create a file geodatabase, you must use either ArcCatalog or the Catalog window in ArcMap. Windows Explorer and My Computer are not capable of building all the components of a file geodatabase.

1 On the Standard toolbar, click the Catalog window button .

2 In the Catalog window, browse to your Chapter4 folder. ▶

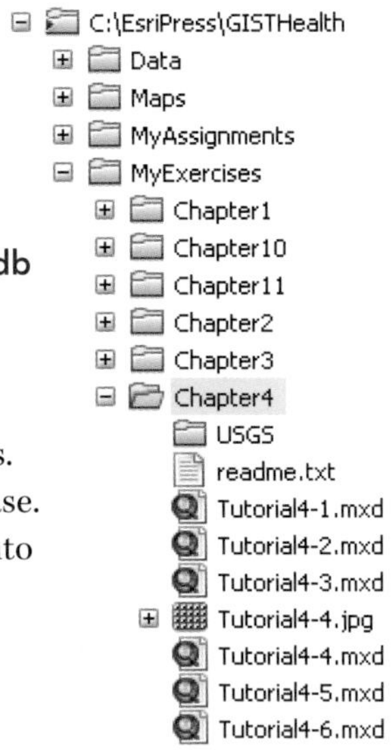

C:\EsriPress\GISTHealth
Data
Maps
MyAssignments
MyExercises
Chapter1
Chapter10
Chapter11
Chapter2
Chapter3
Chapter4
USGS
readme.txt
Tutorial4-1.mxd
Tutorial4-2.mxd
Tutorial4-3.mxd
Tutorial4-4.jpg
Tutorial4-4.mxd
Tutorial4-5.mxd
Tutorial4-6.mxd

3 Right-click Chapter4 in the Catalog window and click New > File Geodatabase.

4 Change the name from New File Geodatabase.gdb to Chapter4.gdb**.**

A file geodatabase is now created that you can populate with feature classes and stand-alone tables. Feature classes are map layers stored in a geodatabase. Next, you will import a map layer in a CAD format into your new file geodatabase as a set of feature classes.

Import a CAD file into a geodatabase

In this exercise, you will import a CAD drawing exchange file (.dxf) showing Pittsburgh's rivers into your file geodatabase. The CAD file was created by a local engineering firm.

1 **In the Catalog window, right-click Chapter4.gdb and click Import > Feature Class (single).**

2 **In the Feature Class to Feature Class dialog box, click the Browse button for Input Features, browse through the Data folder to DataFiles, double-click Rivers.dxf, click Polygon, and click Add.** This step adds the CAD .dxf file to the Input Features box.

3 **For Output Feature Class, type** Rivers **and click OK.** The new Rivers feature class should automatically be added to your table of contents.

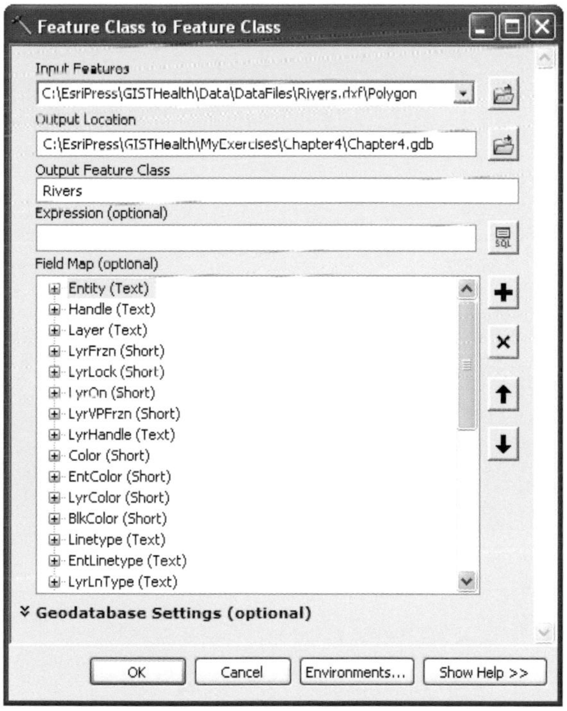

4 **Symbolize the Rivers.dxf polygon layer using a light-blue fill color.**

Export features to CAD files

Detailed features such as sidewalks and topography are sometimes useful for computer-aided design applications. For this purpose, it is necessary to export these features as CAD files. You will not save these files to your file geodatabase because geodatabases are specific to GIS, and CAD files need to be opened directly in CAD software.

1 **In the table of contents, right-click Sidewalks and click Data > Export to CAD.**

2 **In the Export to CAD dialog box, click the Browse button for Output File, browse to your Chapter4 folder, and for Name, type** Sidewalks. **Click Save and OK.** A common format for CAD files is the Autodesk DWG binary format. This format is much smaller and better to use than an ASCII text DXF format.

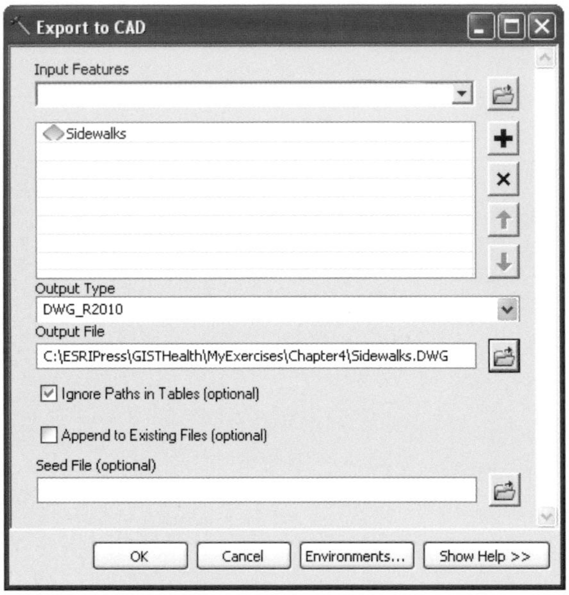

3 **Remove the Sidewalks CAD file from the table of contents.**

Import an ArcInfo interchange file

Some organizations still provide ArcInfo interchange (.E00) files, even though it is an older format. In this exercise, you will import an ArcInfo interchange file downloaded from the US Census Bureau website into an ArcInfo coverage (which has geographic coordinates) and export it to a file geodatabase. You are already familiar with symbolizing area maps, so you will skip that step in this exercise. The 2000 county subdivision layer that you will import is for all of Pennsylvania. In chapter 7, you will learn how to extract a subset of a map layer, such as for the city of Pittsburgh.

1 **On the Standard toolbar, click the ArcToolbox window button .**

2 **Click the plus sign (+) beside Conversion Tools and the plus sign beside To Coverage to expand them.**

3 Double-click Import from E00.

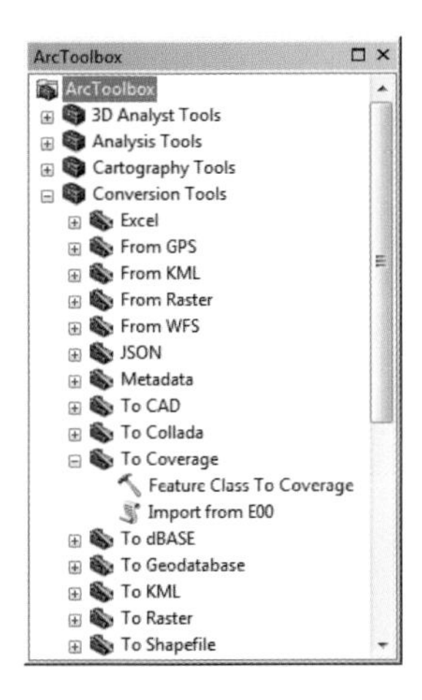

4 In the Import from E00 dialog box, click the Browse button for "Input interchange file", browse through the Data folder to DataFiles, click cs42_d00.e00, and click Open. Choose your Chapter4 folder in MyExercises as the Output folder, click Add, and click OK. This step imports the interchange file as an ArcInfo coverage. Importing the coverage may take a few minutes.

5 Close ArcToolbox.

YOUR TURN

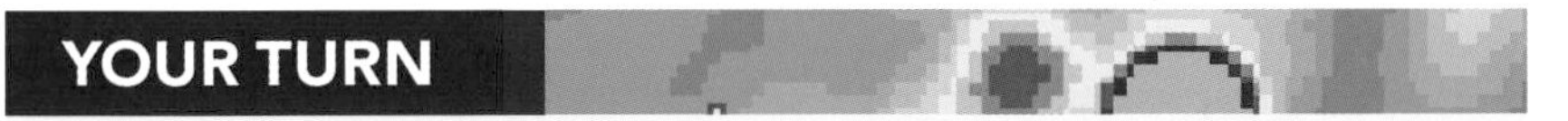

Start My Computer, browse to your Chapter4 folder, and examine the cs42_d00 coverage and its "info" folder. Each coverage has its own folder. Close My Computer.

Export the polygon features of the coverage into your file geodatabase using the Feature Class to Feature Class tool in the Geodatabase toolset. Name the new feature class **PACountySubdivisions**. The county subdivisions should be added to the map document automatically and you will now see the county subdivisions surrounding the city of Pittsburgh. Symbolize PACountySubdivisions as a Hollow symbol and a light-gray outline. Label features using the NAME field and a light-yellow mask.

Examine a layer projection

1 **Right-click PACountySubdivisions, click Properties, and click the Source tab.** Observe that PACountySubdivisions has geographic coordinates, but it still lines up nicely with the other layers, which are displayed in state plane coordinates.

2 **Close the Properties window.**

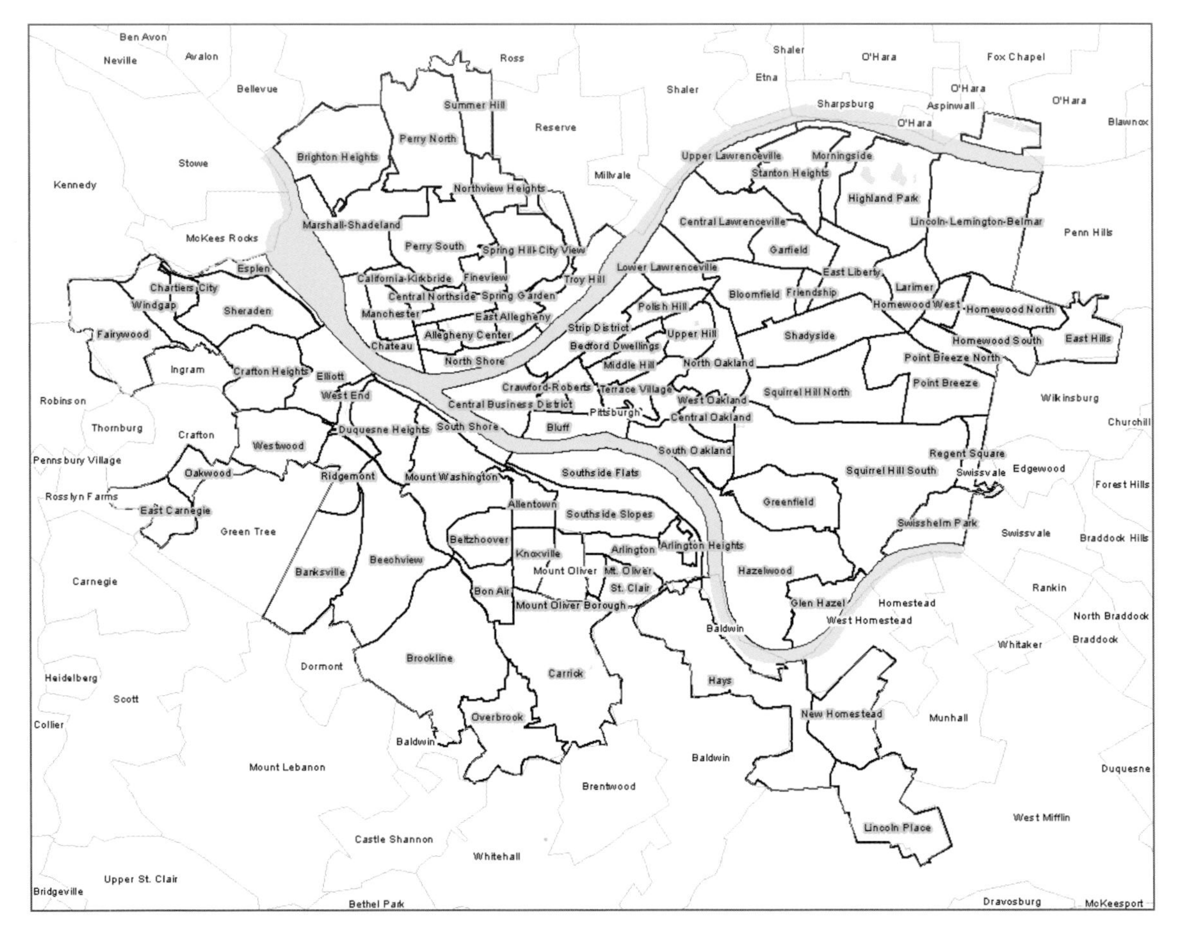

Save the map document

1 **On the File menu, click Save As.**

2 **Save your map document as** Tutorial4-7YourName.mxd **to your Chapter4 folder in MyExercises.** Do not close ArcMap.

Tutorial 4-8
Creating points from x,y coordinates

Event files are tables that have x,y coordinates. The table must contain two fields—one for the x-coordinate and one for the y-coordinate. In this tutorial, you will add a table that has point coordinates in latitude and longitude for schools in Pennsylvania.

Add and examine an XY table

1 On the Standard toolbar, click Add Data, browse through the Data folder to UnitedStates.gdb, and add the table called PASchools.

2 Right-click the PASchools table, click Open, and scroll to the right to examine the LONGITUDE and LATITUDE fields.

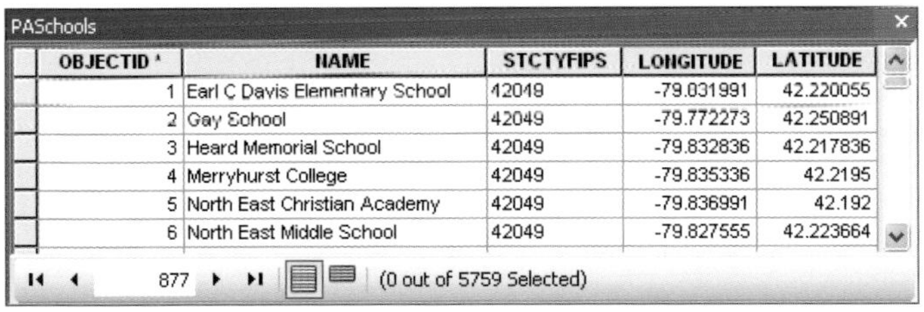

PASchools

OBJECTID *	NAME	STCTYFIPS	LONGITUDE	LATITUDE
1	Earl C Davis Elementary School	42049	-79.831991	42.220055
2	Gay School	42049	-79.772273	42.250891
3	Heard Memorial School	42049	-79.832836	42.217836
4	Merryhurst College	42049	-79.835336	42.2195
5	North East Christian Academy	42049	-79.836991	42.192
6	North East Middle School	42049	-79.827555	42.223664

877 (0 out of 5759 Selected)

3 Close the attribute table.

Assign GCS projection to the XY table

Because the data frame uses state plane coordinates (feet), your points will not appear unless you assign the data frame the geographic coordinate system (GCS), which uses latitude and longitude projection.

1 In the table of contents, right-click PASchools and click Display XY Data. ▶

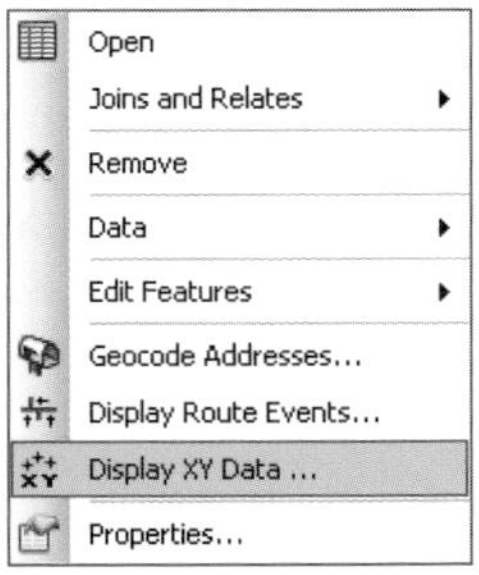

Open
Joins and Relates
Remove
Data
Edit Features
Geocode Addresses...
Display Route Events...
Display XY Data ...
Properties...

2 In the Display XY Data dialog box, click the Edit button.

3 In the Spatial Reference Properties dialog box, browse to Geographic Coordinate Systems > North America > NAD 1983 (GCS_North_American_1983) and click OK twice. ▶

You should now see school points.

A layer called PASchools Events is also created. Notice that the new school point layer nicely overlays the state plane layers, even though the original files use two different coordinate systems.

Spatial Reference Properties

XY Coordinate System

Type here to search

Helle 1954
MARCARIO SOLIS
Mexican Datum of 1993
NAD 1927
NAD 1927 (CGQ77)
NAD 1927 (Definition 1976)
NAD 1983
NAD 1983 (2011)
NAD 1983 (CORS96)
NAD 1983 (CSRS)
NAD 1983 (NSRS2007)
NAD 1983 HARN

Current coordinate system:

GCS_North_American_1983
Authority: Custom

Angular Unit: Degree (0.0174532925199433)
Prime Meridian: Greenwich (0.0)
Datum: D_North_American_1983
Spheroid: GRS_1980
Semimajor Axis: 6378137.0
Semiminor Axis: 6356752.314140356
Inverse Flattening: 298.257222101

OK Cancel

4 Right-click PASchools Events, click Properties, click the Source tab, observe that the map layer now has a spatial reference. Close the Layer Properties dialog box.

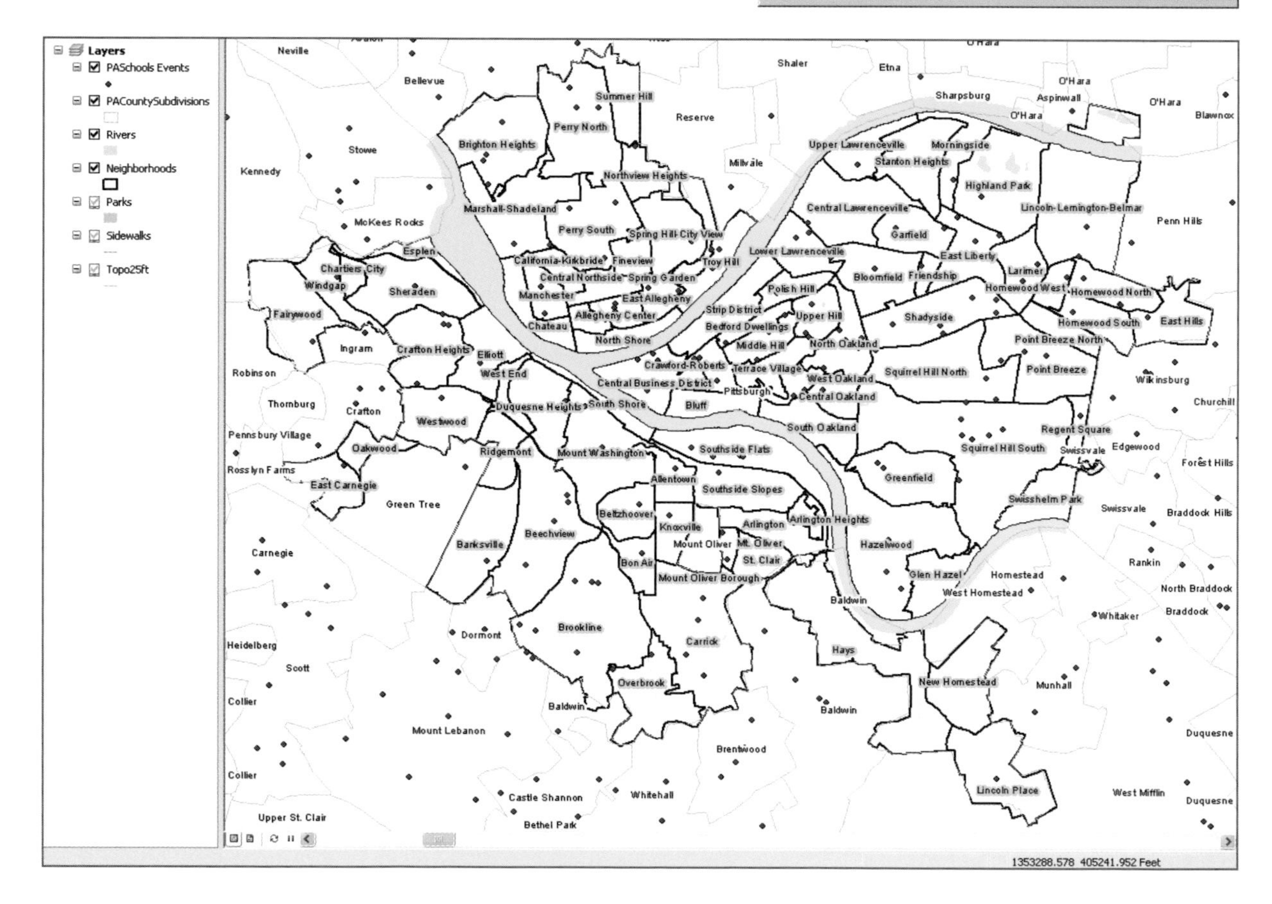

T 4-8

Export events as point features

Many of Pittsburgh's public schools are old, and the building facilities are not equipped for students to participate in physical activities. The school district task force on child obesity can use your map to identify possible off-campus playgrounds. A new schools point feature class could be exported from the event point layer and added to your neighborhood layers to identify the proximity of parks to schools. Such a file is needed to perform certain spatial analysis functions.

1 **Right-click PASchools Events, click Data > Export Data, specify Save as type to be "File and Personal Geodatabase feature classes,"and save the new point feature layer as** PASchools **to Chapter4.gdb in your Chapter4 folder in MyExercises.**

2 **Add the new point features to your map and remove the PASchools Events layer and original PASchools table.**

YOUR TURN

Change the scale to turn the schools off when zoomed beyond 1:24,000. Turn the labels on for the PASchools layer. Add a purple size 1 halo to the PASchools layer labels and set Label Manager to remove duplicate labels. On the Standard toolbar, set the scale bar to a scale of 1:24,000 to see the school details.

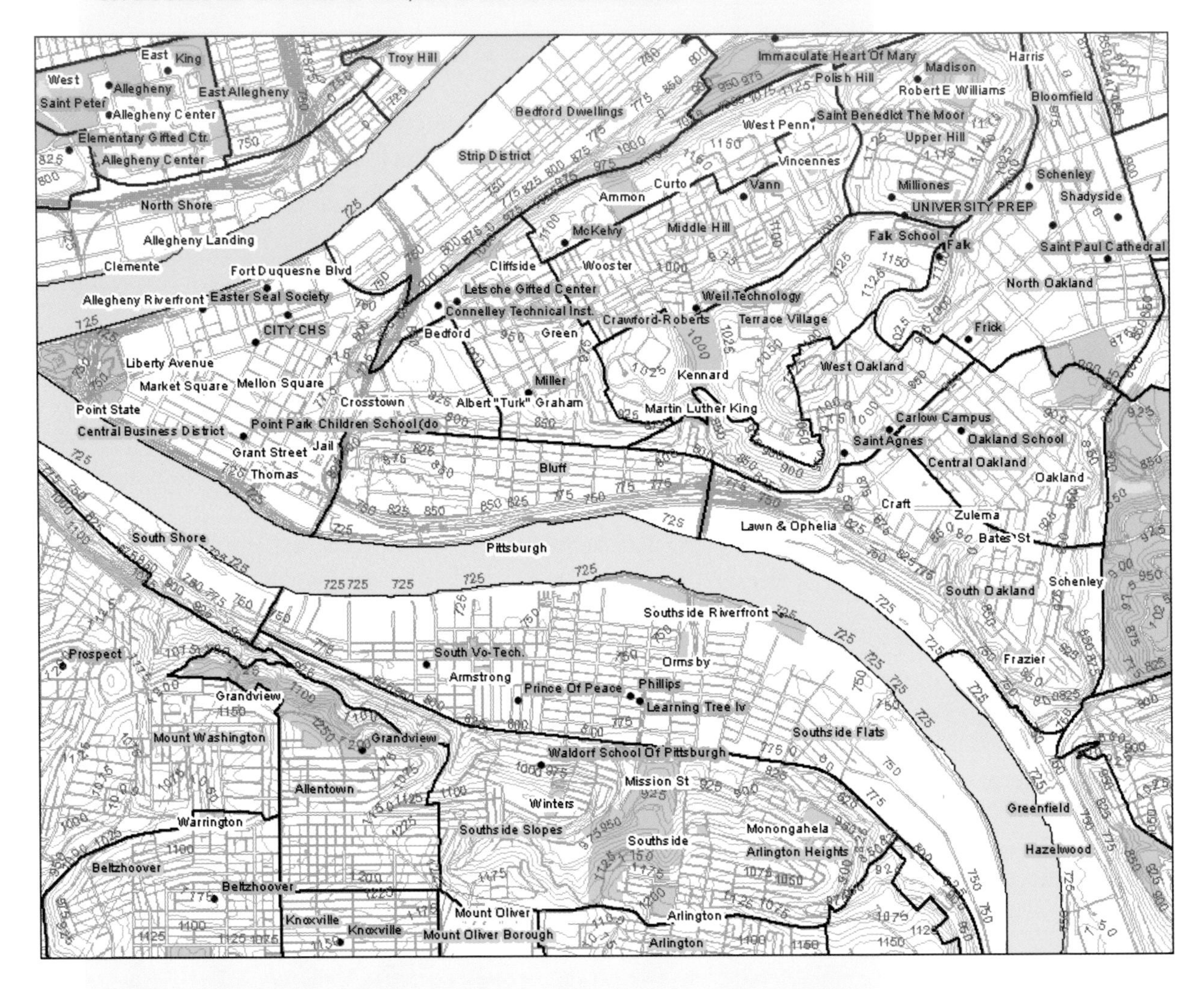

Save the map document

1 On the File menu, click Save As.

2 Save your map document as Tutorial4-8YourName.mxd to your Chapter4 folder in MyExercises. Do not close ArcMap.

Tutorial 4-9
Downloading USGS raster maps

The United States Geological Survey (USGS) has major responsibility for creating, maintaining, and providing basemaps of the United States. It recently launched a new seamless version of The National Map Viewer, which you can use to download GIS basemaps. "Seamless" means that all basemaps are available for viewing across the entire country, so one option for downloading is from the current extent of the viewer, and that extent may cut across several map tiles, counties, or states. The only limitation of the system is that "shipping" of the desired basemap is delayed; you are notified by e-mail when it's ready and given a link to download a compressed file, often with substantial delays. In any event, it's valuable to use a seamless download site for spatial data because of the website's convenience and reliability. If you have trouble downloading the files in this tutorial, copies are saved to the USGS folder in the Chapter4 folder in FinishedExercises.

Use The National Map Viewer

1 **In a web browser, go to** http://viewer.nationalmap.gov/viewer/. USGS recommends using Firefox as the browser. The images in the book may differ from what you see on the website.

2 **At the top of the map, click the Reset Zoom (Initial Extent) button .**

3 **If the Overlays window is not displayed at the left side, click the Overlays expander and click the Content button at the top of the window.** (See next page.)

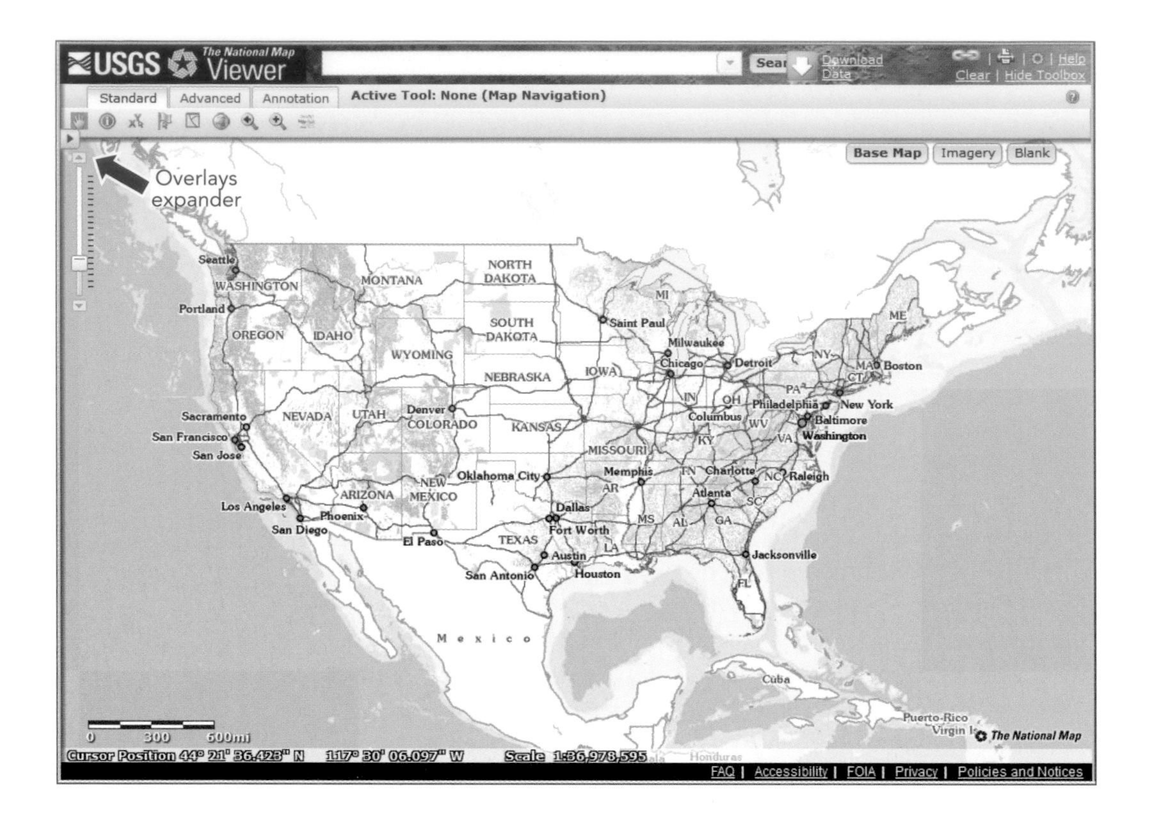

4 **Expand and select Governmental Unit Boundaries, and then expand Labels and then Features. Clear the check boxes for all expanded layers except Unincorporated Place and Unincorporated Place labels (leave these two selected).** ▶

5 **From the GIS Toolbox, click the Standard tab and the Zoom In button. If the toolbox is not displayed, click the Show Toolbox link at the top-right corner of the page.**

Zoom In button

6 **Zoom in on Pennsylvania and then Pittsburgh.**
Pittsburgh is at the western side of the state.

Governmental Unit Boundaries
- Labels
  - Reserve labels
  - Native American Area labels
  - County or Equivalent labels
  - Incorporated Place labels
  - Unincorporated Place labels
  - Minor Civil Division labels
  - Zip Code labels
  - School District labels
  - State or Territory (Low res) labels
  - State or Territory (High res) labels
  - 111th Congressional District labels
- Features
  - Reserve
  - Native American Area
  - County or Equivalent
  - Incorporated Place
  - Unincorporated Place
  - Minor Civil Division
  - Zip Code
  - School District
  - State or Territory (Low res)
  - State or Territory (High res)
  - 111th Congressional District

7 Use the Map Navigation button and other navigation tools to zoom in on downtown Pittsburgh and the North Shore, where Pittsburgh's three rivers meet.

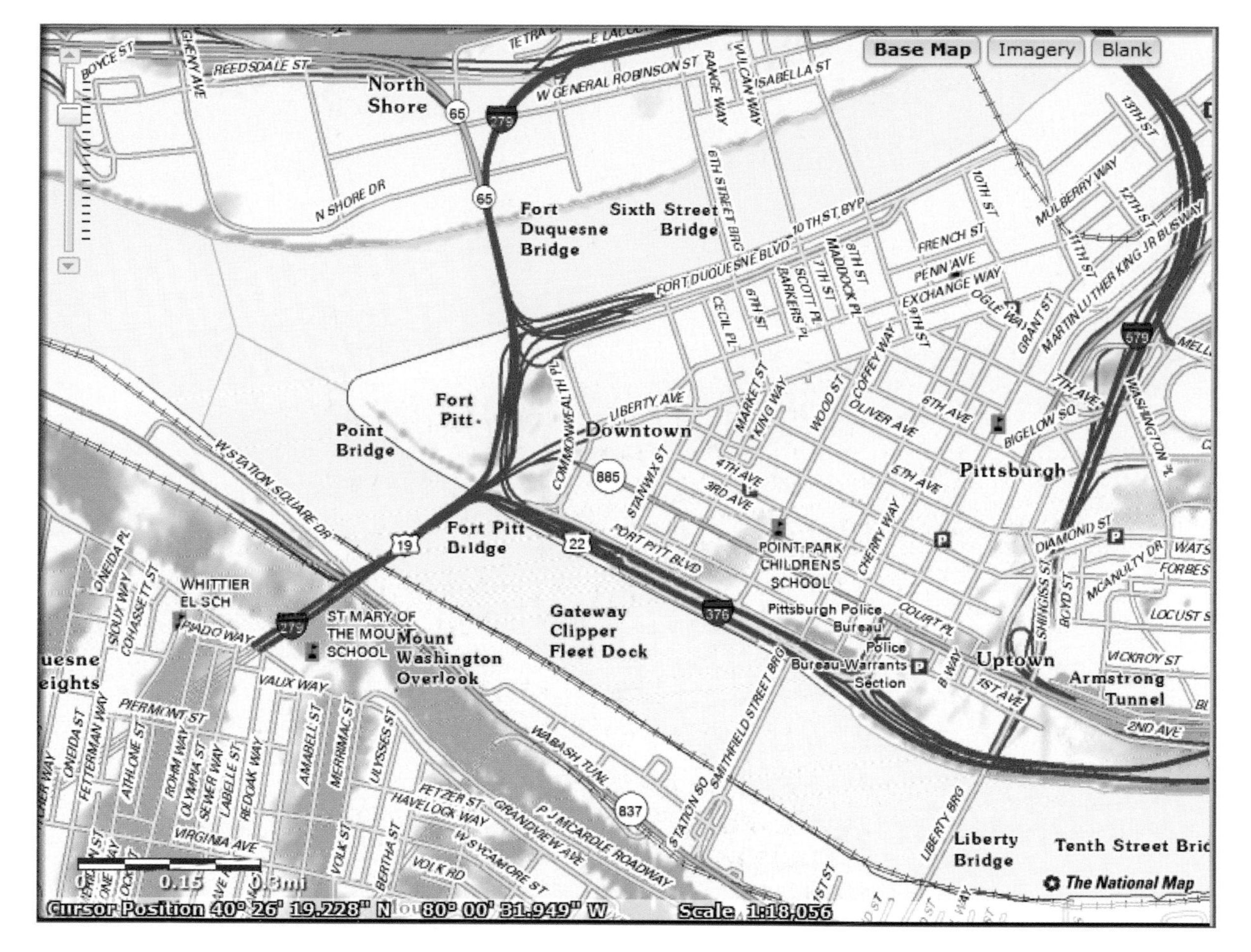

8 At the upper-right corner of the map, click the Imagery button Imagery to see an orthophoto. Make sure your map scale is on the order of 1:24,000 or more (for example, 1:20,000) so that the files you download are not too large. The scale is shown at the bottom of the map. Be sure to include Pittsburgh's football stadium (where the Pittsburgh Steelers play) and the baseball stadium as shown in the figure. (See next page.)

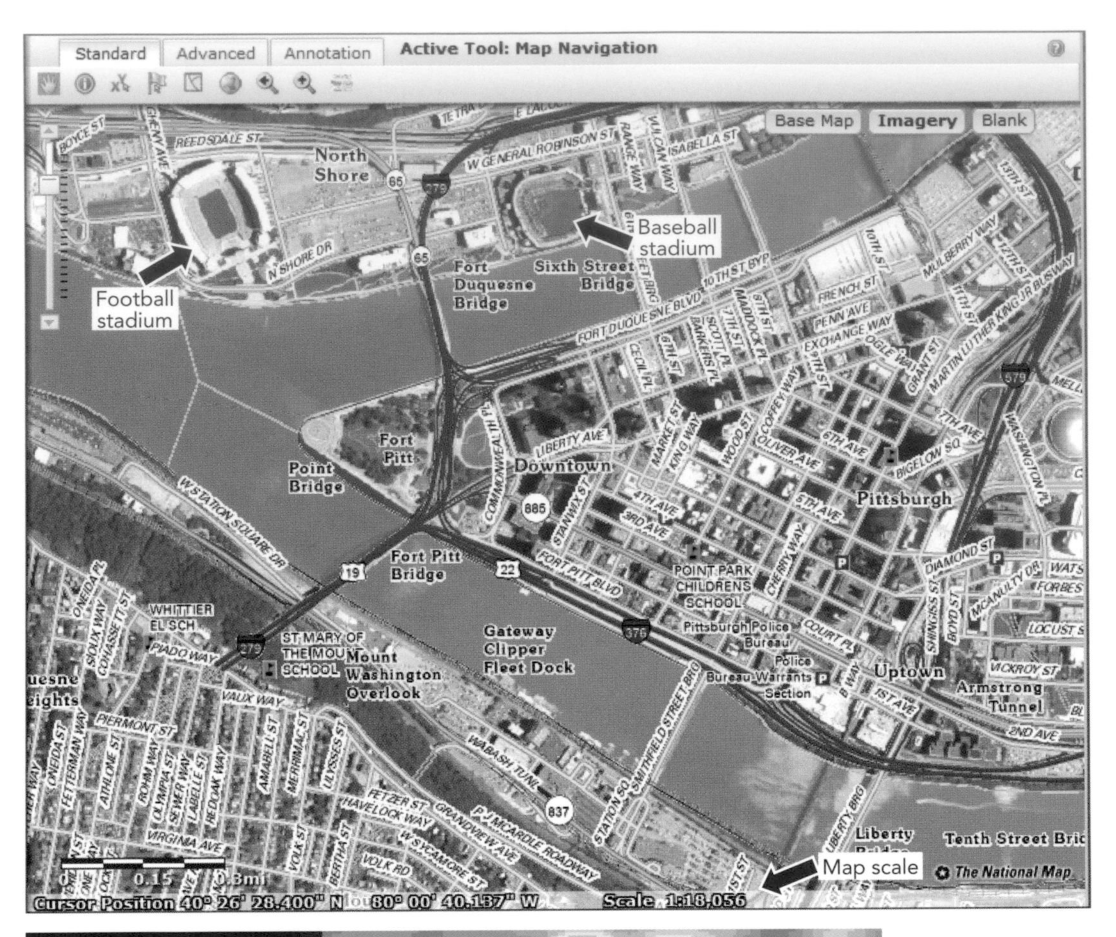

YOUR TURN

Experiment using different Base Data layers, turning them on and off. ***Hint:*** You may need to zoom in to see certain basemaps better. If you do, use the Zoom to Last Extent button to return to your Downtown Golden Triangle/North Shore extent.

Order data for download

There are several options to download data by geographic area. In this exercise, you will use the simplest, by current extent.

1 **Click the Download Data button Download Data .**

2 **In the "Download options" dialog box, click the "Click here" link to download by current map extent.** The default data type for vector maps is File Geodatabase 9.2, which works fine with ArcGIS 10.2.

3 **Select the Orthoimagery check box and click Next.**

4 Select Mar2006 Color Orthoimagery - Allegheny County, PA and click Next.

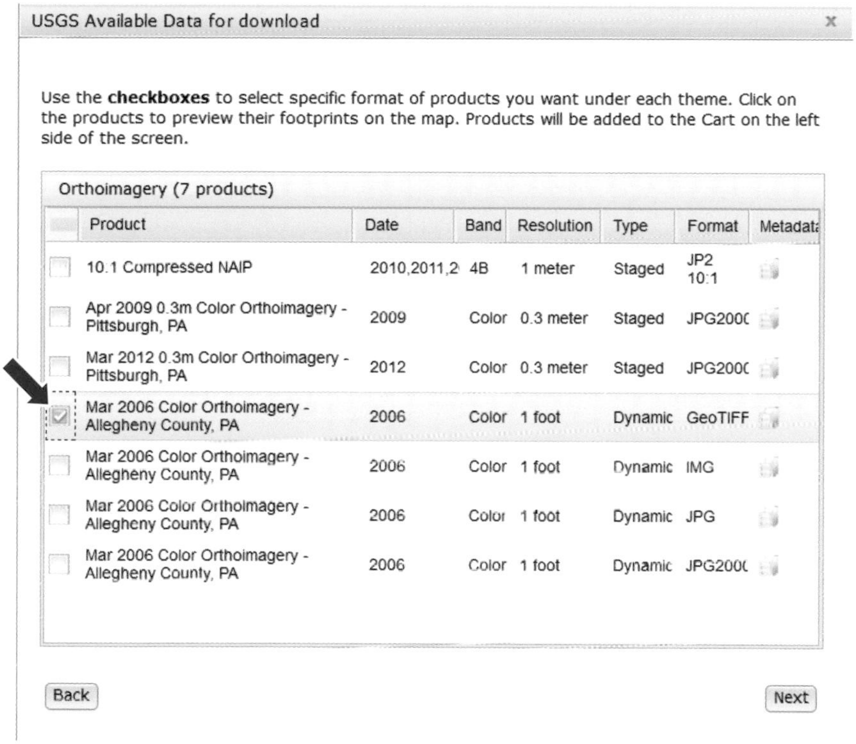

USGS Available Data for download

Use the **checkboxes** to select specific format of products you want under each theme. Click on the products to preview their footprints on the map. Products will be added to the Cart on the left side of the screen.

Orthoimagery (7 products)

	Product	Date	Band	Resolution	Type	Format	Metadata
☐	10:1 Compressed NAIP	2010,2011,2	4B	1 meter	Staged	JP2 10:1	
☐	Apr 2009 0.3m Color Orthoimagery - Pittsburgh, PA	2009	Color	0.3 meter	Staged	JPG2000	
☐	Mar 2012 0.3m Color Orthoimagery - Pittsburgh, PA	2012	Color	0.3 meter	Staged	JPG2000	
☑	Mar 2006 Color Orthoimagery - Allegheny County, PA	2006	Color	1 foot	Dynamic	GeoTIFF	
☐	Mar 2006 Color Orthoimagery - Allegheny County, PA	2006	Color	1 foot	Dynamic	IMG	
☐	Mar 2006 Color Orthoimagery - Allegheny County, PA	2006	Color	1 foot	Dynamic	JPG	
☐	Mar 2006 Color Orthoimagery - Allegheny County, PA	2006	Color	1 foot	Dynamic	JPG2000	

Back Next

5 Click the Checkout button.

6 Type your e-mail address twice and click the Place Order button.

You will get a message saying that your order has been placed and to check your e-mail. Later, you'll get an e-mail message summarizing your order and telling you that a link will arrive in the future, which you can use to download the order.

7 Click OK and close your browser.

Download data

At some point, you'll get an e-mail message containing a link to download the data. It is likely the data is large enough to be divided into multiple "chunks." Your message from the USGS will reflect this. If this is the case, you will download and extract the data one chunk at a time.

1 **Click the link in your e-mail to download the data.** You will see the following messages in succession: "Current order status . . . Adding your request to the queue. . . . Extracting data . . . The data extraction has completed. . . . Please wait for the data to be returned."

2 **Click Save File and save the downloaded file to the USGS folder in your Chapter4 folder in MyExercises.**

3 **In Windows Explorer, double-click the compressed file, click "Extract all files", browse through your Chapter4 folder to the USGS folder, and click OK. Then click Extract.** A folder that has a unique number is created, containing all the files that are needed to display the raster image properly in the correct projections.

4 **Use Windows Explorer to view these files. Close Windows Explorer when you are finished.**

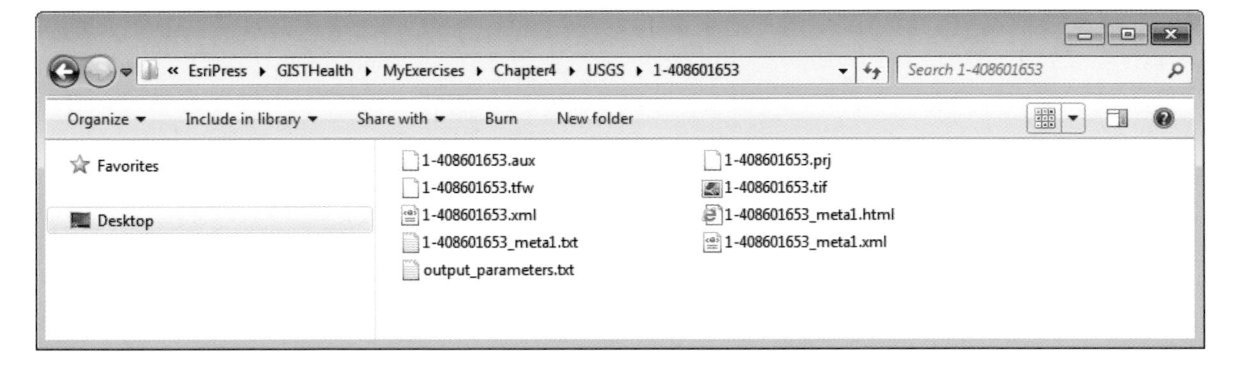

YOUR TURN

If your message from the USGS listed several "chunks," repeat steps 1–4 to download all the remaining files.

Import the raster image into the file geodatabase

In addition to vector files, you can also import raster images into a file geodatabase.

T 4-9

1 **Click the Catalog window button and browse to your Chapter4 folder.**

2 **Right-click Chapter4.gdb and click Import > Raster Datasets.**

3 **In the "Raster To Geodatabase (multiple)" dialog box, click the Browse button for Input Rasters, browse through your Chapter4 folder to the USGS folder, and double-click the first downloaded folder. Click the downloaded .tif file and click Add.** This step adds the TIFF image file to the input panel.

4 Browse to the remaining folders and add each remaining TIFF image file. Click OK. Be patient while the image files are imported.

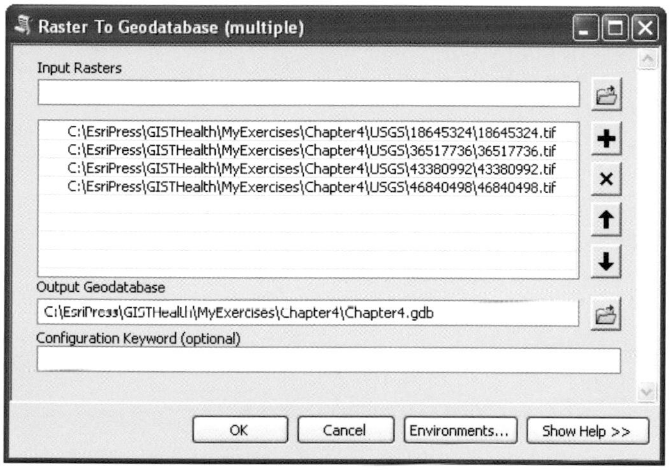

YOUR TURN

Browse through the file geodatabase and notice that ArcMap renamed each TIFF image file.

Add the raster image to the map

The orthophoto raster image you will add next has a spatial reference. So, when you add it to the map document and data frame, ArcMap reprojects it on the fly into state plane coordinates.

1 If necessary, start ArcMap and open Tutorial4-8YourName.mxd.

2 On the Standard toolbar, click Add Data, go to Chapter4.gdb, click the first TIFF image file, and click Add and then Yes if prompted. ArcMap creates raster pyramids for your file. Be patient during this process.

3 In the table of contents, right-click the new image layer and click Zoom To Layer.

4 In the table of contents, right-click the image layer, click Properties, and click the General tab.

5 In the Scale Range box, select the "Don't show layer when zoomed" option, click the "Out beyond" arrow, and click 1:24,000.

6 Click the Source tab, scroll down in the property panel, and observe that the image layer has state plane coordinates. Click OK to close the Properties window.

YOUR TURN

Add the remaining TIFF image files and zoom to the extent of all four. Create a spatial bookmark called **Golden Triangle/North Shore**. Turn off the Rivers layer. Zoom in on small areas to see more details in the orthophoto. Zoom back to the Golden Triangle/North Shore bookmark.

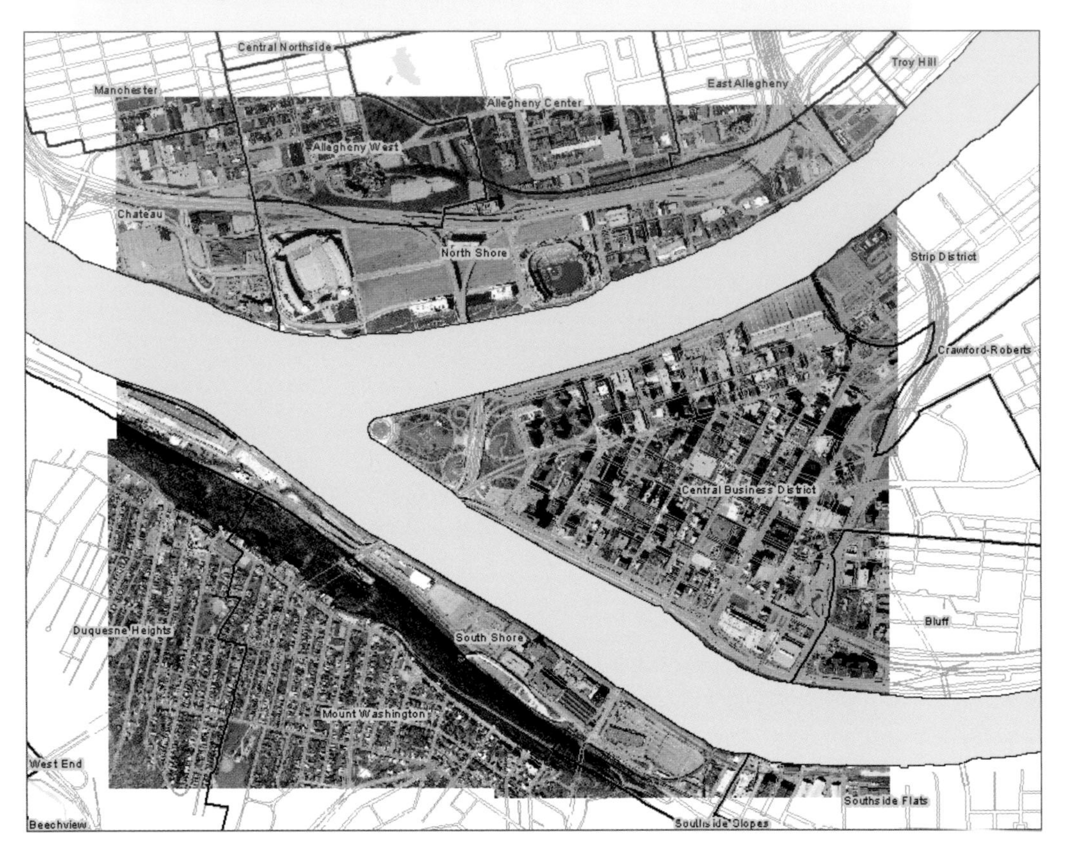

Save the map document

1. **On the File menu, click Save As.**

2. **Save your map document as** Tutorial4-9YourName.mxd **to your Chapter4 folder in MyExercises.** Do not close ArcMap.

YOUR TURN

On the USGS website, try downloading another USGS image from the Orthoimagery folder, NAIP (3 Band) UTM Zone 17N. This image file is much smaller than the orthophoto, but its quality is not as good.

Summary

Small-scale maps, such as those for countries using disease-related data, are best symbolized using size-graduated point markers. The corresponding maps you made for AIDS prevalence clearly depict the parts of the world that are most heavily affected by this disease. The more familiar alternative, the choropleth map, has distortions and creates mixed signals because of variations in the size of the polygons. Bigger polygons appear more important than smaller ones, whereas it is the color value of the polygon fill colors that should be used to communicate meaning.

Large-scale maps for health applications tend to correspond to detailed phenomena and programs, and consequently need to be more detailed. You assembled a map document for Pittsburgh and its neighborhoods that allows a GIS analyst working for a child obesity task force to identify parks and playground areas near schools that could be used for physical education programs. As is typical of large-scale GIS projects, you found that needed GIS layers are available, but from a variety of sources, in a variety of spatial data formats, and in a variety of different projections.

You saw that ArcGIS has all the tools and functionality necessary to handle downloading, importing, transforming, and projecting many types of useful map layers. In addition, you used ArcMap and ArcCatalog, through the Catalog window, to add spatial reference data to map layers and to the data frames that hold them. That way, ArcMap can project map layers on the fly from a mixture of projections to one common projection.

In summary, this chapter has furthered your ability to handle many of the problems that initially confront GIS analysts in real-world projects. You were able to overcome potential stumbling blocks by adding available spatial data into a map document and properly projecting it.

Assignment 4-1

Compare world infant mortality rates with life expectancy

According to the World Health Organization, approximately 10.5 million children under the age of 5 die every year, but great progress has been made since 1970 when this number was 17 million. The highest mortality rates are in developing countries, and almost half of children who die before age 5 live in Africa. A primary cause of these high child mortality rates is the HIV/AIDS epidemic. In this assignment, you will create maps showing infant mortality rates similar to the map you created comparing worldwide AIDS cases. Data was obtained from the US Census International Database (IDB) for the year 2005, and the infant mortality rate is defined as infant deaths per 1,000 live births.

Start with this data

- ***\EsriPress\GISTHealth\Data\World.gdb\Country:*** polygon feature class of world countries with infant mortality rates by country. ***Note:*** *Zero values indicate no data was available for that country.* Field definitions are as follows:
  - IM_Male: infant mortality rate, males
  - IM_Female: infant mortality rate, females
  - LE_Male: life expectancy, males
  - LE_Female: life expectancy, females
- ***\EsriPress\GISTHealth\Data\World.gdb\Ocean:*** graticule lines of constant latitude and longitude at 30-degree intervals

Create maps comparing infant mortality rates with life expectancy

Create a map document called **Assignment4-1YourName.mxd** and save it to your Chapter4 folder in MyAssignments, using relative paths. Use a layout that includes four choropleth maps comparing the following statistics:

- Infant mortality rates of males and females by country
- Life expectancy for males and females by country

Use your judgment as to the break points, color, size, title(s), projection, and so forth.

Export the map to a JPEG image file called **Assignment4-1YourName.jpg** and save it to your Chapter4 folder in MyAssignments.

WHAT TO TURN IN

If your work is to be graded, turn in the following files:

- ***ArcMap document:*** \EsriPress\GISTHealth\MyAssignments\Chapter4\Assignment4-1YourName.mxd
- ***Image file:*** \EsriPress\GISTHealth\MyAssignments\Chapter4\Assignment4-1YourName.jpg

If instructed to do so, instead of individual files, turn in a compressed file, ***Assignment4-1YourName.zip***, that includes all the preceding files. Do not include path information in the compressed file.

Assignment 4-2

Investigate education level and knowledge about HIV by country

Education and awareness about HIV and AIDS is important in the prevention of this disease. Organizations such as USAID, the World Health Organization, and the Centers for Disease Control and Prevention (CDC) have comprehensive strategies that include effective, sustained health education and health promotion programs. The goal of these programs is to reduce the risk of individuals becoming infected with HIV or, if already infected, infecting others. PEPFAR's HIV Spatial Data Repository is part of the effort to provide data for decision making and improve knowledge and understanding of the impact of HIV worldwide. In this assignment, you will compare the educational status and HIV knowledge of females in Indonesia.

Start with this data

- ***Download HIV GIS data for Indonesia:*** DHS 2007 from the HIV Spatial Data Repository website at http://hivspatialdata.net/ and click the Data link. Click Single Country, Indonesia, and the Download Detailed HIV Data link. Save the compressed file IDDHS2007.zip to \EsriPress\GISTHealth\MyAssignments\Chapter4.
- ***\EsriPress\GISTHealth\Data\World.gdb\Ocean:*** graticule lines of constant latitude and longitude at 30-degree intervals.

Create a file geodatabase

Create a file geodatabase called **Assignment4-2YourName.gdb** and save it to your Chapter4 folder in MyAssignments. Import the IDDHS2007 shapefile extracted from IDDHS2007.ZIP into your file geodatabase. Use the Excel spreadsheet to identify the fields used next to create a choropleth and graduated point marker map.

Create a map comparing female education and HIV knowledge

Create a map document called **Assignment4-2YourName.mxd** and save it to your Chapter4 folder in MyAssignments, using relative paths. Include an 11 x 8½ in. landscape layout that has one map including the following:

- A choropleth map layer showing the percentage of ever-married females (age 15–49) who have no education
- A graduated point marker map layer showing the percentage of ever-married females (age 15–49) who have a comprehensive, correct knowledge of AIDS

Use your judgment as to the break points, color, size, title(s), projection, and so forth.

Export the map to a JPEG image file called **Assignment4-2YourName.jpg** and save it to your Chapter4 folder in MyAssignments.

WHAT TO TURN IN

If your work is to be graded, turn in the following files:

- ***File geodatabase:*** \EsriPress\GISTHealth\MyAssignments\Chapter4\Assignment4-2YourName.gdb
- ***ArcMap document:*** \EsriPress\GISTHealth\MyAssignments\Chapter4\Assignment4-2YourName.mxd
- ***Image file:*** \EsriPress\GISTHealth\MyAssignments\Chapter4\Assignment4-2YourName.jpg

If instructed to do so, instead of individual files, turn in a compressed file, **Assignment4-2YourName.zip**, that includes all the preceding files. Do not include path information in the compressed file.

Assignment 4-3
Compare the walkability of neighborhoods

A recent study conducted in San Diego and published in the *American Journal of Public Health* (Saelens et al. 2003) identified 60 percent obesity rates in low-density, unwalkable neighborhoods as compared with 35 percent in walkable neighborhoods. The CDC has determined that obesity is lowest in countries and neighborhoods that allow significant walking and biking. GIS can be used to determine what makes a neighborhood more walkable than others. Layers might include neighborhood amenities such as parks and playgrounds, sidewalk conditions, and public safety. In this assignment, you will compare two Pittsburgh neighborhoods at the same scale. These neighborhoods have a high percentage of children under the age of 18. You will use both vector files and aerial imagery to determine which neighborhood is more "walkable."

Start with this data

- ***\EsriPress\GISTHealth\Data\Pittsburgh.gdb\Buildings:*** polygon feature class of Pittsburgh buildings
- ***\EsriPress\GISTHealth\Data\Pittsburgh.gdb\Neighborhoods:*** polygon feature class of Pittsburgh neighborhoods
- ***\EsriPress\GISTHealth\Data\Pittsburgh.gdb\Playgrounds:*** polyline feature class of Pittsburgh playgrounds (***Note:*** missing a projection file—you must assign this)
- ***\EsriPress\GISTHealth\Data\Pittsburgh.gdb\Sidewalks:*** polyline feature class of Pittsburgh curbs
- ***\EsriPress\GISTHealth\Data\Pittsburgh.gdb\StreetsCL:*** polyline feature class of Pittsburgh streets
  Note: *The preceding data was obtained from the City of Pittsburgh, Department of City Planning (2011).*
- From the USGS server, download and add an aerial orthophoto that is zoomed to the area surrounding the playground called Fort Pitt in the Garfield neighborhood. Save the downloaded image to your file geodatabase.

Create a file geodatabase

Create a file geodatabase called **Assignment4-3YourName.gdb** and save it to your Chapter4 folder in MyAssignments. Export the preceding layers from Pittsburgh.gdb and import them into Assignment4-3YourName.gdb.

Create large-scale neighborhood maps

Create a map document called **Assignment4-3YourName.mxd** and save it to your Chapter4 folder in MyAssignments, using relative paths. Use a 17 x 11 in. landscape layout and include the following:

- Three data frames, approximately 5 x 5 in. each, that have the preceding layers added. Label the neighborhoods using a bright halo label. For the street centerlines, show the lines using no color (making them invisible) but labeled by name. For the neighborhoods, use a Hollow symbol and a black outline width of 2. Use your judgment for the symbology of the other layers.
- In one of the data frames, select and zoom to the Pittsburgh neighborhood of Garfield. In another data frame, select and zoom to the neighborhood of Northview Heights. Use a bright color and thick outline for the selection to draw the focus to these neighborhoods. Make the scale of these data frames 1:14,000.
- In the third data frame, zoom to the Fort Pitt playground in Garfield using a scale of 1:2,000. Label the playground names. Add the aerial image from the USGS server that is zoomed to the area around this playground.
- Add other map layout elements that you think are necessary.

Hints

- *To export files from Pittsburgh.gdb, in the Catalog window right-click each feature class in Pittsburgh.gdb and select Export > To Geodatabase (single). Make sure the Output Location is \EsriPress\GISTHealth\MyAssignments\Chapter4\Assignment4-3YourName.gdb.*
- *Assign projection NAD_1983_StatePlane_Pennsylvania_South_FIPS_3702_Feet to the Playgrounds layer. Import the aerial raster image downloaded from the USGS website.*
- *When downloading the aerial orthophoto, include only the area surrounding the Fort Pitt playground. Use the street names in the GIS map and USGS server to determine the area around the park to download from the USGS website.*

Export your map to a JPEG image file called **Assignment4-3YourName.jpg** and save it to your Chapter4 folder in MyAssignments.

WHAT TO TURN IN

If your work is to be graded, turn in the following files:

- ***File geodatabase:*** \EsriPress\GISTHealth\MyAssignments\Chapter4\Assignment4-3YourName.gdb
- ***ArcMap document:*** \EsriPress\GISTHealth\MyAssignments\Chapter4\Assignment4-3YourName.mxd
- ***Image file:*** \EsriPress\GISTHealth\MyAssignments\Chapter4\Assignment4-3YourName.jpg

If instructed to do so, instead of individual files, turn in a compressed file, **Assignment4-3YourName.zip**, that includes all the preceding files. Do not include path information in the compressed file.

Reference

Saelens, B. E., J. F. Sallis, J. B. Black, and D. Chen. 2003. "Neighborhood-Based Differences in Physical Activity: An Environment Scale Evaluation." *American Journal of Public Health* 92, no. 9: 1552, doi:10.2105/AJPH.93.9.1552.

Chapter 5

Downloading and preparing spatial and tabular data

Objectives

- Download US Census Bureau TIGER/Line map files
- Identify and download data from US Census Bureau data tables
- Prepare census tables for use in mapping
- Join tabular data to boundary map layers
- Create a geodatabase for integration of data
- Build a map for analysis of elevated blood lead levels in children

Health-care scenario

A program manager for the lead hazard program in a county health department wants to create a map to show local pediatricians how lead may be affecting children. He wants a map that shows locations of homes that were built before 1978—when lead was still used in paint—and the number of children who have elevated blood lead levels (BLLs). He can then focus on problem neighborhoods and set up meetings with physicians in those areas to make them aware of populations that are at risk of lead poisoning. He recommends that such populations be screened more carefully.

Solution approach

As the GIS analyst, you need to work with both internally and externally obtained spatial data for this project. The health department has the internal data—a sample of residences in 2005 showing elevated BLLs in children. As explained later in this section, you will also need external data: two basemap layers and corresponding data tables from the US Census Bureau. Chapter 6 covers the geocoding steps needed to produce a map layer from the sample of residential addresses, so you won't have to do geocoding in this chapter. The internal data is already geocoded and your work focuses on the data from the US Census Bureau.

The desired final map is easy enough to design and produce, but as is often the case, you will need to do a lot of preliminary work downloading basemaps and preparing the data for use in ArcMap.

Introduction to US Census Bureau data

Many spatial data sources provide downloading over the Internet. The US Census Bureau maintains a web-based source that can meet many health-related needs. The US Census is a source of major data collections at no cost to users.

The US Census map layers are called TIGER (Topologically Integrated Geographic Encoding and Referencing) files and are available to download at various geographic levels, including state, county, place, tract, block group, and block. Because some of these boundaries, such as tracts and block groups, change over time, these files are available for different years.

Through the year 2000, the US Census Bureau used tabular data called Summary Files. Summary File 1 (SF 1), from the short-form census, is compiled from the questions asked of the total population about every housing unit. Summary File 3 (SF 3), from the long-form census, includes sample data based on questions asked of approximately one household in six, covering income, education, occupation, and mode of travel to work.

In 2005, the US Census Bureau launched a project called the American Community Survey (ACS) that surveys a small sample of housing units in each county, each month. Approximately 3 million housing units receive a survey similar to the old SF 3 long form. Annual or semiannual estimates produced from ACS samples are available at the census tract level and replaced the SF 3 data product starting with Census 2010 data. To learn more about the American Community Survey, visit the website at http://www.census.gov/acs/www/.

For the case at hand, the US Census Bureau provides the needed housing data—namely, the median year structures were built—in the year 2000 SF 3 collection. Because you are interested in housing built before 1978, census data from the year 2000 is sufficient. Census tracts provide a natural unit of analysis, because they are homogeneous neighborhoods of around 4,000 people, so you will download both Census 2000 tract boundaries and the 2000 SF 3 housing data.

To study the current population under age 18, you will use the more recent Census 2010 data. This will require you to download the 2010 tracts and 2010 population data.

The US Census Bureau cannot have the census tabular data already prepared and joined to maps because there are simply too many census variables—over 16,000 of them! Corresponding map files would be too large and cumbersome, if not impossible, to use. Instead, you can join selected census tract data to the attribute table of a census tract map. ArcMap allows you to join data tables if they share a common identifier attribute.

Working with data tables

A data table has a specific format and structure. It is rectangular and is made up of rows of data records that include columns of attributes, which are identifiers or characteristics of data entities. Of course, the data entities in GIS are geographic in nature, such as census tract areas, street centerlines, residences, and so forth. Each column lists data for a single attribute. If viewed in a spreadsheet, the first row of data contains attribute names, and all additional rows contain attribute data. There are no summary rows such as column totals. As you will see, the first two rows in census data tables are identifier, nondata rows. The first row contains cryptic attribute names and the second row carries descriptions of the attributes, providing a built-in data dictionary that defines the attributes. Although convenient, this format is not in a table format that ArcGIS or any other database software package can process. To use it, you will have to "clean" Census Bureau data tables by replacing cryptic names with self-documenting names and deleting the descriptive second row. Then the table will be ready for use in ArcGIS.

At least one attribute of a data table must have a unique, non null identifier value for each row. In database terminology, this is the table's primary key. For example, census tracts have a composite code that is unique across the entire United States and US territories. This code is a composite of state, county, and tract identifying (ID) numbers. In the composite code 42003010300, for example, 42 is the code for Pennsylvania, 003 is the code for Allegheny County, and 010300 is a tract ID number. The county code and tract ID repeat in other states, but as a composite used with the state code, the composite code for each tract is unique. You will use the composite codes for tracts in the lead study. These codes are different for the years 2000 and 2010—hence, you must download both the TIGER layer and the data table for each of these two years.

Overall steps to take

To get the census mapped, you will follow this approach:

1. Download the data.
2. Clean up the data.
3. Place project datasets in a file geodatabase.
4. Join datasets.
5. Create maps.

Once you have completed all the data preparation work, you will create a choropleth map by tract for the housing data, a dot-density map layer for elevated blood lead levels, and a choropleth map showing the percentage of children who have elevated BLLs. A dot-density map is an alternative to using a choropleth map and uses a random distribution of points within polygons to represent the magnitude of an attribute—the more points in a polygon, the larger the magnitude of an attribute.

Tutorial 5-1
Downloading spatial data from the US Census Bureau

You can download census-related map layers that have unique identifiers for polygons such as census tract IDs, but they do not include census attribute data such as population, age, sex, race, income, and so on. You'll need to download the census demographic data separately, from the bureau's American Fact Finder website; do some data preparation; and then join the data to the corresponding map layer.

Download TIGER/Line shapefiles

The end results of this tutorial are downloaded shapefiles. Because Internet sites change often, some of the screen captures that follow may look different from what you find on the website. If you have difficulty downloading the Census TIGER shapefiles, they are available in the Chapter5 folder in FinishedExercises.

1. **From Internet Explorer or another web browser, go to** http://www.census.gov/geo/maps-data/data/tiger.html

2. **On the resulting TIGER Products page, click the TIGER/Line Shapefiles - New 2013 Shapefiles link then the 2010 tab.** The TIGER/LINE Shapefiles link name may vary slightly based on recently uploaded TIGER shapefiles.

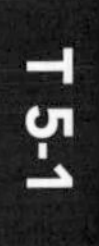

3 Click the Download link under 2010 TIGER/Line Shapefiles.

2013 | 113th CD | 2012 | 2011 | 2010 | 2009 | 2008 | 2007 | 2006SE | Census 2000 | 1992

2010 TIGER/Line Shapefiles

All legal boundaries and names are as of January 1, 2010. Released beginning November 30, 2010. Last update March 26, 2012.

Download

Download by File Type

Web Interface

FTP Site

Download by State

FTP Site

Technical Documentation

File Availability

Special Release - Census Blocks with Population and Housing Unit Counts

User Notes

4 On the 2010 TIGER/Line Shapefiles page under "Download," select Web interface, then under "Select a layer type," click Census Tracts, and then click "submit".

5 Under Census Tract (2010), click Pennsylvania for state, and then click Submit.

6 Click Allegheny County for county, and then click Download.

7 Save the file to your Chapter5 folder in MyExercises and use a compression program to extract all the associated files for the tl_2010_42003_tract10 shapefile to the same folder.

YOUR TURN

Download and extract the tl_2010_42003_tract00 (year 2000) census tract shapefile and the tl_2010_42003_cousub10 (year 2010) county subdivisions shapefile to your Chapter5 folder in MyExercises. You will use these shapefiles in an upcoming tutorial. The county subdivisions will help the director of the lead level program to identify what municipalities have the most cases of children with high blood lead levels.

Tutorial 5-2
Downloading tabular data from American FactFinder

The US Census Bureau American FactFinder website is a good example of a source that provides tabular data including geocodes. In this tutorial, you will download a table that has selected Census 2010 population variables for Allegheny County, Pennsylvania; process them in a spreadsheet; and then join them to the 2010 tract map layer for display. If you have difficulty downloading the file in this exercise, a backup copy called dec_10_PL_QTPL.zip is available in the Chapter5 folder in FinishedExercises.

Download 2010 population data

1 **Using your web browser, go to http://factfinder2.census.gov and click the Advanced Search tab.** This website includes data from both Census 2010 and Census 2000 and lets you build selections to download data about a specific topic tied to a specific geographic location. At the time of this publication, the 2010 SF 1 population data was not yet released, so 2010 Redistricting Data SF (PL 94-171) is used.

2 **On the left navigation bar, click Geographies.**

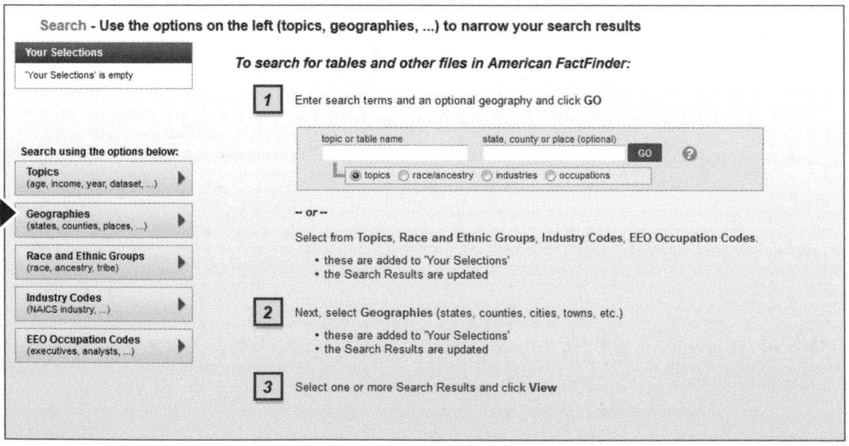

3 **In the Select Geographies Page click on the Name tab. In the "Enter a geography name" text box, type** Pennsylvania**, click Allegheny County, Pennsylvania, and click Go.** ▶

4 **In the Geography Filter Options pane for Geographic Type, click Census Tract (601).** ▶

5 **In the Geography Results pane, select the check box for All Census Tracts within Allegheny County, Pennsylvania, and click Add.** ▶

6 **Close the Select Geographies page.** Your Selections, detailing what you selected, should be indicated in the upper-left corner of the home page as shown in the figure. The search results will display data that is available at the census tract level. ▶

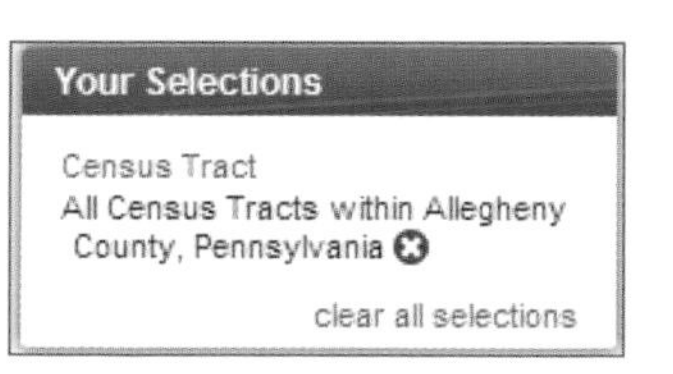

7 **In the Search Results page, search for table QT-PL and then select the check box for QT-PL: Race, Hispanic or Latino, Age, and Housing Occupancy: 2010.** This dataset is the 2010 Redistricting Data SF (PL 94-171).

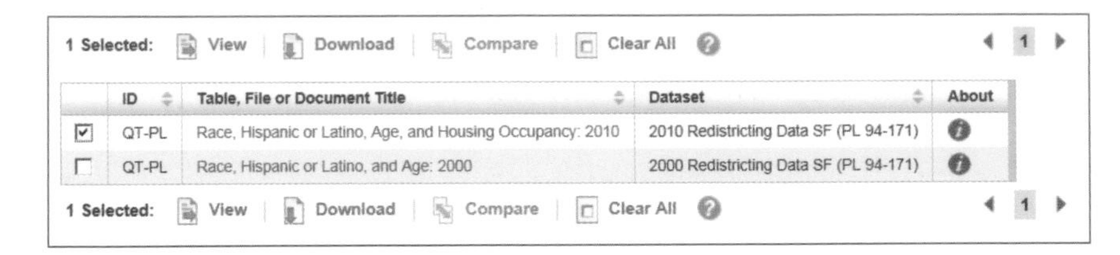

1 Selected: View | Download | Compare | Clear All

	ID	Table, File or Document Title	Dataset	About
☑	QT-PL	Race, Hispanic or Latino, Age, and Housing Occupancy: 2010	2010 Redistricting Data SF (PL 94-171)	
☐	QT-PL	Race, Hispanic or Latino, and Age: 2000	2000 Redistricting Data SF (PL 94-171)	

1 Selected: View | Download | Compare | Clear All

8 **In the Search Results page, click the View button** View **to see the data included in the table.**

Subject	Total		18 years and over	
	Number	Percent	Number	Percent
POPULATION				
Total population	6,600	100.0	6,473	100.0
RACE				
One race	6,513	98.7	6,397	98.8
White	4,345	65.8	4,318	66.7
Black or African American	2,057	31.2	1,971	30.4
American Indian and Alaska Native	13	0.2	13	0.2
Asian	73	1.1	72	1.1
Native Hawaiian and Other Pacific Islander	2	0.0	2	0.0
Some Other Race	23	0.3	21	0.3
Two or More Races	87	1.3	76	1.2
HISPANIC OR LATINO AND RACE				
Hispanic or Latino (of any race)	161	2.4	156	2.4
Not Hispanic or Latino	6,439	97.6	6,317	97.6
One race	6,362	96.4	6,249	96.5
White	4,260	64.5	4,235	65.4
Black or African American	2,004	30.4	1,918	29.6
American Indian and Alaska Native	12	0.2	12	0.2
Asian	72	1.1	71	1.1
Native Hawaiian and Other Pacific Islander	2	0.0	2	0.0
Some Other Race	12	0.2	11	0.2
Two or More Races	77	1.2	68	1.1
HOUSING UNITS				
Total housing units	388	100.0		
OCCUPANCY STATUS				
Occupied housing units	282	72.7		
Vacant housing units	106	27.3		

9 **In the upper-right corner of the Results Page, click Back to Advanced Search.**

10 **Click the Download button Download , click OK, wait for the ZIP file to be created, and click Download again. Save the compressed file to your Chapter5 folder in MyExercises and use a compression program to extract all the associated files to the same folder.** The resulting files include a README text file (readme.txt), two CSV (comma separated value) files, and a text file (.txt) of the data. You will edit this data in Microsoft Excel in an upcoming exercise.

Download 2000 housing data

Health officials are interested in areas of a city that have housing units built before 1978. This is the year when highly toxic lead-based paint was banned. According to the Centers for Disease Control and Prevention, lead remains in about 24 million housing units, many of which are older homes. Data for the median year houses were built can be downloaded from the US Census Bureau American FactFinder website. Because you are interested in older houses, this data can be downloaded using the 2000 census tables. If you have difficulty downloading the file in this exercise, a backup copy called dec_00_SF3_H035.zip is available in the Chapter5 folder in FinishedExercises.

1 **If you are not already there, go to** http://factfinder2.census.gov and click Advanced Search.

2 **If it is not already in Your Selections, click Geographies, and then click All Census Tracts within Allegheny County, Pennsylvania. Click Add. Remove table QT-PL from the selection.**

3 **On the left navigation bar, click Topics (if its pane is closed) and click the plus sign (+) for Housing and then for Physical Characteristic.**

4 **Click Year Structure Built.** The search results change to show only the datasets that have data about when housing units were built. At the time of this publication, data was only available for the year 2000 so your numbers might differ from the screen capture in the book.

5 **Close the Select Topics window and type** H035 **in the topic or table search box.**

6 **In the ID column, select the check box for H035: MEDIAN YEAR STRUCTURE BUILT and click the View button.** The resulting table shows each census tract and the median year structures were built. Note that housing units built before 1941 are displayed as "1940-".

«‹ 1 - 18 of 416 ›»

	Census Tract 103, Allegheny County, Pennsylvania	Census Tract 201, Allegheny County, Pennsylvania	Census Tract 203, Allegheny County, Pennsylvania	Census Tract 305, Allegheny County, Pennsylvania	Census Tract 402, Allegheny County, Pennsylvania	Census Tract 403, Allegheny County, Pennsylvania
Median year structure built	1940-	1,960	1940-	1,979	1,945	1940-

7 **Click Back to Advanced Search.**

8 **Click the Download button, click OK, and click Download again. Save the compressed file to your Chapter5 folder in MyExercises and use a compression program to extract all the associated files to the same folder.**

You will edit this data in a spreadsheet in an upcoming exercise.

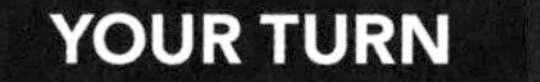

YOUR TURN

Explore other datasets that are available on the American FactFinder and American Community Survey websites. Files are periodically updated, so be sure to check back often. Close the websites when you are finished.

Tutorial 5-3
Processing tabular data

Many downloaded files contain unnecessary text or text that needs to be edited. In this tutorial, you will do some cleanup work using Microsoft Excel. If you have difficulty in this section, a copy of the finished product called Tracts2010.xlsx is available in the Chapter5 folder in FinishedExercises.

Open and clean population data using Microsoft Excel

1 **Start Microsoft Excel.**

2 **Click the File > Open.**

3 **Click the "Files of type" arrow and click All Files (*.*).**

4 **Browse for your Chapter5 folder, click DEC_10_PL_QTPL_with_ann.csv, and click Open.**

5 **Click in the cells to rename each of the following: B(Geo.id2) to** GEOID10, **D (SUBHD0101_S01) to** TOT_POP, **F (SUBHD0201_S01) to** POP_OVR18, **CB (SUBHD0101_S20) to** TOT_HOUSING, **CD (SUBHD0101_S21) to** OCCUPIED, **and CF (SUBHD0101_S22) to** VACANT.

6 **Delete all other columns.**

The resulting spreadsheet should contain 403 rows and six columns, which you will rename in the next exercise. The first population column is the total population and the second population column is the population over age 18.

The first column of the spreadsheet (GEOID10) is the one you will join to census tract polygons. ▶

	A	B	C	D	E	F
1	GEOID10	TOT_POP	POP_OVR18	TOT_HOUSING	OCCUPIED	VACANT
2	42003010300	6600	6473	388	282	106
3	42003020100	3629	3561	2342	1906	436
4	42003020300	616	567	473	403	70
5	42003030500	2256	1793	1270	1154	116
6	42003040200	2604	2369	687	594	93

Change the identifier data type to text

The final problem is that the tract identifier in the tracts TIGER layer you downloaded has a data type of text, although the matching GEOID10 column in the Microsoft Excel spreadsheet has a numeric data type. Text cells in Excel have a prefix character of a single quotation mark that is generally not visible but is there nonetheless. So you will add a single quotation mark to each GEOID10 value to make it a text value.

1 Click the A column selector cell to select that column.

2 On the Home ribbon in Excel, click the Find & Select button and click Replace.

3 Type values as shown in the figure (note the single quotation mark in the "Replace with" text box). ▶

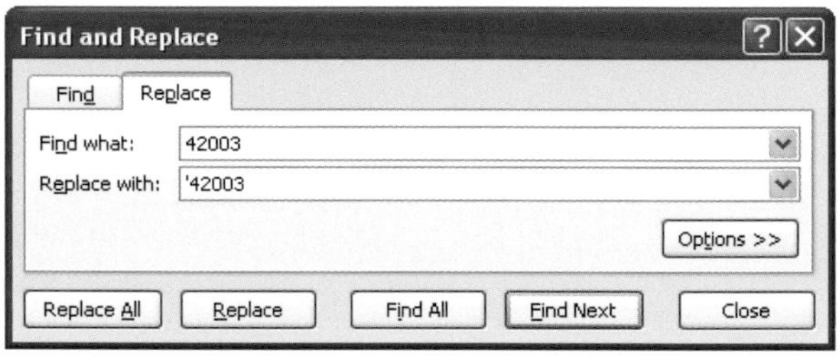

Find and Replace

Find | Replace

Find what: 42003

Replace with: '42003

Options >>

Replace All | Replace | Find All | Find Next | Close

4 Click Replace All. All cells get a note, indicated by a small green triangle, that numbers are stored as text.

5 At the bottom of the spreadsheet, double-click the lower-left tab that has the text DEC_10_PL_QTPL, and type Tracts2010 **to rename the tab.**

	A	B	C	D	E	F
1	GEOID10	TOT_POP	POP_OVR18	TOT_HOUSING	OCCUPIED	VACANT
2	42003010300	6600	6473	388	282	106
3	42003020100	3629	3561	2342	1906	436
4	42003020300	616	567	473	403	70
5	42003030500	2256	1793	1270	1154	116
6	42003040200	2604	2369	687	594	93
7	42003040400	2488	2467	1480	1369	111
8	42003040500	3694	3660	1379	1300	79

Tracts2010

Now you have stripped the table to only the data you need. One more column is needed for the study—a column that calculates the population under age 18. This can be done by subtracting the population over age 18 from the total population. Although this can be done in Microsoft Excel, you will do this calculation in ArcMap to avoid having a column that contains an Excel calculation and also to gain practice creating and calculating columns in ArcMap.

Save the spreadsheet as a Microsoft Excel file

1 **Click File and click Save As. Change "Save as type" to Excel Workbook and save your spreadsheet as** Tracts2010.xlsx **to your Chapter5 folder in MyExercises.**

YOUR TURN

Open the CSV file called DEC_00_SF3_H035_with_ann.csv, which has the median year houses were built. Delete columns A and C. Add a single quotation mark to each ID value in column A. Rename column A 'Id' and column B 'Median year structure built.'

Many cells in the new column B have 1940-values. These are homes that were built before 1940. Replace these values with the value **1939**. This step is necessary to create a choropleth map that has a range of years when houses were built (choropleth maps using quantities must have numeric values). Change the name of the worksheet to **Tracts2000**.

Save your spreadsheet as **Excel Workbook, Tracts2000.xlsx** to your Chapter5 folder in MyExercises. If you have trouble completing this task, a copy is available in the Chapter5 folder in FinishedExercises. Close Microsoft Excel when you are finished.

	A	B	C	D	E
1	Id	Median year structure built			
2	42003010300	1939			
3	42003020100	1960			
4	42003020300	1939			
5	42003030500	1979			
6	42003040200	1945			
7	42003040300	1939			
8	42003040400	1953			

Tracts2000

Tutorial 5-4
Using ArcCatalog utilities

In this tutorial, you will use ArcCatalog to build and maintain a file geodatabase. After you create a file geodatabase, you can start using ArcCatalog utilities.

Open ArcCatalog

1 On the taskbar, click Start, and then click All Programs > ArcGIS > ArcCatalog 10.2.

2 On the ArcCatalog toolbar, click the Connect To Folder button, expand the folder and file tree for EsriPress, click the GISTHealth folder icon to select it, and click OK.

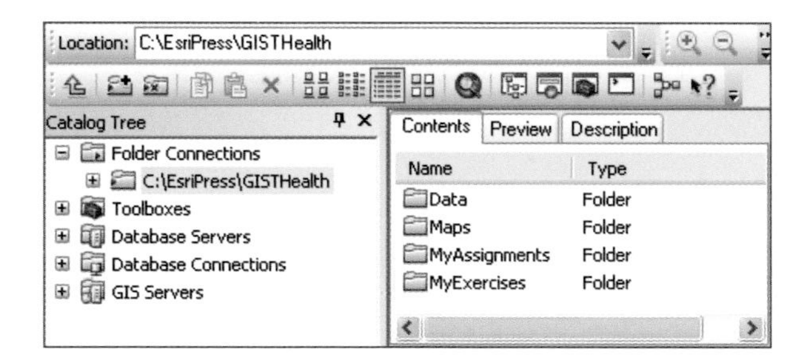

Create a file geodatabase

To create a file geodatabase, you must use ArcCatalog or Catalog. Windows Explorer and My Computer do not have the capability to build all the parts needed for a file geodatabase.

1 In the Catalog Tree panel, expand the MyExercises folder for GISTHealth.

2 Click the Chapter5 folder to display its contents in the right panel of ArcCatalog.

3 In the Catalog Tree panel, right-click the Chapter5 folder and click New > File Geodatabase.

4 **Change the name from New File Geodatabase.gdb to** Chapter5.gdb.

ArcCatalog creates a file geodatabase that you can now populate with feature classes and stand-alone tables. Feature classes are the map layers stored in a geodatabase. In the next exercise, you will import map layers into your new file geodatabase.

Import shapefiles

1 **In the right panel of ArcCatalog, right-click Chapter5.gdb and click Import > Feature Class (multiple).** The multiple import option allows you to import several features at the same time.

2 **In the Feature Class to Geodatabase (multiple) dialog box, click the Browse button for Input Features, double-click your Chapter5 folder to open it, and select tl_2010_42003_cousub10.shp, tl_2010_42003_tract00.shp, and tl_2010_42003_tract10.shp. Click Add.** The shapefiles are added to the input panel.

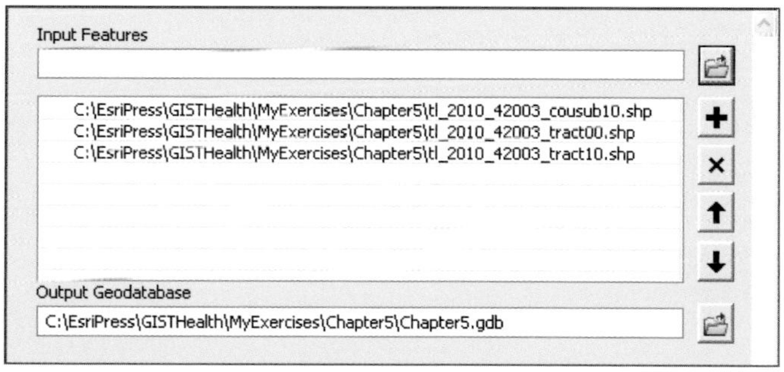

Input Features
C:\EsriPress\GISTHealth\MyExercises\Chapter5\tl_2010_42003_cousub10.shp
C:\EsriPress\GISTHealth\MyExercises\Chapter5\tl_2010_42003_tract00.shp
C:\EsriPress\GISTHealth\MyExercises\Chapter5\tl_2010_42003_tract10.shp
Output Geodatabase
C:\EsriPress\GISTHealth\MyExercises\Chapter5\Chapter5.gdb

3 **Click OK.** Wait while ArcCatalog imports the shapefiles into the file geodatabase.

Import data tables

In this exercise, you will import the census spreadsheets you downloaded from American FactFinder at the tract level.

1 **Right-click Chapter5.gdb and click Import > Table (single).**

2 **In the Table to Table dialog box, click the Browse button for Input Rows, browse through the Chapter 5 folder, click Tracts2000.xls > Tracts2000$, and click Add twice.**

3 **In the Output Table box, type** TractsData2000.

T 5-4

4 Click OK. ▶

Input Rows
C:\EsriPress\GISTHealth\MyExercises\Chapter5\Tracts2000.xlsx\Tracts2000$
Output Location
C:\EsriPress\GISTHealth\MyExercises\Chapter5\Chapter5.gdb
Output Table
TractsData2000
Expression (optional)
Field Map (optional)
Id (Text)
Median_year_structure_built (Double)

YOUR TURN

Import the Tracts2010$ worksheet from the Tracts2010 spreadsheet, naming the output table **TractsData2010**.

Rename features

Because a file geodatabase has a special file format, ArcCatalog is needed for many of the file management tasks, such as renaming and copying items.

1 **In the Catalog Tree panel, expand Chapter5.gdb, right-click tl_2010_42003_cousub10, click Rename, and type** CountySubdivisions2010.

2 **Repeat step 1 to rename tl_2010_42003_tract00 to** CensusTracts2000 **and tl_2010_42003_tract10 to** CensusTracts2010. Your resulting geodatabase will include the five files shown in the figure—three polygon feature classes and two data tables. ▶

Chapter5
Chapter5.gdb
CensusTracts2000
CensusTracts2010
CountySubdivisions2010
TractsData2000
TractsData2010

Copy and delete features

1 **In the Catalog tree, expand Chapter5.gdb, right-click CountySubdivisions2010, and click Copy. Then right-click Chapter5.gdb and click Paste. Click OK.** ArcCatalog creates a copy of the polygon feature class, CountySubdivisions2010_1. ▶

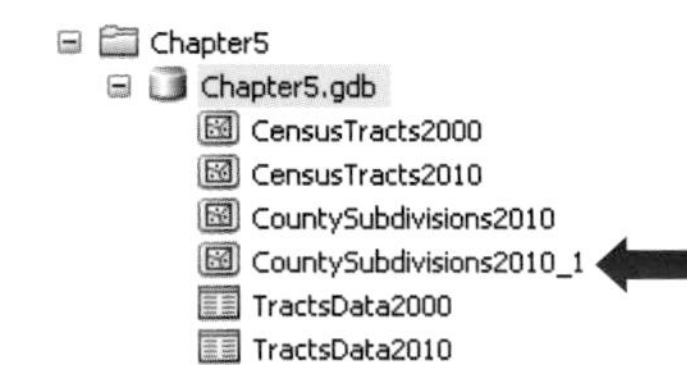

2 **Right-click CountiesSubdivisions2010_1 and click Delete. Click Yes.**

YOUR TURN

Open a Computer window, browse for Chapter5.gdb, right-click the folder, and click Properties to get the properties and size of the geodatabase. Take a look at the files inside of it comprising the county subdivisions, census tracts, and census tract data. You should find that the folder size on the disk is about 2.68 MB and that the files are incomprehensible. You'll need ArcCatalog or the Catalog window in ArcMap to use and manipulate these files. Leave the Computer window open for use in the following exercise.

Compress a file geodatabase

1 **In ArcCatalog in the Catalog tree, right-click Chapter5.gdb, click Administration > Compress File Geodatabase, and click OK.**

2 **Use a Computer window to check the size of the Chapter5.gdb folder.**

In this case, there is hardly a reduction in file size (about 2.46 MB). Although ArcMap can display compressed feature layers by uncompressing them on the fly, you will use the next step to uncompress the folder and get the layers back to original size.

3 **In the Catalog tree, right-click Chapter5.gdb, click Administration > Uncompress File Geodatabase, and click OK.**

Examine metadata

Spatial data needs a lot of documentation for interpretation and proper use. "Metadata" is the term for this documentation. It describes the context, content, and structure of GIS data. In ArcGIS for Desktop, ArcCatalog is used by data providers for creating and viewing this metadata.

1 **In ArcCatalog in the Catalog Tree panel, locate and select the CensusTracts2010 layer from Chapter5.gdb. In the right pane, click the Description tab.** It might take a few minutes to generate the description. Wait for it to appear. Metadata is available in a number of styles, fitted to various metadata standards. The style you see in the Description tab is the default style: a simple description of the layer. Other styles have more information. To see them, you need to change your metadata style in the options for ArcCatalog. You will change to the Federal Geographic Data Committee (FGDC) style to see how this works. ▶

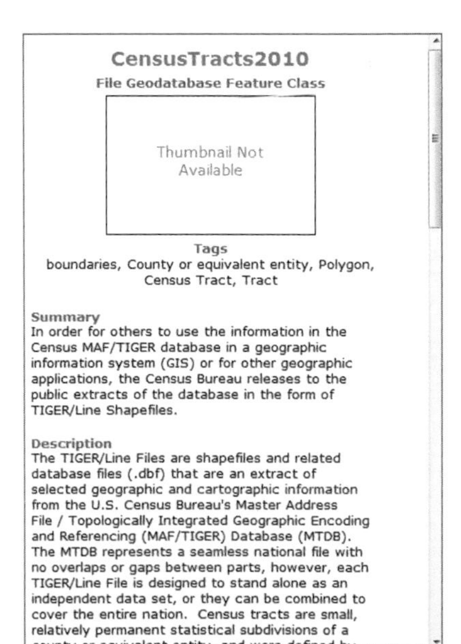

2 Click Customize > ArcCatalog Options. In the ArcCatalog Options dialog, click the Metadata tab. Click the dropdown arrow for Metadata Style and pick FGDC CSDGM Metadata. Click OK. For the new metadata to take effect, you will have to close and reopen ArcCatalog. ▶

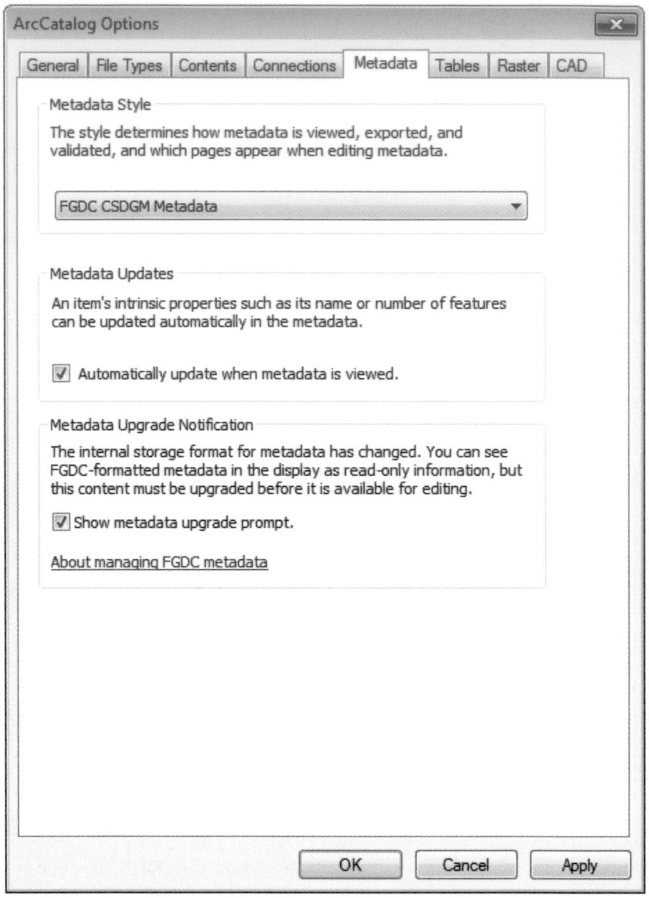

ArcCatalog Options

General | File Types | Contents | Connections | Metadata | Tables | Raster | CAD

Metadata Style

The style determines how metadata is viewed, exported, and validated, and which pages appear when editing metadata.

FGDC CSDGM Metadata

Metadata Updates

An item's intrinsic properties such as its name or number of features can be updated automatically in the metadata.

☑ Automatically update when metadata is viewed.

Metadata Upgrade Notification

The internal storage format for metadata has changed. You can see FGDC-formatted metadata in the display as read-only information, but this content must be upgraded before it is available for editing.

☑ Show metadata upgrade prompt.

About managing FGDC metadata

OK | Cancel | Apply

3 Close ArcCatalog. Open ArcCatalog and navigate to Chapter5.gdb. In the Catalog tree, locate and select the CensusTracts2010 layer. In the right pane, click the Description tab.

4 Scroll through it until you find the Field labeled GEOID10. You will see that this attribute is a concatenation of state, county, and tract codes.

FIELD GEOID10 ▶
* ALIAS GEOID10
* DATA TYPE String
* WIDTH 11
* PRECISION 0
* SCALE 0
FIELD DESCRIPTION
Census tract identifier; a concatenation of 2010 Census state FIPS code, county FIPS code, and census tract code

DESCRIPTION SOURCE
U.S. Census Bureau

CODED VALUES
NAME OF CODELIST INCITS.38-200x (R2004), Codes for the Identification of the States, the District of Columbia, Puerto Rico, and the Insular Areas of the United States (Formerly FIPS 5-2), INCITS.31-200x (R2007), Codes for the Identification of the Counties and Equivalent Areas of the United States, Puerto Rico, and the Insular Areas of the United States (Formerly FIPS 6-4), and the census tract code found in TRACTCE10
SOURCE U.S. Census Bureau

YOUR TURN

Examine other metadata for the CensusTracts2010 layer, including Citation (includes citation and contacts), Spatial Reference (includes coordinate system and reference system identifier), and Distribution (includes contact and format information).

Examine the metadata for other layers that are in the geodatabases in the Data folder for GISTHealth.

Edit metadata

Metadata can be edited in ArcCatalog, which makes the data easier to work with. In an earlier exercise, for example, you entered a value of 1939 for housing units built before 1940. This edit should be explained in the metadata. You can also use metadata to add more descriptive information about attributes.

1 **In the Catalog tree, locate and select the TractsData2000 table in Chapter5.gdb. Click the Description tab and then the Edit button** Edit **.**

2 **In the Summary pane, type** Database of median year structure was built.

3 **In the Description pane, type** PLEASE NOTE: Year 1939 should be interpreted as structures built before 1940.

4 **At the top of the Edit window, click the Save button** Save **.**

YOUR TURN

Edit the field metadata for TractsData2010. At the bottom of the leftmost panel, click Fields. In the right panel, open New Entity and Attribute Details. Click the down arrow for Details: TractsData2010. Click the attributes TOT_POP and POP_OVR18 and add the alias descriptions **Total Population** and **Population Over Age 18**, respectively. Save the metadata.

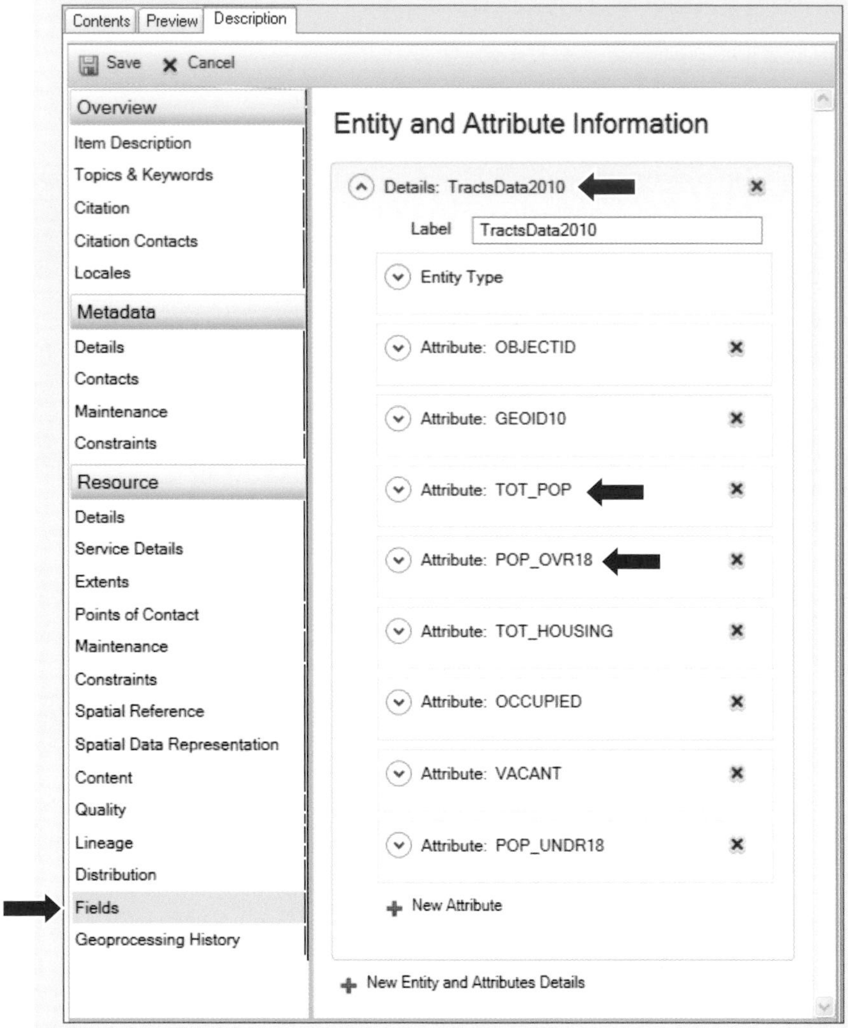

Contents Preview Description
Save Cancel
Overview
Item Description
Topics & Keywords
Citation
Citation Contacts
Locales
Metadata
Details
Contacts
Maintenance
Constraints
Resource
Details
Service Details
Extents
Points of Contact
Maintenance
Constraints
Spatial Reference
Spatial Data Representation
Content
Quality
Lineage
Distribution
Fields
Geoprocessing History
Entity and Attribute Information
Details: TractsData2010
Label TractsData2010
Entity Type
Attribute: OBJECTID
Attribute: GEOID10
Attribute: TOT_POP
Attribute: POP_OVR18
Attribute: TOT_HOUSING
Attribute: OCCUPIED
Attribute: VACANT
Attribute: POP_UNDR18
New Attribute
New Entity and Attributes Details

5 Close ArcCatalog.

Tutorial 5-5

Joining housing and elevated blood case tables to a census tract map

Now that you have downloaded and prepared the census and housing data, you are ready to join the data.

Join data to census tracts

1. **Start ArcMap, click File > New > My Templates > Blank Map, and click OK to begin a new map document.**

2. **On the Standard toolbar, click Add Data, browse through Chapter5.gdb, select CensusTracts2000 and TractsData2000, and click Add.**

3. **Click Add Data, browse through the Data folder to ACHD.gdb, click ElevatedBloodCases_00, and click Add.**

4. **In the table of contents, right-click CensusTracts2000 and click Open Attribute Table.** Notice that the number of records is 416 and the field CTIDFP00 includes the state, county, and tract codes. Close the table when you are finished.

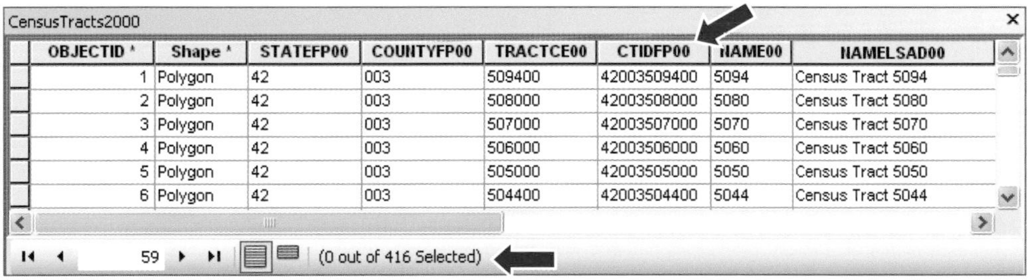

CensusTracts2000

OBJECTID *	Shape *	STATEFP00	COUNTYFP00	TRACTCE00	CTIDFP00	NAME00	NAMELSAD00
1	Polygon	42	003	509400	42003509400	5094	Census Tract 5094
2	Polygon	42	003	508000	42003508000	5080	Census Tract 5080
3	Polygon	42	003	507000	42003507000	5070	Census Tract 5070
4	Polygon	42	003	506000	42003506000	5060	Census Tract 5060
5	Polygon	42	003	505000	42003505000	5050	Census Tract 5050
6	Polygon	42	003	504400	42003504400	5044	Census Tract 5044

59 (0 out of 416 Selected)

T 5-5

5 In the table of contents, right-click TractsData2000 and click Open. Notice that the number of records is 416 and the field Id includes the state, county, and tract codes. Close the table when you are finished. ▶

TractsData2000

OBJECTID *	Id *	Median_year_structure_built
1	42003010300	1939
2	42003020100	1960
3	42003020300	1939
4	42003030500	1979
5	42003040200	1945
6	42003040300	1939

150 (0 out of 416 Selected)

6 In the table of contents, right-click ElevatedBloodCases_00 and click Open. Notice that the number of records is 416 and the field TRACT_00 includes the state, county, and tract codes. Although the field names are different in all three tables, the data and field types are the same. Close the table when you are finished. ▶

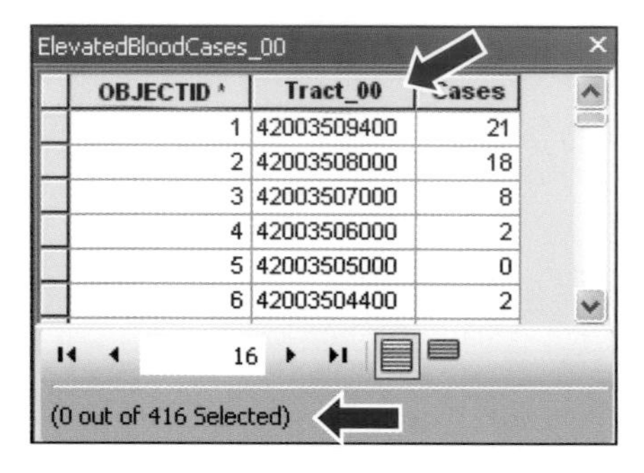

ElevatedBloodCases_00

OBJECTID *	Tract_00	Cases
1	42003509400	21
2	42003508000	18
3	42003507000	8
4	42003506000	2
5	42003505000	0
6	42003504400	2

16

(0 out of 416 Selected)

7 In the table of contents, right-click CensusTracts2000 and click "Joins and Relates" > Join.

In the next step, you will join the housing data containing the median year houses were built to the 2000 census tract polygons.

8 In step 1 of the Join Data dialog box, click CTIDFP00 in the drop-down list. In step 2, click TractsData2000. In step 3, click Id. You have just set up the process for joining the two related fields from the attribute tables of the two layers you are working with. The CTIDFP00 field is the census tract from the tracts layer, and the Id field is the same census tract from the TractsData2000 table. Both of these fields must be the same data type (that is, either both numbers or both text). Otherwise, the fields might not appear in the list. ▶

Join Data

Join lets you append additional data to this layer's attribute table so you can, for example, symbolize the layer's features using this data.

What do you want to join to this layer?

Join attributes from a table

1. Choose the field in this layer that the join will be based on:

CTIDFP00

2. Choose the table to join to this layer, or load the table from disk:

TractsData2000

Show the attribute tables of layers in this list

3. Choose the field in the table to base the join on:

Id

Join Options

Keep all records

All records in the target table are shown in the resulting table. Unmatched records will contain null values for all fields being appended into the target table from the join table.

Keep only matching records

If a record in the target table doesn't have a match in the join table, that record is removed from the resulting target table.

Validate Join

About Joining Data OK Cancel

T 5-5

9 Click OK and then Yes if prompted to create an index.

10 Open the attribute table for CensusTracts2000 and scroll to the right.
Fields from the attribute table of TractsData2000 are now joined to the CensusTracts2000 attribute table.

YOUR TURN

Join ElevatedBloodCases_00 to CensusTracts2000. Use the TRACT_00 field in step 3 of the dialog box.

Join tables permanently

Table joins are temporary. To permanently join these tables, you will export the joined layer as a new feature class. The resulting layer will have all the attributes from the joined tables as permanent attributes.

1 In the table of contents, right-click CensusTracts2000 and click Data > Export Data.

2 Save the output to Chapter5.gdb and name it HousingLeadStudy**, but do not add the exported data to your map.**

3 Close ArcMap, but do not save your changes.

Tutorial 5-6
Building a lead study comparison map

Now that you have prepared the spatial and attribute data, you are ready to build a map that compares children with elevated blood lead levels to the housing data.

Add map layers

1. **Start ArcMap, click File > New > My Templates > Blank Map, and click OK to begin a new map document.**

2. **On the Standard toolbar, click Add Data, browse through the Data folder to ACHD.gdb, and add Municipalities and Rivers.** These layers are used as a visual reference to orient the map reader. Note that the coordinate system for the data frame is state plane (feet).

3. **Click Add Data, browse through Chapter5.gdb, and add HousingLeadStudy.**

4. **Add another copy of HousingLeadStudy.**

Symbolize lead levels as a dot-density map

1. **Move Rivers to the top of the table of contents and symbolize it using a light-blue fill color.**

2. **Move Municipalities below Rivers and symbolize it using a Hollow symbol and a black outline width of 1.15.**

3. **Right-click the top copy of HousingLeadStudy, click Properties, click the Symbology tab, and in the Show pane, click Quantities > Dot density.**

4. **Under Field Selection, click Cases, and click the top arrow button (>) to transfer that column to the right panel of the Field Selection area.**

5. **In the right panel of the Field Selection area, double-click the dot in the Symbol tab and change the symbol color to red. Then click OK.**

6 **Under Background, click the line symbol button and change the color to No Color. Click OK.**

7 **Change the dot size to** 1.5 **and the dot value to 1. Click OK.** A dot value of 1 means that there is one randomly placed dot in a tract for every case that occurred in the tract.

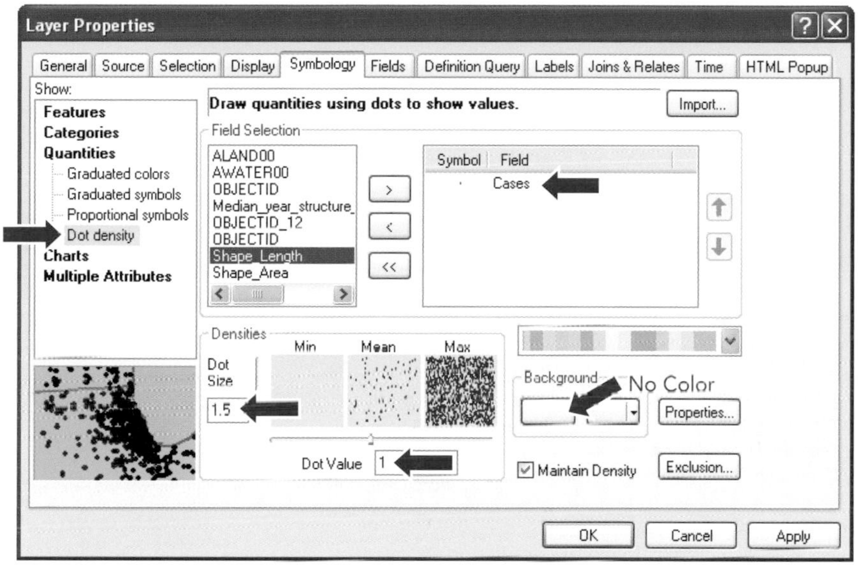

Symbolize housing as a choropleth map

1 **Symbolize the second copy of HousingLeadStudy as a choropleth map using the field Median_year_structure_built and five classes of 1939-1950, 1951-1960, 1961-1970, 1971-1980, and 1981-1996.**

2 **Label the classes as follows:**

- 1950 and before
- 1951-1960
- 1961-1970
- 1971-1980
- 1981 and later

3 **Use a gray color ramp and reverse it so that the highest color value is for the oldest category of median year built. (To reverse the color ramp, right-click the first symbol in the list and click Flip Symbols.)**

4 **Double-click each of the five symbols and change Outline Color to No Color. Click OK.** (See next page.)

As expected, you can see a correlation between houses built before 1980 (remember, highly toxic lead was removed in 1978) and cases of elevated

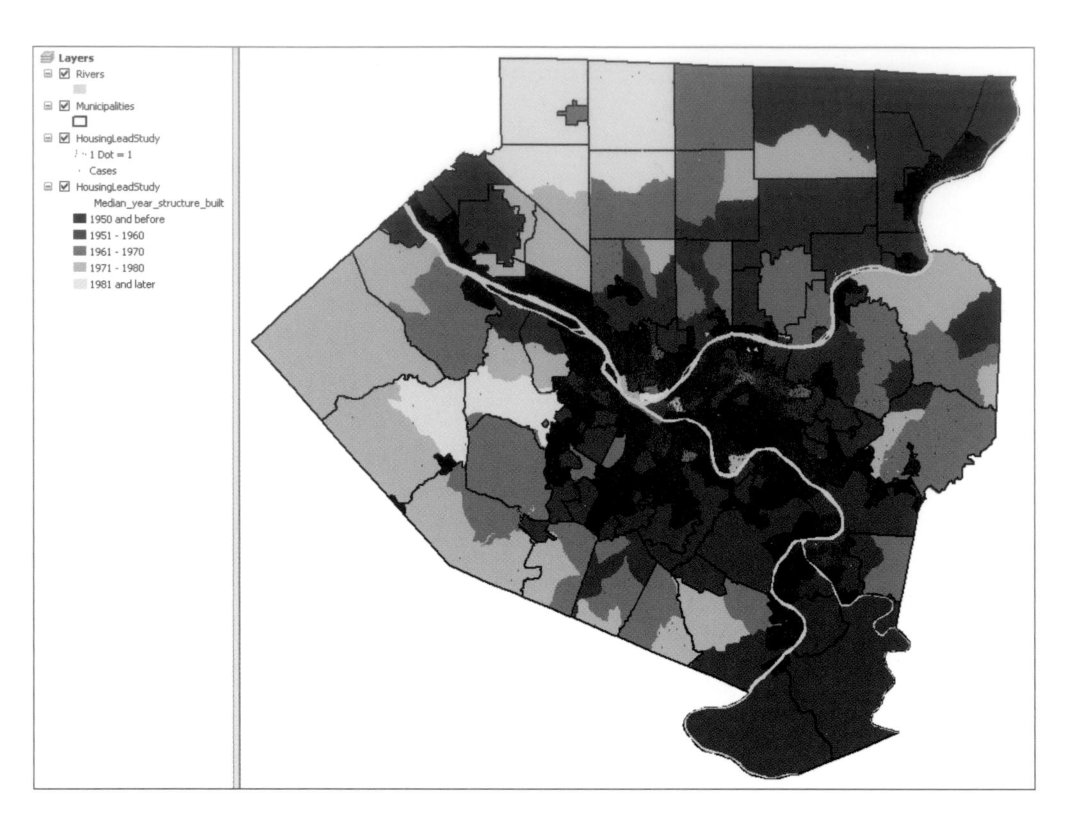

blood lead levels in children. Other factors probably affect the frequency of elevated BLLs. Poverty could also be a factor and could be an additional US Census variable to download and compare.

Using the attribute table, you can derive statistics about the number of kids who have elevated BLLs and the mean of the median year houses were built.

YOUR TURN

Right-click one of the HousingLeadStudy layers and open the attribute table. Right-click the Cases field and click Sort Descending. Select the 35 records of census tracts that have elevated blood lead levels of 50 and over. Right-click the Median_year_structure_built field and click Statistics. Notice that the mean of the median year houses were built for these records is 1941. Select the records for census tracts that have five or fewer cases and notice that the mean of the median year houses were built was 1956.

Save the map document

1 **On the File menu, click Save As.**

2 **Save your map document as** Tutorial5-6YourName.mxd **to your Chapter5 folder in MyExercises.** Do not close ArcMap.

Tutorial 5-7

Showing elevated blood lead levels by tract

Although it is useful to observe census tracts that have a high number of cases of children who have elevated levels of lead in their blood, a better study is to look at the percentage of children who have elevated blood lead levels.

Calculate the number of children under age 18 per tract

1 **Create a new empty map document.**

2 **On the Standard toolbar, click Add Data, browse through the Data folder to ACHD.gdb, select ElevatedBloodCases_10 and Rivers, and click Add.**

3 **Click Add Data, browse through Chapter5.gdb, and add CensusTracts2010, CountySubdivisions2010, and TractsData2010. Click Add.**

4 **Right-click the TractsData2010 layer and open the attribute table.**

5 **Click the Table Options arrow and Add Field. Add a field called** POP_UNDR18 **with data type Double.**

6 **Right-click the field POP_UNDR18 and click Field Calculator. Click Yes to continue.**

7 **In the Field Calculator dialog box, subtract the field POP_OVR18 from TOT_POP.** The POP_UNDR18 field now shows the number of children under age 18 per census tract. This field will be used to calculate the percentage of children who have elevated blood lead levels.

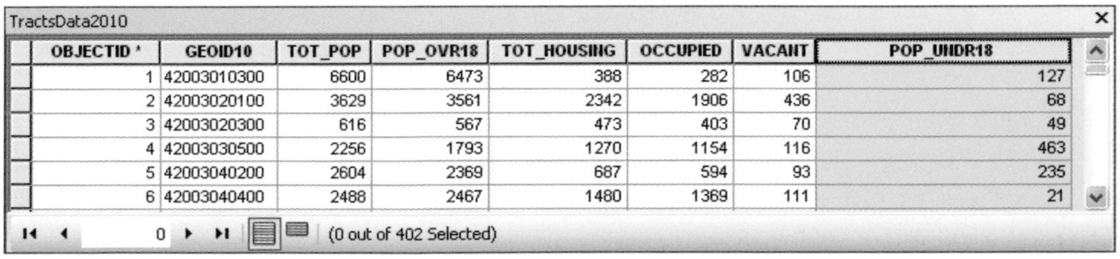

TractsData2010

OBJECTID *	GEOID10	TOT_POP	POP_OVR18	TOT_HOUSING	OCCUPIED	VACANT	POP_UNDR18
1	42003010300	6600	6473	388	282	106	127
2	42003020100	3629	3561	2342	1906	436	68
3	42003020300	616	567	473	403	70	49
4	42003030500	2256	1793	1270	1154	116	463
5	42003040200	2604	2369	687	594	93	235
6	42003040400	2488	2467	1480	1369	111	21

(0 out of 402 Selected)

T 5-7

Join tables to tract polygons

1 In the table of contents, right-click CensusTracts2010 and click Joins and Relates > Join.

2 In step 1 of the Join Data dialog box in the drop-down list, click GEOID10. In step 2, click TractsData2010. In step 3, click GEOID10.

Join Data

Join lets you append additional data to this layer's attribute table so you can, for example, symbolize the layer's features using this data.

What do you want to join to this layer?

Join attributes from a table

1. Choose the field in this layer that the join will be based on:

GEOID10

2. Choose the table to join to this layer, or load the table from disk:

TractsData2010

Show the attribute tables of layers in this list

3. Choose the field in the table to base the join on:

GEOID10

Join Options

Keep all records

All records in the target table are shown in the resulting table. Unmatched records will contain null values for all fields being appended into the target table from the join table.

Keep only matching records

If a record in the target table doesn't have a match in the join table, that record is removed from the resulting target table.

Validate Join

About Joining Data | OK | Cancel

3 Click OK and then Yes.

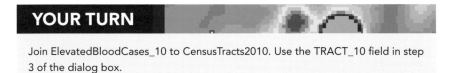

Join ElevatedBloodCases_10 to CensusTracts2010. Use the TRACT_10 field in step 3 of the dialog box.

Show the percentage of children who have elevated blood lead levels by tract

1 Right-click the CensusTracts2010 layer, click Properties, and click the Symbology tab. In the Show pane, click Quantities > Graduated Colors.

2 In the Fields pane, in the Value list, click Cases and in the Normalization list, click POP_UNDR18. Choose a yellow to brown color ramp. By choosing these fields, you are showing the percentage of children who have elevated blood lead levels.

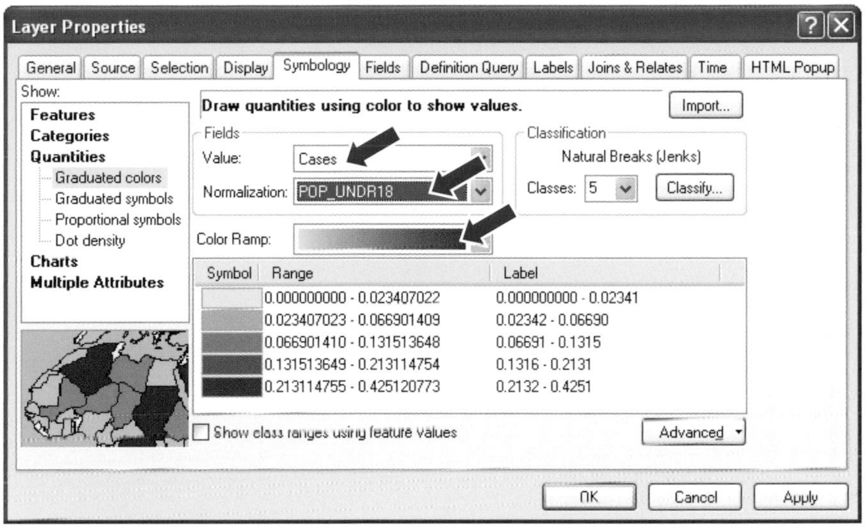

3 In the bottom panel, click the Label tab, click Format labels >. In the Category pane, click Percentage, and click "The number represents a fraction. Adjust it to show a percentage." Click the Numeric Options button and set the options to two decimal places. Click OK twice.

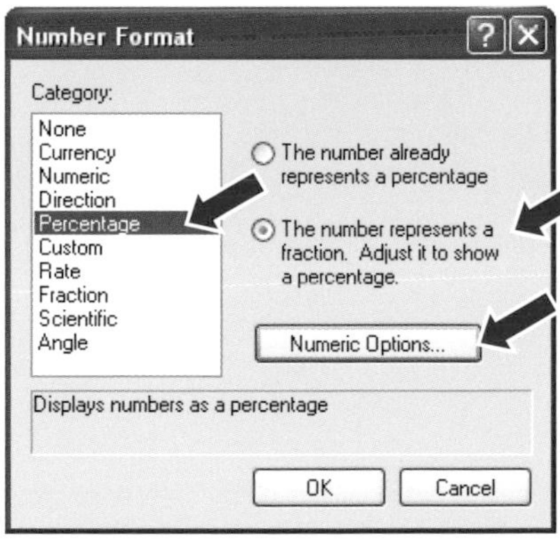

4 **Classify the data using five classes and the following break values:** 3%, 6%, 9%, 18%, 42.51%. **Click OK.**

5 **Symbolize Rivers as light blue and CountySubdivisions2010 using a Hollow symbol and an outline width of** 1.15.

6 **Label the CountySubdivisions2010 layer using the field NAME10 and a halo mask.** Although the highest percentage of children who have elevated blood lead levels are within the municipality of Pittsburgh, there are other municipalities, especially along the rivers, that also have high percentages of children with elevated blood lead levels.

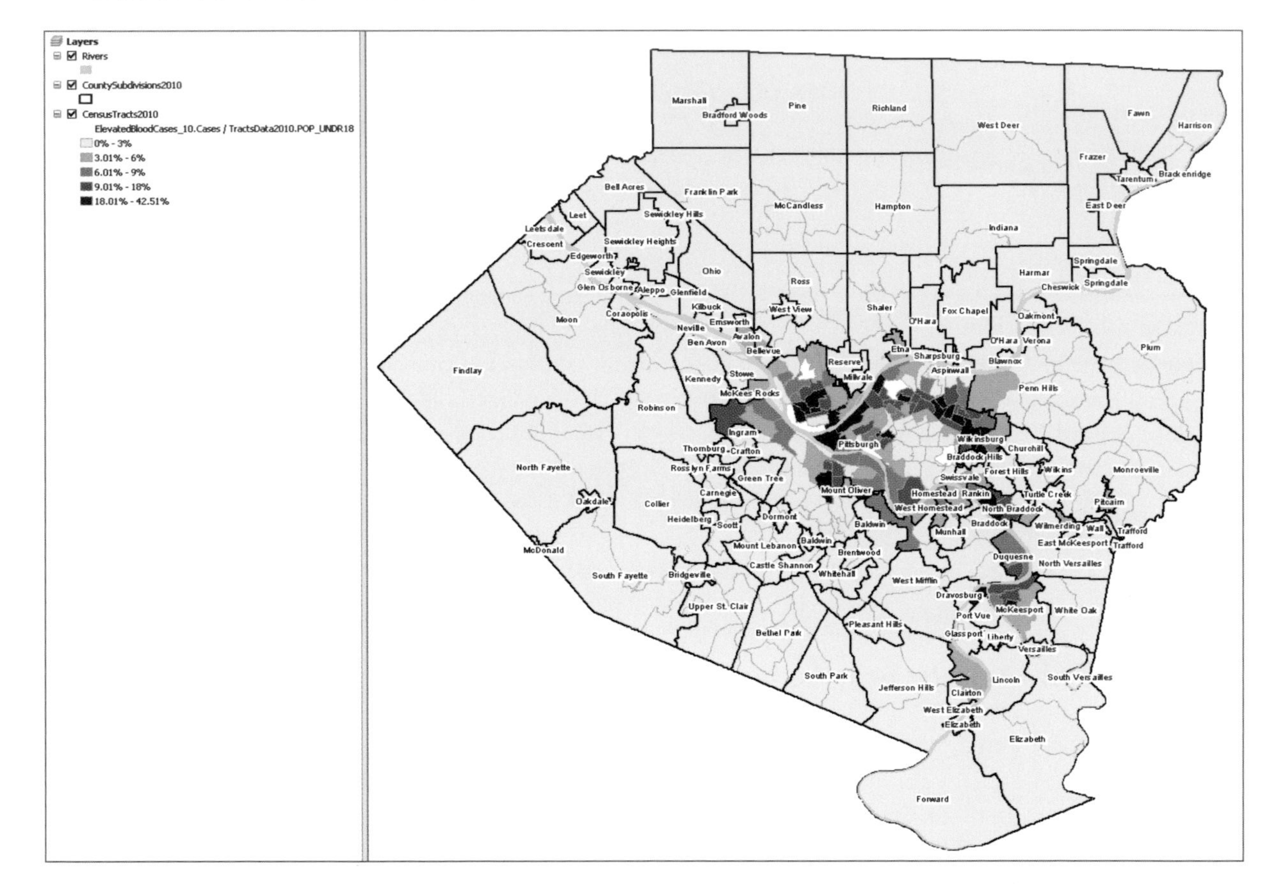

Save the map document

1 **On the File menu, click Save As.**

2 **Save your map document as** Tutorial5-7YourName.mxd **to your Chapter5 folder in MyExercises.** Do not close ArcMap.

Tutorial 5-8
Showing elevated blood lead levels by municipality and neighborhood

In this tutorial, you will display the cases of children with elevated BLLs by Allegheny County subdivisions and by Pittsburgh neighborhoods, making the map more meaningful for a health official or a local pediatrician who likely is not familiar with census tract numbers. To do this, you will create point centroids of census tract polygons. The centroid of a polygon is the point at which the polygon would balance on a pencil point if the polygon were cut out of cardboard. Together, polygons and their centroids give you the ability to aggregate data (for example, the number of cases of BLLs and the number of children who are under 18) to county subdivisions and neighborhoods.

Point centroids can also be used to display two attributes from the same map layer, one as a choropleth map and the other as size-graduated point markers. ArcMap has an algorithm that calculates and adds centroid coordinates to an attribute table, thus allowing you to create a new point layer.

Add x,y coordinates to a polygon attribute table

1 **In the CensusTracts2010 table, click the Table Options arrow and click Add Field.**

2 **For Name, type** X **and for Type, click Double. Click OK.**

3 **Repeat steps 1 and 2, only this time call the new field** Y.

4 **Scroll to the right in the CensusTracts2010 table, right-click the CensusTracts2010. X column heading, click Calculate Geometry, and click Yes. In the Property box, select "X Coordinate of Centroid." In Coordinate System, select "Use coordinate system of the data source." In Units, select "Decimal Degrees." Click OK and Yes.** The attribute name is fully qualified to CensusTracts2010.X to indicate that of the joined set of tables in the display, ArcMap identifies the X attribute as being in the CensusTracts2010 table.

5 **Repeat step 4, only this time right-click CensusTracts2010.Y and click Y Coordinate of Centroid.** The result is longitude and latitude coordinates for X and Y. (See next page.)

CensusTracts2010

OBJECTID *	GEOID10 *	TOT_POP	POP_OVR18	TOT_HOUSING	OCCUPIED	VACANT	POP_UNDR18	CensusTracts2010.PCT_ELEVBL	CensusTracts2010.X	CensusTracts2010.Y
396	42003980800	0	0	0	0	0	0	<Null>	-79.964131	40.431971
392	42003980400	21	21	15	14	1	0	<Null>	-80.02002	40.481939
398	42003981000	4	4	2	2	0	0	<Null>	-79.948876	40.473082
400	42003981200	0	0	0	0	0	0	<Null>	-80.010801	40.446457
394	42003980600	11	11	4	4	0	0	<Null>	-80.028012	40.451987
391	42003980300	1	1	1	1	0	0	<Null>	-79.905723	40.43255
397	42003980900	1797	1796	0	0	0	1	0	-80.041947	40.466541
399	42003981100	7	6	4	4	0	1	0	-79.906331	40.442042
395	42003980700	19	18	15	10	5	1	0	-80.011803	40.437742
390	42003980100	18	15	8	8	0	3	0	-79.914416	40.481103
393	42003980500	27	24	16	14	2	3	0	-79.942194	40.434375
402	42003982200	4816	4811	169	165	4	5	20	-79.954765	40.444488
6	42003040400	2488	2467	1480	1369	111	21	0	-79.949373	40.447348
401	42003981800	461	434	43	43	0	27	0	-79.897221	40.480383
7	42003040500	3694	3660	1379	1300	79	34	14.705882	-79.955953	40.439623
203	42003459202	661	621	493	471	22	40	2.5	-80.101093	40.428245
3	42003020300	616	567	473	403	70	49	20.408163	-79.9815	40.454254

0 (0 out of 402 Selected)

Export a table

When you export joined tables as a table, you get all the attributes of the joined tables stored together permanently in one table. The resulting table can have several uses—for example, you can make a new point layer based on the centroid coordinates.

1 **In the CensusTracts2010 table, click the Table Options arrow and click Export.**

2 **In the Export Data dialog box, for the "Output table" box, click the Browse button, and in the Saving Data dialog box, change "Save as type" to File Geodatabase tables, browse for Chapter5.gdb, change Name to** CensusTract2010XYTable, **and click Save > OK > Yes.** Open the table to see that it has all the columns of both joined tables. Then close the table.

3 **Close the CensusTracts2010 attribute table.**

Create a feature class from an XY table

1 **On the ArcMap Windows menu, click Catalog.** A version of ArcCatalog opens as a Catalog window in ArcMap, providing quick access to GIS utility programs.

2 **In the Catalog tree, expand the GISTHealth folder connection to MyExercises > Chapter5, and then expand the contents of Chapter5.gdb.**

3 **Right-click CensusTract2010XYTable and click Create Feature Class > From XY Table.**

4 **In the Create Feature Class From XY Table dialog box, click the Coordinate System of Input Coordinates button, click Geographic Coordinate Systems > North America > NAD 1983, and click OK.**

5 **Under Output, click the Browse button, change "Save as type" to "File and Personal Geodatabase feature classes," browse for Chapter5.gdb, change Name to** CensusTract2010Centroids, **and click Save and then OK.** ▶

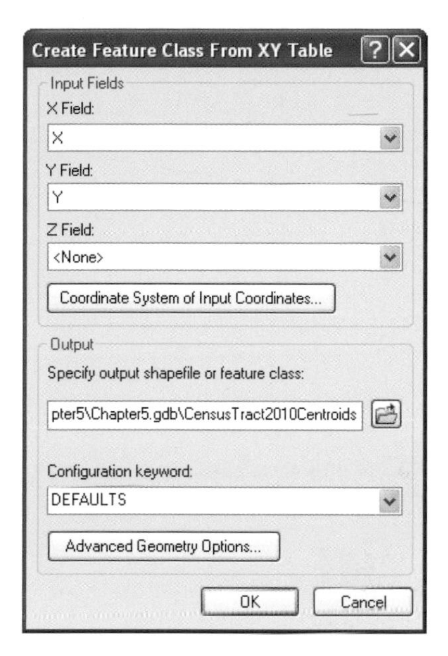

6 **Close the Catalog window in ArcMap.**

7 **On the Standard toolbar, click Add Data, browse through Chapter5.gdb, and double-click CensusTract2010Centroids.**

8 **Turn off the CensusTracts2010 layer and the labels for County-Subdivisions2010.** Now you can get a better look at the centroids point layer you just created. Notice that many county subdivisions have multiple centroids. Each of these points has data about the number of cases of elevated blood lead levels and the number of children who are under age 18.

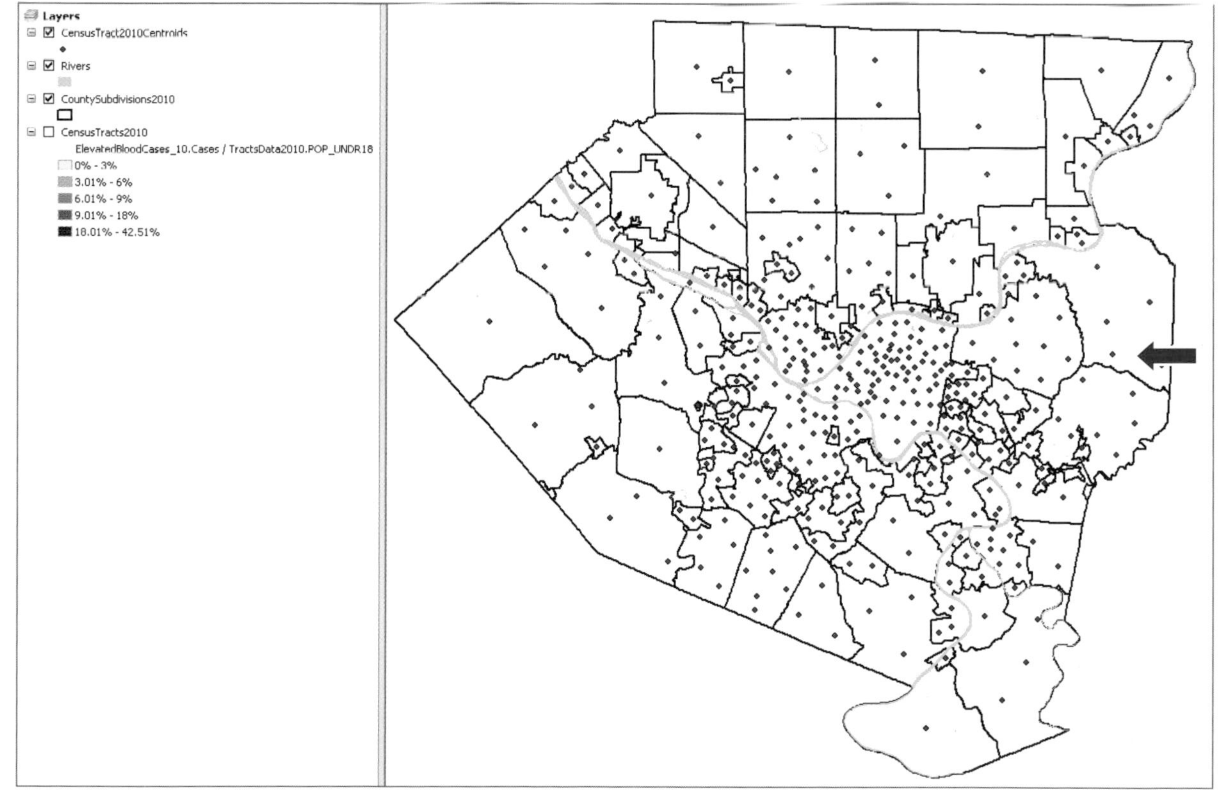

T 5-8

Spatially join tract centroids to county subdivisions

In this exercise, you will count, or aggregate, points within county subdivisions, and then display the results on a map. Before aggregating the data, you must do some preliminary tasks.

1. **Right-click CountySubdivisions2010 and click Joins and Relates > Join.**

2. **In the Join Data dialog box, for "What do you want to join to this layer?" click "Join data from another layer based on spatial location."**

3. **In the number 2 setting, select the Sum check box.** This option is needed because it adds the number of cases and children under age 18 for every census tract centroid in a county subdivision.

4. **Save the newly joined file as** CountySubdivision-TractJoin **to Chapter5.gdb in your Chapter5 folder in MyExercises.** ▶

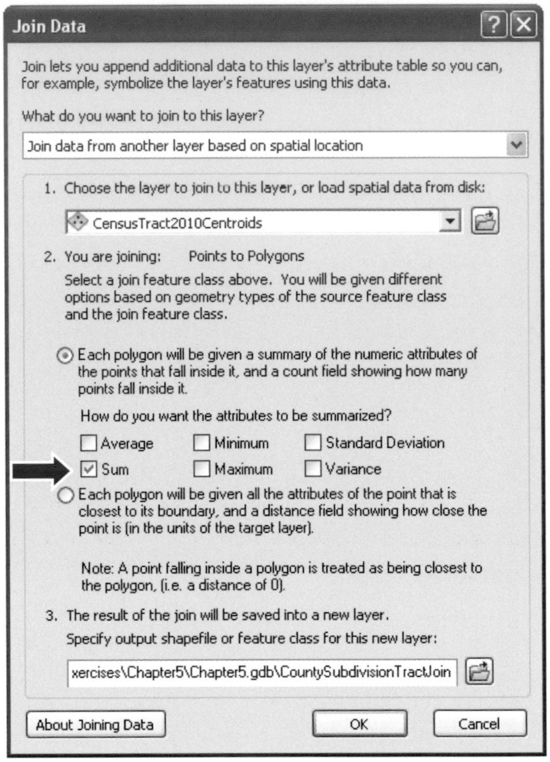

Join Data

Join lets you append additional data to this layer's attribute table so you can, for example, symbolize the layer's features using this data.

What do you want to join to this layer?

Join data from another layer based on spatial location

1. Choose the layer to join to this layer, or load spatial data from disk:

CensusTract2010Centroids

2. You are joining: Points to Polygons

Select a join feature class above. You will be given different options based on geometry types of the source feature class and the join feature class.

Each polygon will be given a summary of the numeric attributes of the points that fall inside it, and a count field showing how many points fall inside it.

How do you want the attributes to be summarized?

Average Minimum Standard Deviation

Sum Maximum Variance

Each polygon will be given all the attributes of the point that is closest to its boundary, and a distance field showing how close the point is (in the units of the target layer).

Note: A point falling inside a polygon is treated as being closest to the polygon, (i.e. a distance of 0).

3. The result of the join will be saved into a new layer.

Specify output shapefile or feature class for this new layer:

xercises\Chapter5\Chapter5.gdb\CountySubdivisionTractJoin

About Joining Data OK Cancel

5. **Right-click CountySubdivisionTractJoin and open the attribute table.**

6. **Scroll to the right and notice the new fields that sum up the number of cases and the population under age 18 per county subdivision.**

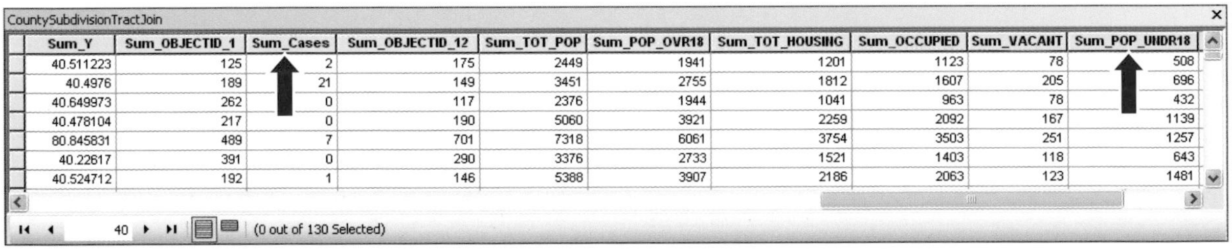

CountySubdivisionTractJoin

Sum_Y	Sum_OBJECTID_1	Sum_Cases	Sum_OBJECTID_12	Sum_TOT_POP	Sum_POP_OVR18	Sum_TOT_HOUSING	Sum_OCCUPIED	Sum_VACANT	Sum_POP_UNDR18
40.511223	125	2	175	2449	1941	1201	1123	78	508
40.4976	189	21	149	3451	2755	1812	1607	205	696
40.649973	262	0	117	2376	1944	1041	963	78	432
40.478104	217	0	190	5060	3921	2259	2092	167	1139
80.845831	489	7	701	7318	6061	3754	3503	251	1257
40.22617	391	0	290	3376	2733	1521	1403	118	643
40.524712	192	1	146	5388	3907	2186	2063	123	1481

40 (0 out of 130 Selected)

7. **In the table of contents, remove the CensusTracts2010 and CensusTract-2010Centroids layers.**

8. **In the table of contents, right-click CountySubdivisionTractJoin, click Properties, and click the Symbology tab.**

9. **In the Show pane, click Quantities > Graduated colors, and under Fields, for Value, click Sum_Cases, and for Normalization, click Sum_POP_Under18.**

10 Change the classes and labels to read as follows:

- 0% - 2%
- 2.01% - 4%
- 4.01% - 8%
- 8.01% - 20.33%

The resulting map shows a high percentage of cases east and south of Pittsburgh.

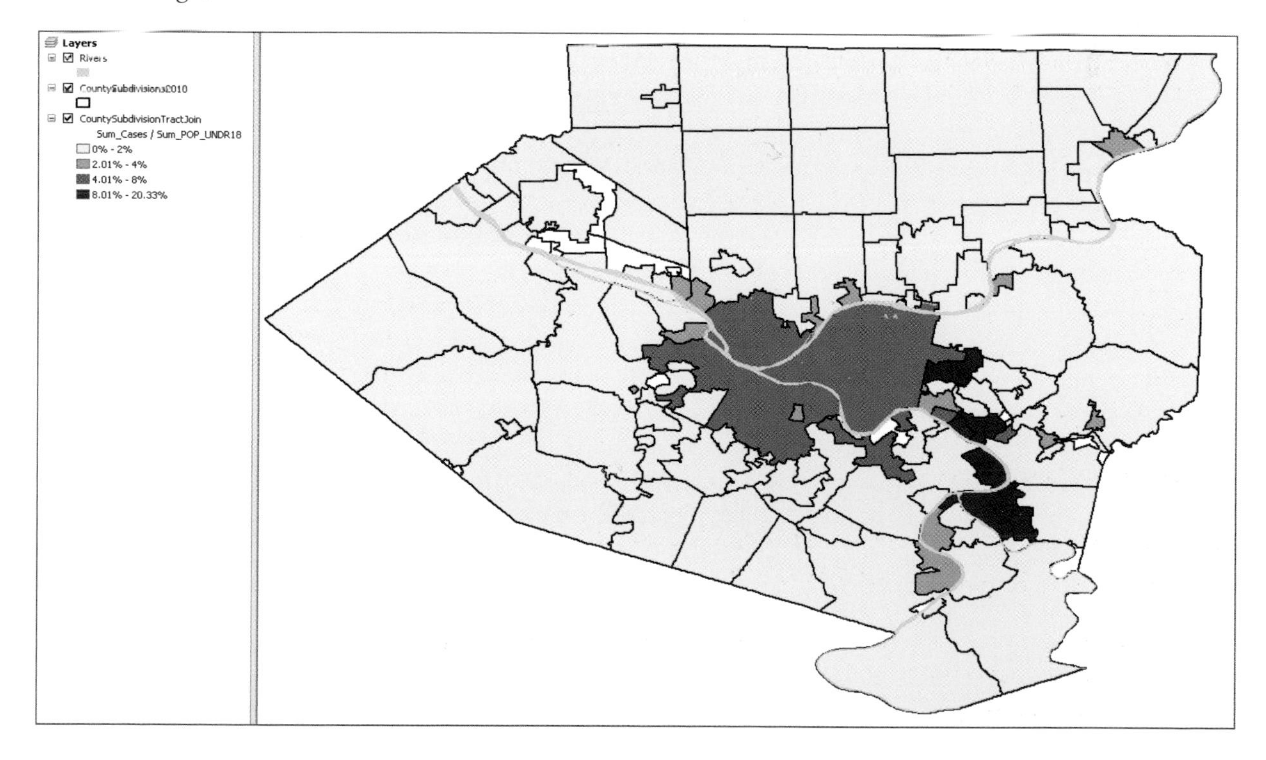

11 On the Tools toolbar, use the Identify tool to determine the county subdivisions that have the highest percentage of kids with elevated BLLs.

YOUR TURN

Add the Neighborhoods layer from Pittsburgh.gdb in the Data folder and repeat the spatial join process in steps 1–4 to determine the percentage of children in Pittsburgh neighborhoods with elevated BLLs. Then use the Identify tool to find the neighborhoods that have the highest percentage of children with elevated BLLs.

Save the map document

1 On the File menu, click Save As.

2 Save your map document as Tutorial5-8YourName.mxd **to your Chapter5 folder in MyExercises.** Close ArcMap.

Summary

Preparing data to do analytic work for GIS-based studies takes multiple skills, and it almost always takes more time than anticipated. This chapter focused on the skills you need for obtaining external data—from US Census Bureau websites, in this case—and for getting the data into the right table format for use in ArcMap. You had to find and download needed census data, fix several problems with the data values to make the data usable, and then join the data to a census tract map layer. With the skills learned in chapters 3 and 4, you could produce the map in just a few steps.

As far as the substantive knowledge gained, you provided evidence that the built environment affects children's health. Parts of Allegheny County that predominantly have houses built before 1978 tend to have concentrations of cases of elevated blood lead levels in children. The tutorials in this chapter asked you to add additional census variables to the map in an attempt to further explain the geographical concentrations of elevated blood lead levels in children.

Next, in chapter 6, you will prepare internal data for use in GIS. If internal records contain street addresses or geocodes such as ZIP Codes or county IDs, you can use geocoding to spatially process these records as map features.

Assignment 5-1

Map housing gross rent compared with elevated blood lead levels

In this chapter, you mapped the locations of children with elevated blood lead levels compared with the age of housing structures. The map clearly showed that these cases were clustered in Pittsburgh neighborhoods that have older structures. Other census variables you might want to compare are poverty, low educational attainment, or other low socioeconomic status indicators. Some studies show that financial housing statistics are a better indicator of the economic status of a city than poverty rates. It can also be argued that homeowners might take better care of their homes than those who rent. In this assignment, you will download US Census data for median and gross rents and compare this data with elevated blood lead levels.

Start with this data

- ***U.S. Census 2000 SF 3 Table (H063):*** downloaded for Allegheny County Census Tracts from http://factfinder2.census.gov/ using Topics > Housing > Financial Characteristic > Gross Rent > H063: MEDIAN GROSS RENT (DOLLARS) [1]: 2000 SF 3 Sample Data.
- ***tl_2010_42003_tract00.shp:*** polygon shapefile of Allegheny County Census Tract polygons, downloaded from http://www.census.gov (also available in the Chapter5 folder in FinishedExercises in the compressed file tl_2010_42003_tract00.zip).
- ***\EsriPress\GISTHealth\Data\ACHD.gdb\ElevatedBloodCases_00:*** the number of cases of children who have elevated blood lead levels aggregated to census tracts (2000). The elevated blood data for this study was provided by the Allegheny County Health Department (2005).
- ***\EsriPress\GISTHealth\Data\ACHD.gdb\Rivers:*** Allegheny County water features.
- ***\EsriPress\GISTHealth\Data\ACHD.gdb\Municipalities:*** Allegheny County municipalities.

Create a file geodatabase

Create a file geodatabase called **Assignment5-1YourName.gdb** and save it to your Chapter5 folder in MyAssignments. Using ArcCatalog, export Elevated BloodCases_00 from ACHD.gdb into your file geodatabase as a table of the same name. Export Rivers and Municipalities from ACHD.gdb into your file geodatabase as polygon feature classes using the same names. Import the tracts 2000 shapefile tl_2010_42003_tract00 as a polygon feature class called **CensusTracts2000**.

Edit data in spreadsheet software

In Microsoft Excel, prepare the DEC_00_SF3_H063 spreadsheet to join to census tract polygons. Import the newly prepared spreadsheet into your file geodatabase. Rename the DEC_00_SF3_H063 spreadsheet as a table called **MedianGrossRent2000**.

Create a comparison map for financial housing data and elevated blood lead levels

Create a map document called **Assignment5-1YourName.mxd** and save it to your Chapter5 folder in MyAssignments, using relative paths. Use a map layout that includes a choropleth map for median gross rents (US dollars) per census tract and size-graduated point markers for the number of elevated blood lead level cases per census tract. Use your judgment on the break points, color, size, title(s), and so on. Add Rivers and Municipalities for visual reference.

Hints

- *Add Rivers or Municipalities first to set the data frame projection to NAD_1983_StatePlane_Pennsylvania_South_FIPS_3702_Feet.*
- *Add CensusTracts2000 twice and join MedianGrossRent2000 and ElevatedBloodCases_00 to both layers.*
- *To show the number of cases as graduated symbols, click the Symbology tab and in the Show pane, click "Graduated symbols"; for Background, click No Color.*

Export the map as a JPEG image file called **Assignment5-1YourName.jpg** and save it to your Chapter5 folder in MyAssignments.

Create a Word document

Create a Microsoft Word document called **Assignment5-1YourName.docx** and save it to your Chapter5 folder in MyAssignments. Insert your map layout image and describe any visual patterns you see.

Using the attribute table CensusTracts2000, determine the mean of the median gross rent (dollars) of census tracts that have 50 or more cases of elevated blood lead levels. Find the mean of the median gross rent (dollars) of census tracts that have zero cases. Include a sentence detailing your statistical findings. Add a few sentences describing other US Census tables that you could add to the study.

WHAT TO TURN IN

If your work is to be graded, turn in the following files:

- ***File geodatabase:*** \EsriPress\GISTHealth\MyAssignments\Chapter5\Assignment5-1YourName.gdb
- ***ArcMap document:*** \EsriPress\GISTHealth\MyAssignments\Chapter5\Assignment5-1YourName.mxd
- ***Microsoft Word document:*** \EsriPress\GISTHealth\MyAssignments\Chapter5\Assignment5-1YourName.docx

If instructed to do so, instead of individual files, turn in a compressed file, **Assignment5-1YourName.zip**, that includes all the preceding files. Do not include path information in the compressed file.

Assignment 5-2

Map housing complaints compared with elevated blood lead levels

The local health department investigates complaints from landlords and tenants about unsafe or unsanitary housing conditions. This data can also be mapped and used to compare with locations showing elevated blood lead levels. In this assignment, you will create a map of housing complaints by census tract and compare this with elevated blood lead levels.

Start with this data

- *\EsriPress\GISTHealth\Data\ACHD.gdb\HousingComplaints:* a table of the number of housing complaints aggregated to census tracts (2000) in Allegheny County. The housing complaint data for this study was provided by the Allegheny County Health Department (2005).
- *\EsriPress\GISTHealth\Data\ACHD.gdb\ElevatedBloodCases_00:* the number of cases of children who have elevated blood lead levels aggregated to census tracts (2000). The elevated blood lead level data for this study was provided by the Allegheny County Health Department (2005).
- *\EsriPress\GISTHealth\Data\ACHD.gdb\Rivers:* Allegheny County water features.
- *\EsriPress\GISTHealth\Data\ACHD.gdb\Municipalities:* Allegheny County municipalities.
- *tl_2010_42003_tract00.shp:* polygon shapefile of Allegheny County census tract polygons, downloaded from http://www.census.gov (also available in the Chapter5 folder in FinishedExercises in compressed file tl_2010_42003_tract00.zip).

Create a file geodatabase

Create a file geodatabase called **Assignment5-2YourName.gdb** and save it to your Chapter5 folder in MyAssignments. Using ArcCatalog, export HousingComplaints, ElevatedBloodCases_00, Rivers, and Municipalities from ACHD.gdb and import them into your file geodatabase. Import the shapefile tl_2010_42003_tract00 into your file geodatabase, renaming it **CensusTracts2000**.

Create a comparison map for housing complaints and elevated blood lead levels

Create a map document called **Assignment5-2YourName.mxd** and save it to your Chapter5 folder in MyAssignments, using relative paths. Use a map layout that includes a choropleth map for housing complaints per census tract and size-graduated point markers for the number of elevated blood lead levels per census tract. Use your judgment on the break points, color, size, title(s), and so forth. Add Rivers and Municipalities for visual reference.

Hints

- *Add Rivers or Municipalities first to set the data frame projection to NAD_1983_StatePlane_Pennsylvania_South_FIPS_3702_Feet.*
- *Add CensusTracts2000 twice and join HousingComplaints and ElevatedBloodCases_00 to both layers.*
- *To show the number of cases as graduated symbols, click the Symbology tab. In the Show pane, click "Graduated symbols" and for Background, click No Color.*

Export the map layout as a JPEG image file called **Assignment5-2YourName.jpg** and save it to your Chapter5 folder in MyAssignments.

Create a Word document

Create a Microsoft Word document called **Assignment5-2YourName.docx** and save it to your Chapter5 folder in MyAssignments. Insert your map layout image and describe any visual patterns you see. Using the CensusTracts2000 attribute table, determine the mean and total number of housing complaints for census tracts that have 50 or more cases of elevated blood lead levels and the mean and total number of housing complaints for census tracts that have zero cases. Include a sentence detailing your statistical findings.

In your Microsoft Word document, answer the following questions:

- What municipality has the census tract with the highest number of housing complaints?
- What three municipalities in the northeast part of the county have a high number of housing complaints (over 50)?

WHAT TO TURN IN

If your work is to be graded, turn in the following files:

- ***File geodatabase:*** \EsriPress\GISTHealth\MyAssignments\Chapter5\Assignment5-2YourName.gdb
- ***ArcMap document:*** \EsriPress\GISTHealth\MyAssignments\Chapter5\Assignment5-2YourName.mxd
- ***Microsoft Word document:*** \EsriPress\GISTHealth\MyAssignments\Chapter5\Assignment5-2YourName.docx

If instructed to do so, instead of individual files, turn in a compressed file, **Assignment5-2YourName.zip**, that includes all the preceding files. Do not include path information in the compressed file.

Chapter 6
Geocoding tabular data

Objectives

- Create new health-care map layers using internal and local data
- Geocode ZIP Code data
- Spatially join and aggregate point data to create choropleth maps
- Batch geocode address data
- Interactively rematch address data to fix input errors

Health-care scenario

Top management at a major hospital in Pittsburgh, Pennsylvania, has recently hired you as a GIS analyst. You have downloaded basemaps and data from the US Census Bureau and Esri website to use as GIS data. Now you need to spatially process some of the hospital's internal data, using ArcMap geocoding tools. (Patient data used in this tutorial is fictional data created by the book's authors.)

One of your future projects is to evaluate alternative locations for a satellite hospital clinic. You will create two new layers to make a good starting point for this endeavor. The two datasets you will work with are (1) all other hospitals in the county and (2) a multistate sample of patient data. You will need to locate the hospitals as precisely as possible to assess the local competition. Your own hospital clinic, however, will have a number of specialties that have no local competitors, so you will need to visualize patient demand patterns not only locally, but also in the multistate area. For this purpose, you will not plot individual residential locations of patients. Instead, counts of patients by ZIP Code will best meet your needs.

Solution approach

The most common form of geocoding uses sophisticated programs to match tabular street address data to street address attributes in a line map layer of streets. Such programs use "fuzzy matching" to account for variations in abbreviations and spellings of address data, just as your postal delivery person does when getting the mail to you.

TIGER/Line street files, available from the US Census Bureau, are limited. They do not have data and separate points for each street address, such as 33 Pine Ave. Instead, each TIGER/Line feature is a block-long street segment that has street numbers for only the start and the end of the block on both odd and even sides of the street. For Pine Avenue, for instance, the data might be odd–even street numbers 1, 2 and 99, 98 if the street has blocks broken up by house numbers in the hundreds. The ArcMap geocoding program for TIGER/Line formatted streets finds the relevant street segment for a street address and approximates a point location using simple interpolation of starting and ending street numbers and points.

Geocoding is not always successful; for example, the input address data in a tabular file may have errors, or the TIGER/Line street map may be missing streets or attribute data. When geocoding addresses, ArcMap provides a report that gives the number of matched addresses that result in points on the map, as well as the number of unmatched addresses. It is often possible to improve the match rate by using the ArcMap interactive rematching interface and making the corrections, record by record.

Typically, given good input data, you can expect about an 85 percent match rate in urban areas, without any rematching. The range of successfully matched addresses, however, is quite high, typically from 50 percent to 99 percent, depending on both the quality of the input address data and of the street maps used. Street maps from commercial vendors generally provide better address match rates than the free TIGER/Line maps.

For this study, the competitor hospitals need to be located on your map as points, so you plan to geocode hospital data to a street network. The number of hospitals is relatively low, so the manual steps needed to correct nonmatching addresses will not be very time consuming. Your goal is to geocode all the hospitals.

In some cases, you will not need, or even want, very fine detail, such as for estimating demand patterns and protecting the privacy of data. Geocoding to ZIP Code polygons, as you will do in the next tutorial, may be sufficient. Generally, tabular ZIP Code data is accurate, so you can expect match rates in the 90th percentile by placing points at ZIP Code centroids. Although you could geocode patient residences to the street network, you decide that ZIP Code counts of patients will be sufficiently detailed for studying location patterns, especially over a tri-state region.

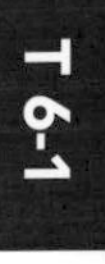

Polygon address matching

Tutorial 6-1
Geocoding patients to ZIP Codes

Suppose you have a table that contains the addresses of patients and their ZIP Codes. Using the ArcMap geocoding program, you can create a point layer from the ZIP Code list. The point features use the centers, or centroids, of ZIP Code polygons. The data you will use in this section contains fictitious ZIP Code locations that are analogous to actual locations for individual patients in a hospital.

Open an existing map

You will begin by opening the map document Tutorial6-1.mxd, which contains polygon features of ZIP Codes for three US states: Pennsylvania, Ohio, and West Virginia. This is a region where most patients for a western Pennsylvania hospital are clustered.

1 **Start ArcMap and open Tutorial6-1.mxd.** The map opens with US state and ZIP Code boundaries for the tri-state area.

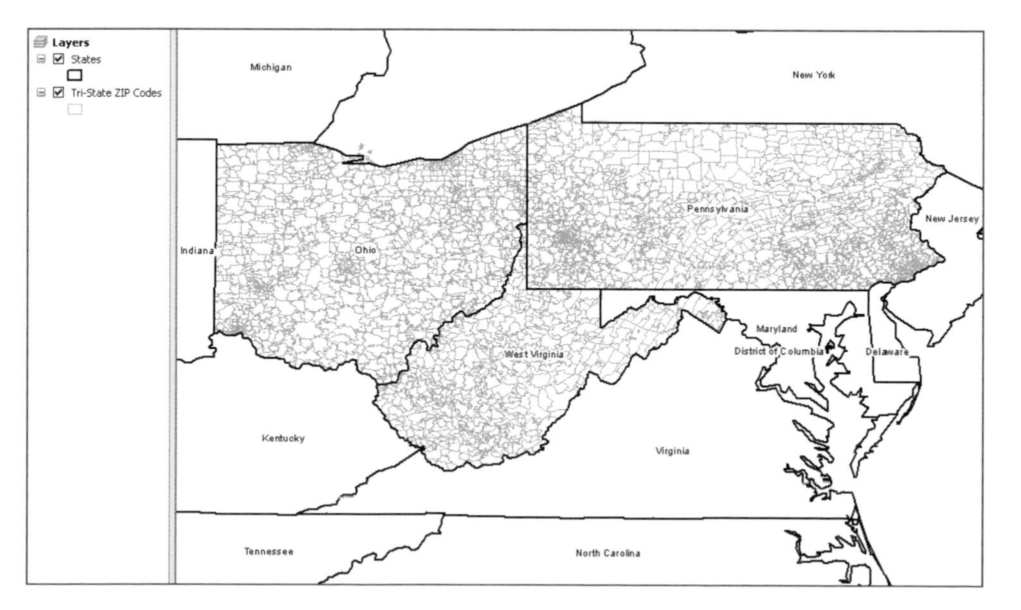

Add a patient database and open the attribute table

The input data is a table of patients by ZIP Code. You will geocode this to a reference layer, ZIP Code polygons. For now, you will open the input table and observe its attributes.

1 **On the Standard toolbar, click Add Data, browse through the Data folder to SiteSelection.gdb, and click Patients. Then click Add.**

2 **In the table of contents, right-click Patients and click Open.** The table lists ZIP Codes for each patient. ▶

Patients

OBJECTID *	SeqNum	ZipCode
1	1	15219
2	2	16123
3	3	15019
4	4	15227
5	5	15668
6	6	26055

18

(0 out of 9251 Selected)

3 **Close the table.**

Create a file geodatabase

1 **On the Standard toolbar, click the Catalog window button.**

2 **In the Catalog window, right-click your Chapter6 folder in MyExercises and click New > File Geodatabase.**

3 **Change the geodatabase name to** Chapter6.gdb.

Build an address locator for ZIP Codes

Before you can geocode the patient locations, you have to tell ArcMap which data is the reference data (ZIP Code polygons), and then define a set of parameters to tell it how to read the input data table (Patients). This is done by creating an address locator, which is a stored set of specifications for carrying out the geocoding process. After you create and store an address locator, you can reuse it in other geocoding projects.

1 **Right-click Chapter6.gdb and click New > Address Locator.**

2 **In the Create Address Locator dialog box, click the Browse button for Address Locator Style, and in the Select Address Locator Style dialog box, scroll down, click US Address - ZIP 5-Digit, and click OK.** ▶

Ignore the error message that appears at the top of the dialog box. The warning disappears once you fill in the reference data information in the next step.

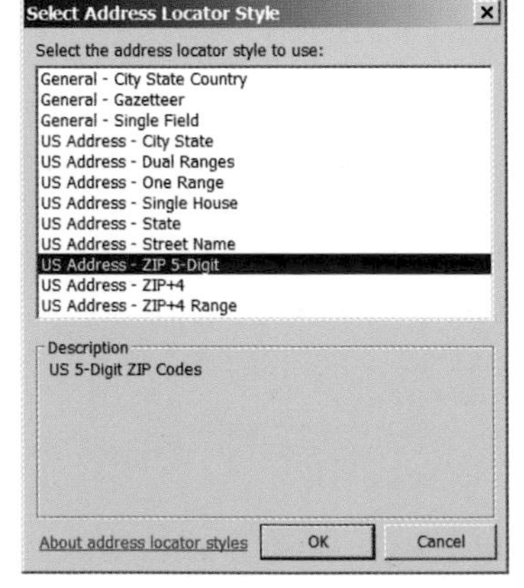

3 **Click the Reference Data arrow and click Tri-State ZIP Codes.**

4 **For Output Address Locator, click the Browse button, double-click Chapter6.gdb, type** TriStateZIPCodes **for Name, and click Save.**

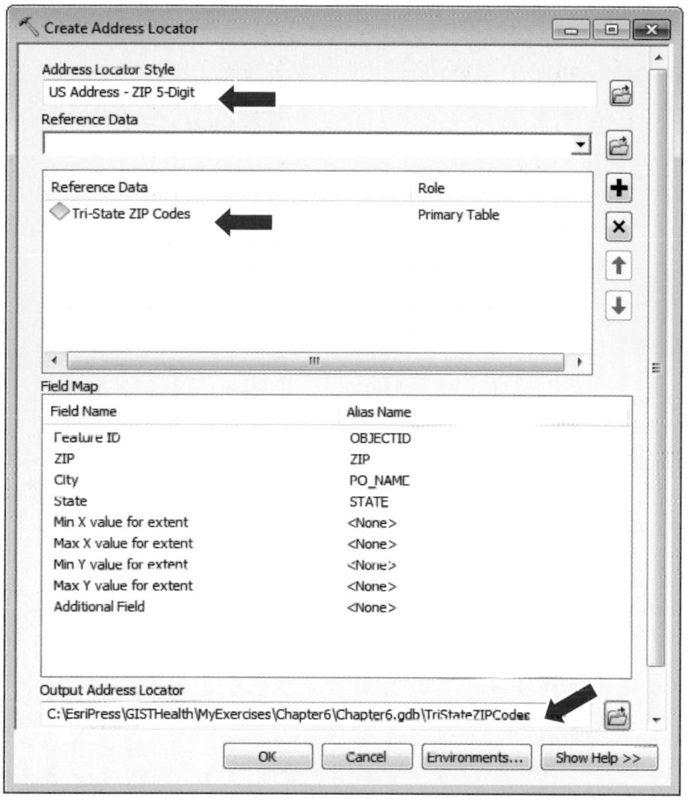

5 **Click OK and wait until Catalog informs you that the address locator is created.** The TriStateZIPCodes address locator appears as an address locator under an expanded Chapter6.gdb in the Catalog panel.

6 **Close the Catalog window.**

Geocode patients by ZIP Code

1 **On the ArcMap Menu bar, click Customize > Toolbars > Geocoding.** The Geocoding toolbar appears.

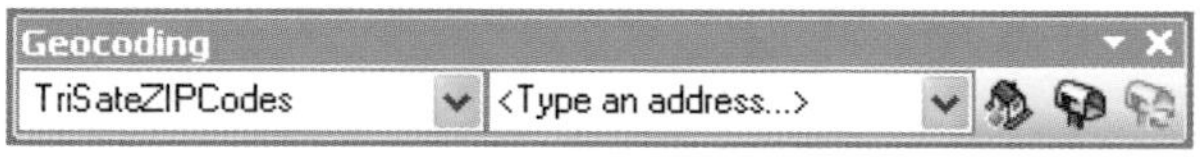

2 **On the Geocoding toolbar, click the Geocode Addresses button, click TriStateZIPCodes to select it, and click OK.**

3 **In the Geocode Addresses: TriStateZipCodes dialog box, for "Address table," click Patients; under Address Input Fields, click the ZIPCode arrow and click ZipCode; and for "Output shapefile or feature class," click the Browse button, double-click Chapter6.gdb, type** GeocodedPatients **for Name, and click Save.** ▶

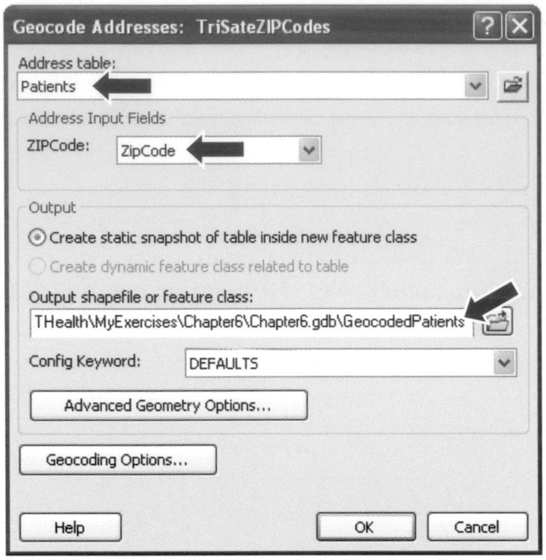

4 **In the dialog box, click Geocoding Options, and under Output Fields at the bottom, select the "X and Y coordinates" check box and click OK.** Selecting this option adds x,y coordinates to the attribute table, making the resulting data useful in other application software. ▶

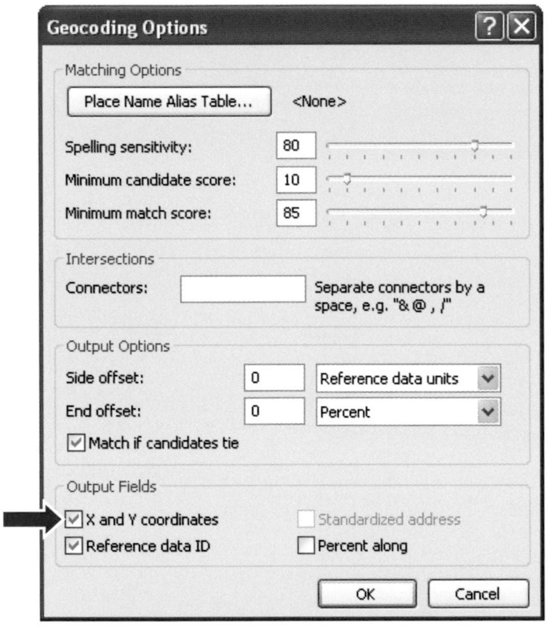

5 **Click OK again.** ArcMap geocodes the addresses by ZIP Code, which results in 8,457 of the records (91 percent) matched and 794 of the records (9 percent) unmatched. This is a very good match rate. Your result may vary slightly from these numbers and percentages depending on the software version used. ▶

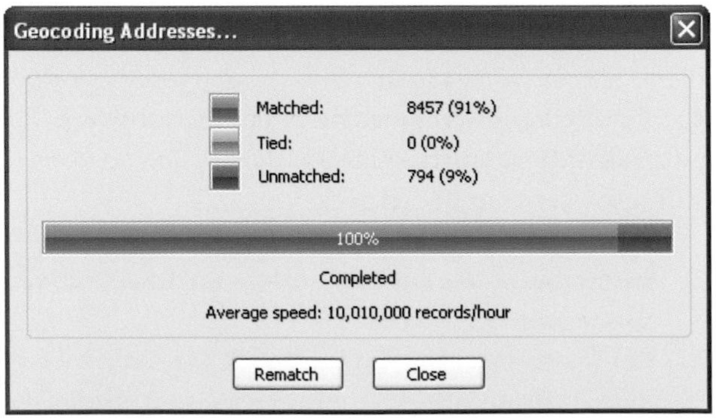

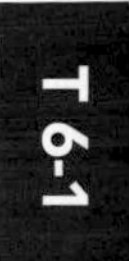

6 **Click Close.** ArcMap adds the geocoding results to the map using point markers at the centroids of ZIP Codes that have one or more patients.

7 **In the table of contents, click the List By Drawing Order button.**

8 **Right-click Geocoding Result: Geocoded Patients and click Zoom To Layer.** As you might expect, patient locations are clustered around southwestern Pennsylvania near the location of the hospital, but patients also come from other areas of Pennsylvania as well as the other two states in your study, Ohio and West Virginia. Notice that some patients travel quite a distance to the hospital in Pittsburgh. Because hospital administrators are focusing on a new regional site, you will focus only on patients in western Pennsylvania.

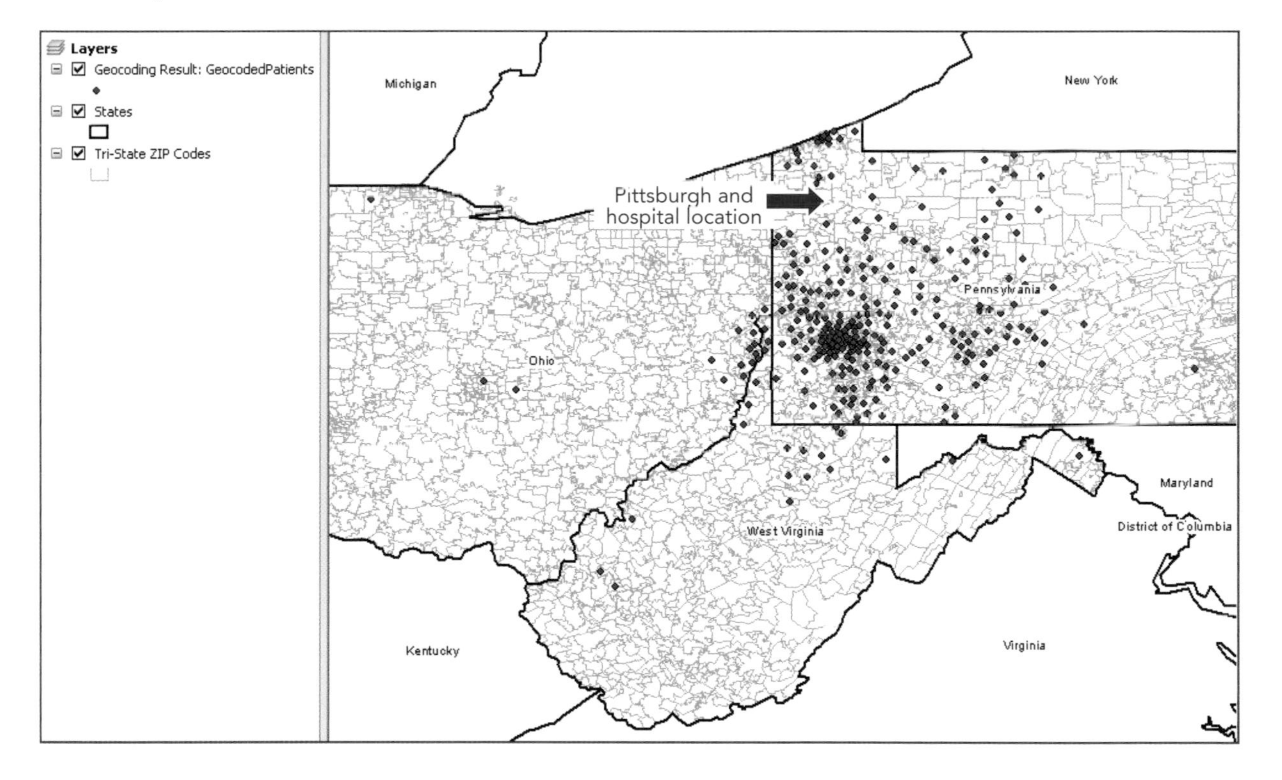

Check unmatched patients

Records that did not match likely contained incorrect ZIP Code values, or else ArcMap could not find matching records in the ZipCodes layer. These could be patients outside the tri-state study area. The attribute table of GeocodedPatients will show the unmatched patients.

1 **In the table of contents, right-click the GeocodedPatients layer and click Open Attribute Table.**

2 **Right-click the Status field and click Sort Descending.** The status will be "U" for unmatched. Scroll to the right to see the ZIP Codes that did not match. Because this is a high match rate and fine for the purpose of site selection, you will not rematch any of the unmatched records in this exercise.

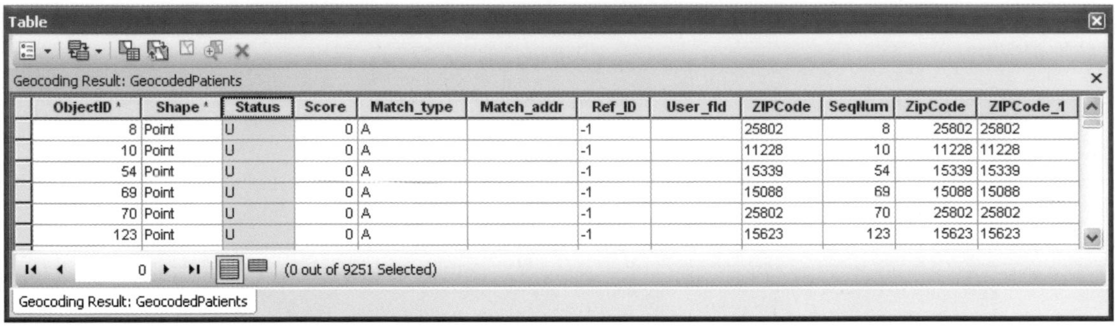

Table

Geocoding Result: GeocodedPatients

ObjectID *	Shape *	Status	Score	Match_type	Match_addr	Ref_ID	User_fld	ZIPCode	SeqNum	ZipCode	ZIPCode_1
8	Point	U	0	A		-1		25802	8	25802	25802
10	Point	U	0	A		-1		11228	10	11228	11228
54	Point	U	0	A		-1		15339	54	15339	15339
69	Point	U	0	A		-1		15088	69	15088	15088
70	Point	U	0	A		-1		25802	70	25802	25802
123	Point	U	0	A		-1		15623	123	15623	15623

0 (0 out of 9251 Selected)

Geocoding Result: GeocodedPatients

3 **Close the GeocodedPatients table.**

Save the map document

1 **On the File menu, click Save As.**

2 **Save your map document as** Tutorial6-1YourName.mxd **to your Chapter6 folder in MyExercises.** Do not close ArcMap.

Tutorial 6-2

Spatially joining patient and ZIP Code layers

A map that shows ZIP Code centroids is misleading because several patients could be at the same point, yet the points themselves do not indicate that. A better way to visualize patients is to create a graduated-point or choropleth map that displays the number of patients by ZIP Code. To spatially process the map, you can count patients by ZIP Code using a process known as a spatial join. In this tutorial, you will spatially join the patient points to ZIP Codes in Ohio, Pennsylvania, and West Virginia. This will give hospital administrators a good idea of the location patterns for regional patients.

Spatially join points to polygons

1 **In the table of contents, right-click the Tri-State ZIP Codes layer and click Joins and Relates > Join.**

2 **Click the "What do you want to join to this layer?" arrow and click "Join data from another layer based on spatial location."**

3 **For step 1 of the Join Data dialog box in the drop-down list, click GeocodedPatients.**

4 **Accept the default settings for step 2. For step 3, name the output** TriStatePatients **and save it to Chapter6.gdb.** ▶

5 **Click OK.** The output is a new polygon feature class containing ZIP Code boundaries and attributes for a count of patients by ZIP Code.

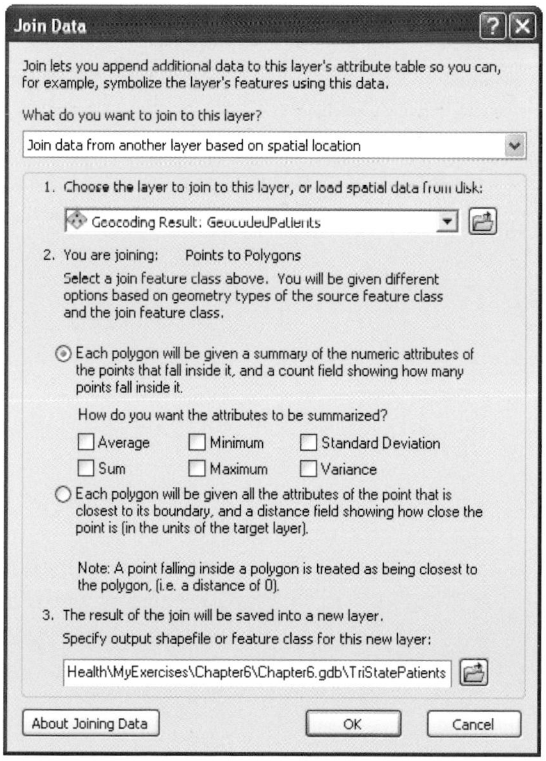

Join Data

Join lets you append additional data to this layer's attribute table so you can, for example, symbolize the layer's features using this data.

What do you want to join to this layer?

Join data from another layer based on spatial location

1. Choose the layer to join to this layer, or load spatial data from disk:

Geocoding Result: GeocodedPatients

2. You are joining: Points to Polygons

Select a join feature class above. You will be given different options based on geometry types of the source feature class and the join feature class.

Each polygon will be given a summary of the numeric attributes of the points that fall inside it, and a count field showing how many points fall inside it.

How do you want the attributes to be summarized?

Average Minimum Standard Deviation

Sum Maximum Variance

Each polygon will be given all the attributes of the point that is closest to its boundary, and a distance field showing how close the point is (in the units of the target layer).

Note: A point falling inside a polygon is treated as being closest to the polygon, (i.e. a distance of 0).

3. The result of the join will be saved into a new layer.

Specify output shapefile or feature class for this new layer:

Health\MyExercises\Chapter6\Chapter6.gdb\TriStatePatients

About Joining Data OK Cancel

6 **Open the TriStatePatients attribute table and note that ArcMap added a count field that has the number of patients in each ZIP Code.** Some ZIP Codes have a null value, meaning that no patients were located in that ZIP Code.

TriStatePatients

ObjectID	ZIP	PO_NAME	STATE	SUMBLKPOP	POP2004	POP04_SQMI	SQMI	Count_	Shape_Length	Shape_Area
4125	15001	ALIQUIPPA	PA	35954	35189	591.7	59.46	90	0.849248	0.016386
4126	15003	AMBRIDGE	PA	12907	12501	1935	6.46	82	0.216508	0.001779
4127	15005	BADEN	PA	9343	9451	624.2	15.14	97	0.538926	0.004174
4128	15007	BAKERSTOWN	PA	229	245	844.7	0.28	<Null>	0.044535	0.00008
4129	15009	BEAVER	PA	14933	14674	680.6	21.55	1	0.390381	0.005949
4130	15010	BEAVER FALLS	PA	29728	29293	565.2	51.82	62	0.866791	0.014318
4131	15012	BELLE VERNON	PA	17631	17839	479.3	37.21	58	0.647455	0.010189
4132	15014	BRACKENRIDGE	PA	3514	3390	6163.6	0.55	<Null>	0.050298	0.000151

1 (0 out of 3079 Selected)

7 **Close the attribute table.**

Save the map document

1 **On the File menu, click Save As.**

2 **Save your map document as** Tutorial6-2YourName.mxd **to your Chapter6 folder in MyExercises.** Do not close ArcMap.

Tutorial 6-3

Creating a choropleth map showing patient counts by ZIP Code

You can now create a choropleth map based on the patient counts in each ZIP Code.

1 **Turn off the GeocodedPatients layer.**

2 **Right-click the new TriStatePatients layer and click Properties.**

3 **Click the Symbology tab, and in the Show panel, click Quantities > Graduated Colors. Under Fields for Value, click Count_.**

4 **Use four classes that are of equal interval and a gray color ramp.**

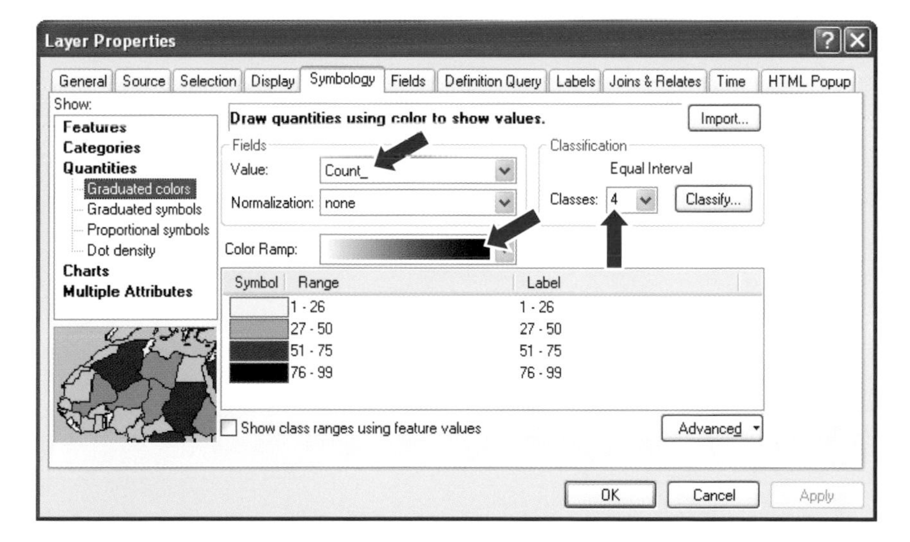

5 **Click OK.**

6 **Add the USCounties layer from UnitedStates.gdb in the Data folder to your map. If a Geographic Coordinate Systems warning appears, close it. Symbolize the layer using a Hollow fill and dark-blue outline of width 1.15.**

7 **Zoom to southwestern Pennsylvania as shown in the figure.** You can now see clearly where most of the health-care organization's patients are clustered.

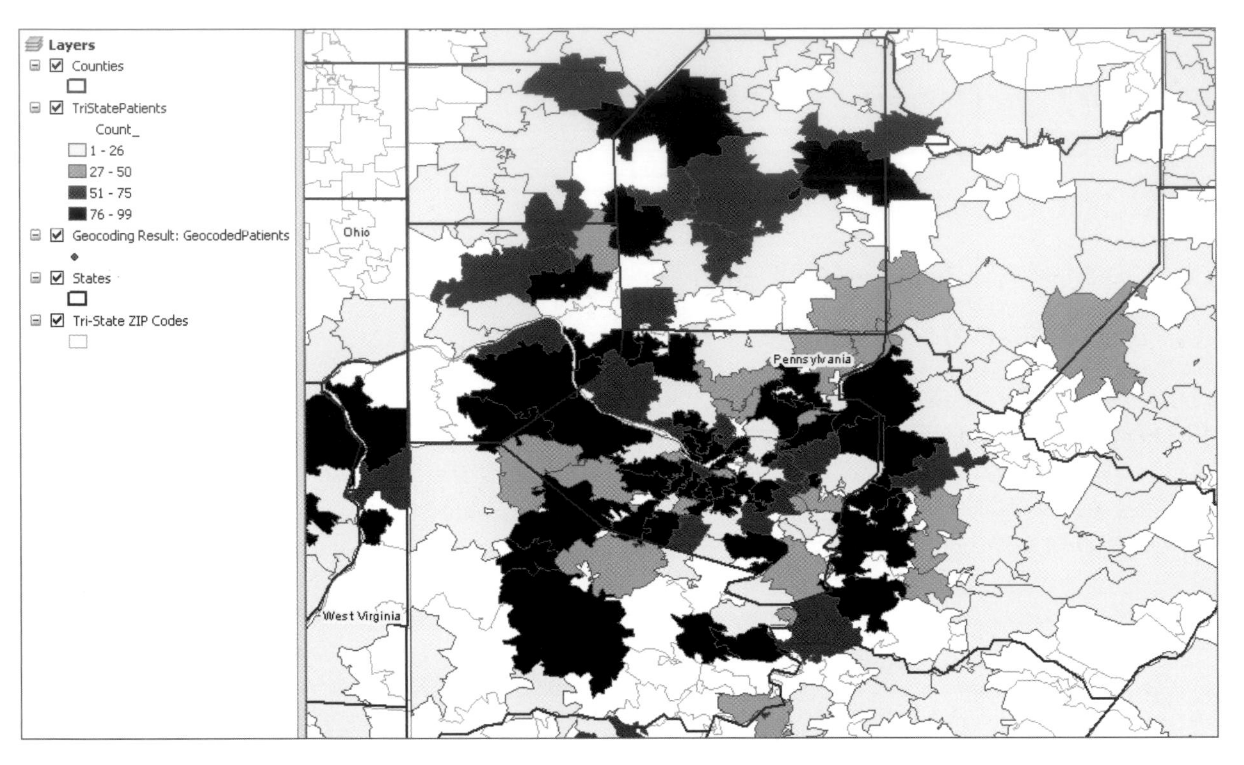

YOUR TURN

Add and symbolize two additional layers:

- \EsriPress\GISTHealth\Data\UnitedStates.gdb\USCities
- \EsriPress\GISTHealth\Data\UnitedStates.gdb\USInterstates

Label the cities using a nice halo label. Zoom to Allegheny County, Pennsylvania. Based on the number of patients and their proximity to interstates, in what city or cities would you recommend opening satellite clinics?

Save the map document

1 **On the File menu, click Save As.**

2 **Save your map document as** Tutorial6-3YourName.mxd **to your Chapter6 folder in MyExercises.** Do not close ArcMap.

Linear address matching

Tutorial 6-4

Geocoding hospital addresses to streets for competitive analysis

In this tutorial, you will address match the locations of existing hospitals to Allegheny County streets. The streets used here are Census 2000 TIGER/Line street centerlines. Esri StreetMap Premium for ArcGIS 10.2, which comes with ArcGIS 10.2, is another good resource for street centerlines, especially if you are geocoding across multiple counties or states.

Begin a new health-care map

1 Start ArcMap using a new empty map. If ArcMap is already open, on the Standard toolbar, click the New (Create a new map document) button, Select a Blank Map and click OK.

Add a Streets layer

The Streets layer is the reference layer to which you will match hospital addresses.

1 On the Standard toolbar, click Add Data, browse through the Data folder to SiteSelection.gdb, and double-click Streets. This step adds the street centerlines feature class for Allegheny County using Pennsylvania south state plane coordinates. This map layer has over 80,000 block-long street segments.

2 Symbolize streets using a light-brown hue.

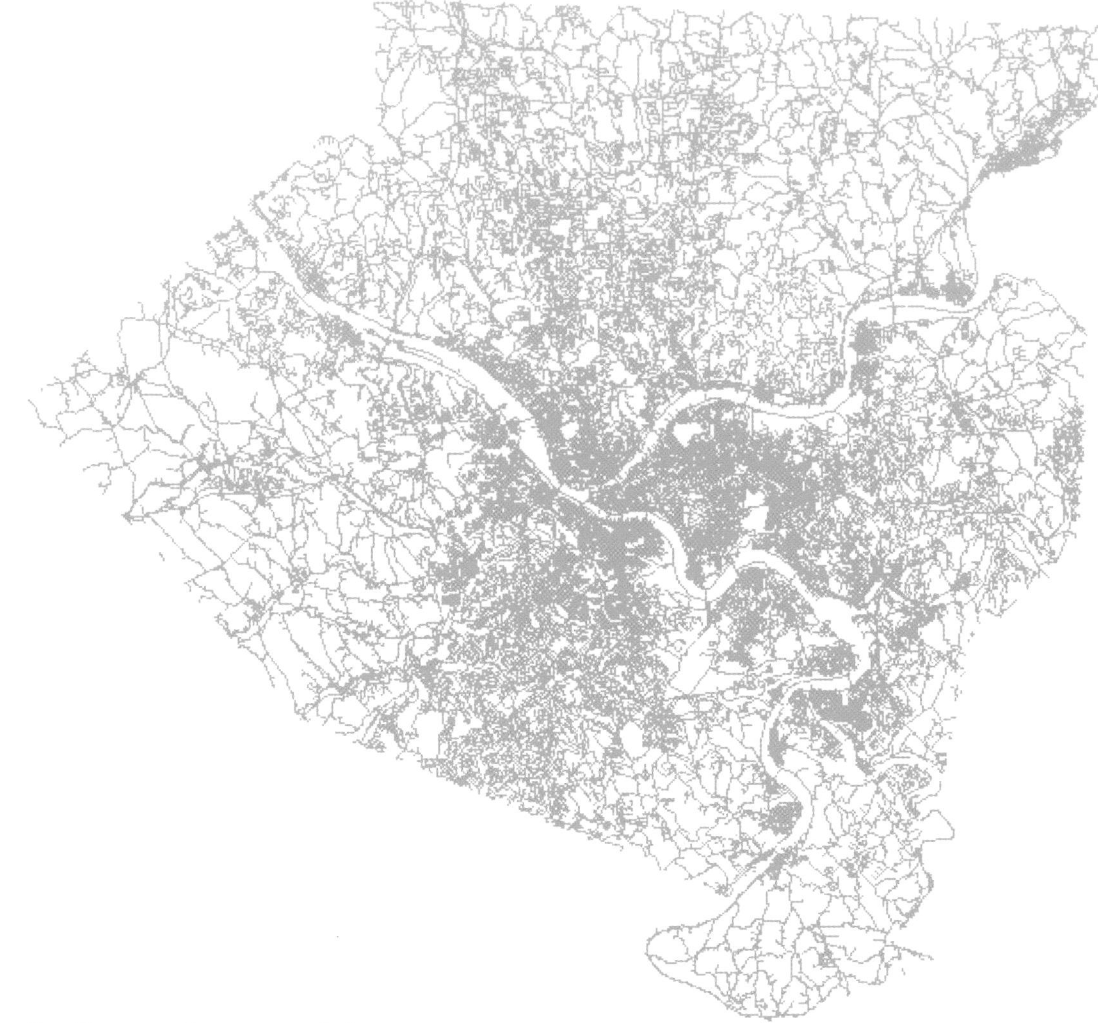

3 Zoom to the center of the map.

4 Using the Identify tool on the Tools toolbar, click a line segment and note the fields listed for each line segment. The fields used in address matching include FENAME (street name), FETYPE (street type), FRADDL (from address left), TOADDL (to address left), FRADDR (from address right), TOADDR (to address right), and ZIPL and ZIPR (ZIP Codes). (See facing page.)

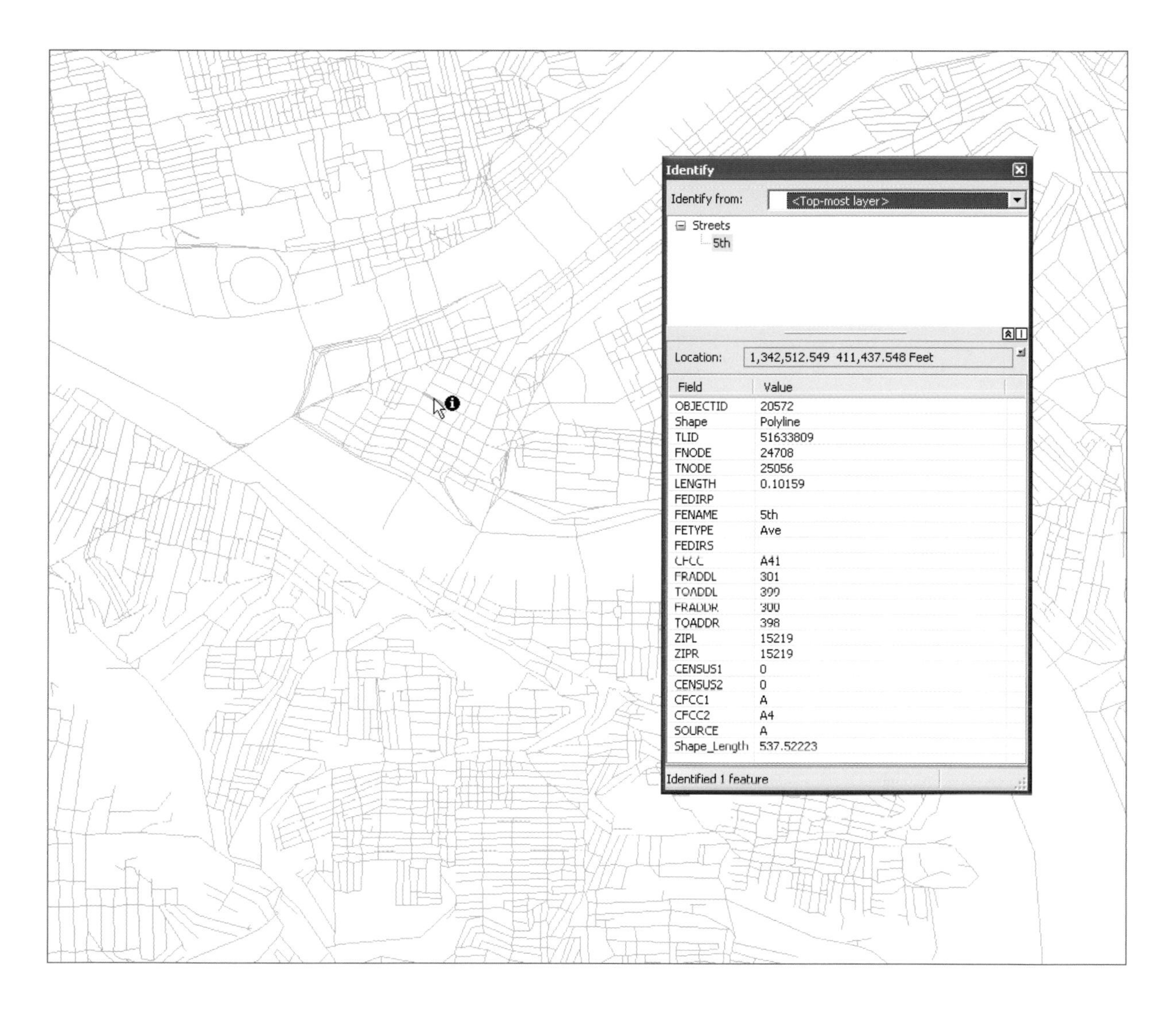

5 Close the Identify window and zoom to the full map extent.

Add the hospital database

The hospital database is the input database you will use to create point features for each hospital address.

1 On the Standard toolbar, click Add Data, browse through the Data folder to SiteSelection.gdb, and double-click Hospitals. This is a database of hospitals located in Allegheny County.

2 **In the table of contents, right-click Hospitals and click Open.** The attribute table lists hospital names, street addresses, ZIP Codes, and the number of beds for each hospital. The address locator will use the ADDRESS and ZIPCODE fields to geocode each record.

Hospitals

OBJECTID *	NAME	ADDRESS	ZIPCODE	BEDS
1	Allegheny General Hospital	320 East North Avenue	15212	420
2	Children's Home of Pittsburgh	5618 Kentucky Avenue	15232	11
3	Children's Hospital Of Pittsburgh	4401 Penn Ave	15224	296
4	Children's Institute of Pittsburgh	6301 Northumberland Street	15217	39
5	Jefferson Regional Medical Center	565 Coal Valley Road	15236	343
6	LifeCare Hospitals of Pittsburgh	225 Penn Avenue	15221	107
7	Magee-Womens Hospital of UPMC	3324 Forbes Ave	15213	202
8	Mercy Hospital Of Pittsburgh	14001 Blvd of the Allies	15111	448
9	Mercy Hospital Of Pittsburgh	1400 Locust Street	15219	448
10	Mercy Hospital-North Shore Campus	1004 Arch Street	15212	132
11	Select Specialty Hospital	200 Lothrop Street	15213	41
12	Southwood Psychiatric Hospital	2575 Boyce Plaza Road	15241	102
13	St. Clair Memorial Hospital	1000 Bower Hill Road	15243	290
14	UPMC Passavant	9100 Babcock Boulevard	15237	258
15	UPMC Presbyterian	200 Lothrop Street	15213	1320
16	UPMC Shadyside	5230 Centre Avenue	15232	486
17	UPMC South Side	2000 Mary Street	15203	136
18	UPMC St. Margaret	815 Freeport Road	15215	198
19	Va Medical Center	3850 O Hara St	15213	146
20	Veterans Affairs Pittsburgh Healthcare System	Delafield Road	15260	692
21	West Penn Hospital	4800 Friendship Ave	15224	457

1 (0 out of 21 Selected)

3 **Close the Hospitals table.**

Build an address locator for streets

The steps used to set up the address locator for streets are the same as the ones used in tutorial 6-1 for ZIP Codes, but some of the parameters differ because you are geocoding at the street level.

1 **Click the Catalog window button.**

2 **In the Catalog window, browse to Chapter6.gdb.**

3 **Right-click Chapter6.gdb and click New > Address Locator.**

4 **In the Create Address Locator dialog box, click the Browse button for Address Locator Style, and in the Select Address Locator Style dialog box, scroll down, click US Address - Dual Ranges, and click OK.**

Ignore the error message that appears at the top of the dialog box. The warning disappears once you fill in the reference data information in the next step.

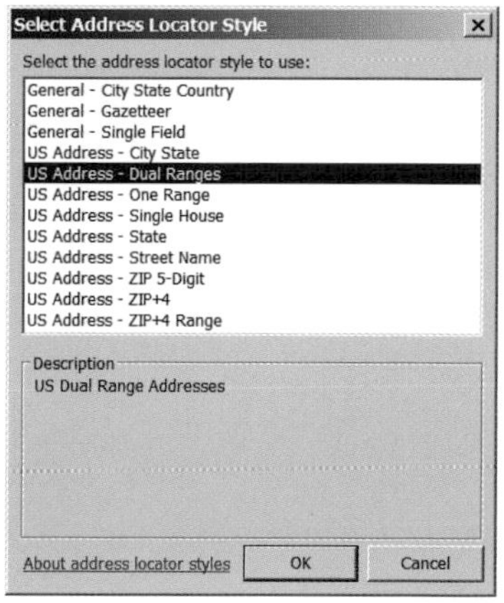

Select Address Locator Style

Select the address locator style to use:

General - City State Country
General - Gazetteer
General - Single Field
US Address - City State
US Address - Dual Ranges
US Address - One Range
US Address - Single House
US Address - State
US Address - Street Name
US Address - ZIP 5-Digit
US Address - ZIP+4
US Address - ZIP+4 Range

Description
US Dual Range Addresses

About address locator styles | OK | Cancel

T 6-4

5 Click the Reference Data arrow and click Streets.

6 For Output Address Locator, click the Browse button, double-click Chapter6.gdb, type AlleghenyCountyStreets **for Name, and click Save and then OK. Wait until Catalog informs you that the address locator is created.**

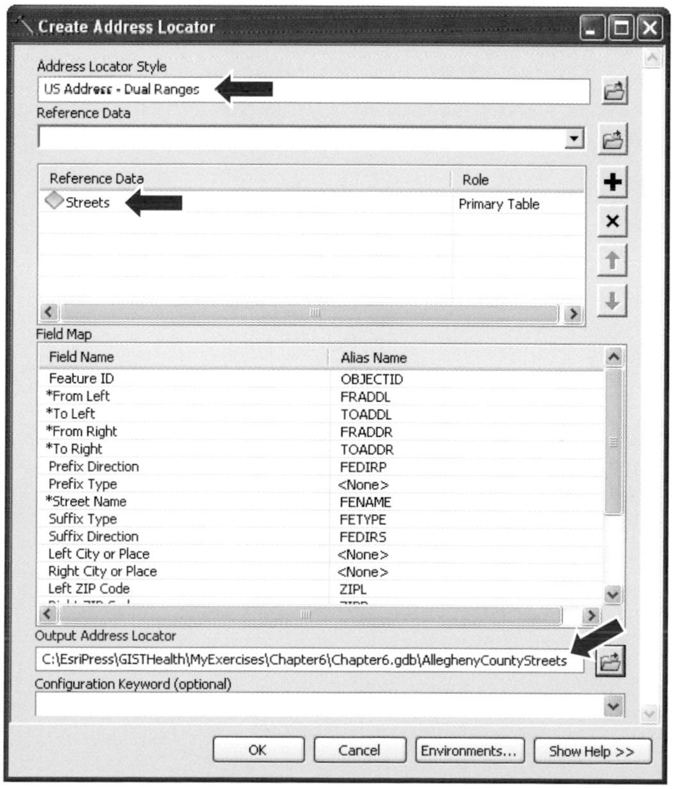

Create Address Locator

Address Locator Style
US Address - Dual Ranges

Reference Data

Reference Data	Role
Streets	Primary Table

Field Map

Field Name	Alias Name
Feature ID	OBJECTID
*From Left	FRADDL
*To Left	TOADDL
*From Right	FRADDR
*To Right	TOADDR
Prefix Direction	FEDIRP
Prefix Type	<None>
*Street Name	FENAME
Suffix Type	FETYPE
Suffix Direction	FEDIRS
Left City or Place	<None>
Right City or Place	<None>
Left ZIP Code	ZIPL

Output Address Locator
C:\EsriPress\GISTHealth\MyExercises\Chapter6\Chapter6.gdb\AlleghenyCountyStreets

Configuration Keyword (optional)

OK | Cancel | Environments... | Show Help >>

7 Close Catalog.

Geocode hospitals to streets

1 **In the table of contents, right-click Hospitals and click Geocode Addresses.** This step is an alternative to using the Geocoding toolbar. ▶

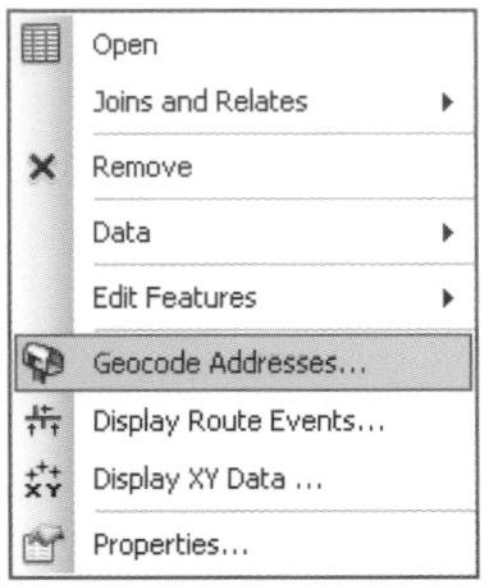

2 **Click AlleghenyCountyStreets as the address locator and click OK.** ▶

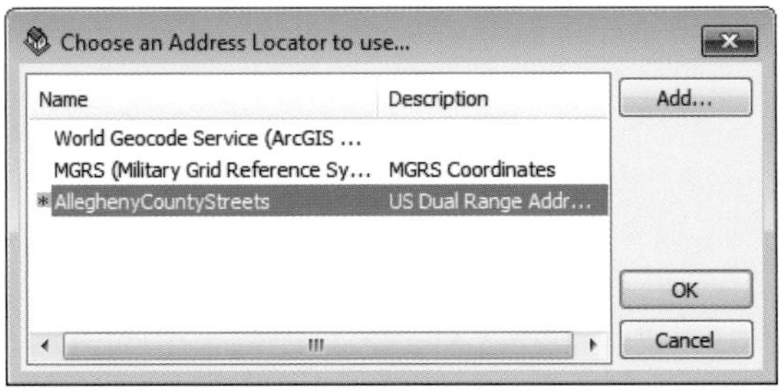

3 **Check that Hospitals is selected for "Address table"; under Address Input Fields, click ADDRESS for the Street or Intersection field and click ZIPCODE for the ZIP Code field. Change the name of the output to** GeocodedHospitals **and save it to Chapter6.gdb.** ▶

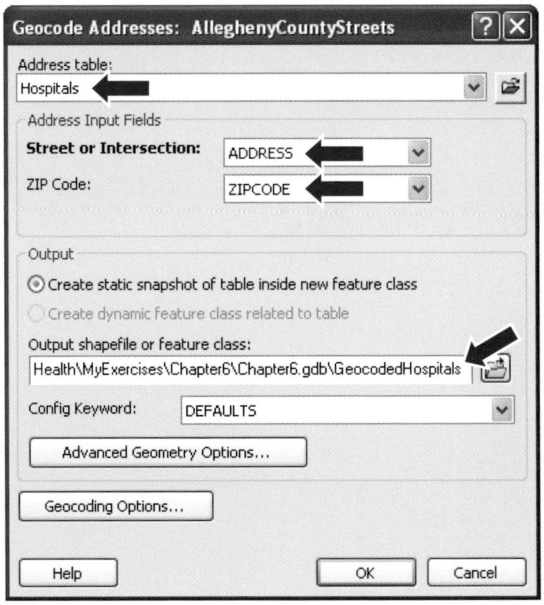

4 In the dialog box, click Geocoding Options. In the Geocoding Options dialog box, select the "X and Y coordinates" check box and click OK. Notice that the side offset is 20 ft. This offset places each hospital on the correct side of the street centerline. ▶

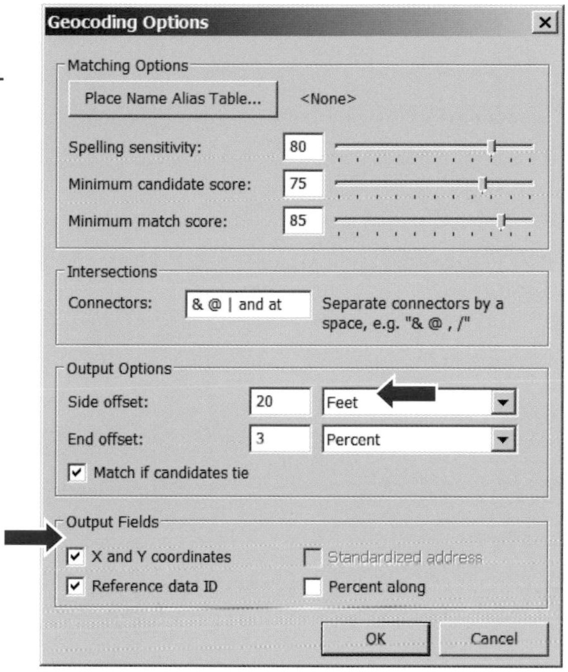

5 Click OK again. ArcMap geocodes the addresses by ZIP Code with 16 (76 percent) of the records matched and 5 (24 percent) of records unmatched. Your result may vary slightly from these numbers and percentages depending on the software version used. ▶

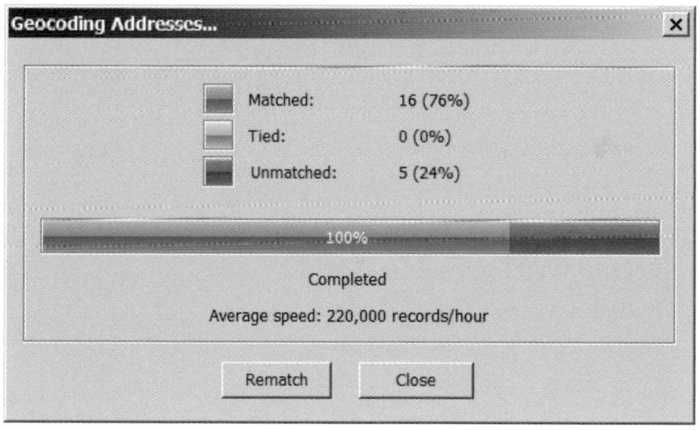

6 Click Close. ArcMap adds the geocoding results to the map, placing the point markers for each hospital offset along street centerlines.

7 In the table of contents, click List By Drawing Order.

The map shows the hospitals that are a successful match. Matched points appear offset 20 ft along the street centerlines where hospitals are located in Allegheny County. In the next exercise, you will investigate why some addresses did not match.

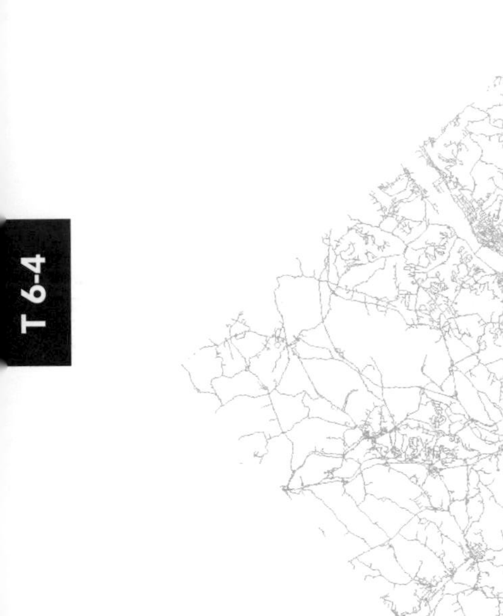

Check unmatched hospitals

1 In the table of contents, right-click the Geocoding Result: GeocodedHospitals layer and click Open Attribute Table.

2 Right-click the Status field and click Sort Descending. The three hospitals that did not match are listed as U (unmatched). You might have more or fewer unmatched addresses, depending on the software version you are using. The Score column indicates whether an address completely matched (100) or matched but not completely (95). Also note that the x,y coordinates are state plane. This is because the street centerline map is in state plane coordinates.

Geocoding Result: GeocodedHospitals

FID	Shape	Status	Score	Match_type	Match_addr	Side	Ref_ID	X	Y	User_fld	Addr_type	ARC_Street	ARC_ZIP	NAME
4	Point	U	0	A			-1	0	0			565 Coal Valley Road	15236	Jefferson Regional Medical Center
7	Point	U	0	A			-1	0	0			14001 Blvd of the Allies	15111	Mercy Hospital Of Pittsburgh
13	Point	U	0	A			-1	0	0			9100 Babcock Boulevard	15237	UPMC Passavant
18	Point	U	0	A			-1	0	0			3850 O Hara St	15213	Va Medical Center
19	Point	U	0	A			-1	0	0			Delafield Road	15260	Veterans Affairs Pittsburgh Healthcare System
0	Point	M	100	A	320 E North Ave, 15212	L	15245	1341489.572238	417062.806002	0	StreetAddress	320 East North Avenue	15212	Allegheny General Hospital
1	Point	M	100	A	5618 Kentucky Ave, 15232	R	29922	1361519.374006	414397.879241	0	StreetAddress	5618 Kentucky Avenue	15232	Children's Home of Pittsburgh

3 Close the table.

Save the map document

1 On the File menu, click Save As.

2 Save your map document as Tutorial6-4YourName.mxd **to your Chapter6 folder in MyExercises.** Do not close ArcMap.

Tutorial 6-5
Rematching addresses

Unmatched records are the result of errors in either the reference data or the input data. To match records that didn't match, you'll need to do some cleanup work. This is common for the geocoding process. The ability to make corrections to the address data depends on the user's knowledge of local streets and addresses. One approach is to change the settings of the Address Locator in batch mode, the initial process for matching addresses all at once, and then rerun the process. Another approach is to use an interactive rematching interface where you can examine and fix unmatched records case by case. In this tutorial, you will use the ArcMap interactive review process to correct and then match a few of the unmatched records.

Interactively rematch an address

1 **In the table of contents, click Geocoding Result: Geocoded Hospitals to select that layer.**

2 **If the toolbar is not already open, on the Menu bar, click Customize > Toolbars > Geocoding.**

3 **On the Geocoding toolbar, click the Review/Rematch Addresses button** . You can increase the width of the address statistics panel by pressing ALT+2.

4 **In the Interactive Rematch - GeocodedHospitals dialog box, click the "Show results" arrow and click Unmatched Addresses. Scroll horizontally across the fields so you can see the Name, Address, and Zip_Code fields.** (See facing page.)

Interactive Rematch - GeocodedHospitals

Show results: Unmatched Addresses | Manage result sets... | Refresh | Rematch Automatically

Matched: 16 (76%)
Tied: 0 (0%)
Unmatched: 5 (24%)

NAME	ADDRESS	ZIPCODE	BEDS
Jefferson Regional Medical Center	565 Coal Valley Road	15236	343
Mercy Hospital Of Pittsburgh	14001 Blvd of the Allies	15111	448
UPMC Passavant	9100 Babcock Boulevard	15237	258
Va Medical Center	3850 O Hara St	15213	146

2 (of 5)

Address:
Street or Intersection 14001 BLVD OF T
ZIP Code 15111

0 Candidates

Score	Side	Match_addr	FromAddr	ToAddr	PreDir	PreType	StreetName	SufType

Candidate details:
FromAddr
ToAddr
PreDir
PreType
StreetName
SufType
SufDir
City
State
ZIP
Ref_ID
X
Y
User_fld
Addr_type
Score
Match_addr
Side

Geocoding Options... | Zoom to Candidates | Pick Address from Map | Search | Match | Unmatch | Save Edits | Close

5 **Click the record selector button on the left end of the record that contains the value 14001 Blvd of the Allies.** This address has two problems resulting in an unmatched score. The first is, the street number should be 1401. The second is, the Blvd of the Allies spans two ZIP Codes: 15219 and 15213.The data has the incorrect ZIP Code, 15111. The Interactive Rematch dialog box allows you to examine and repair these types of errors so that you can geocode the unmatched addresses for a better matching score.

6 **In the Street or Intersection box of the Address area, change 14001 to 1401.**

7 In the ZIP Code box of the Address area, type 15219 **and press ENTER.** As you make these settings, keep your eye on the Score field under "Candidate details" in the table of unmatched records. Once you apply the changes, the value for the selected record changes to 100, indicating that a perfect match has been made.

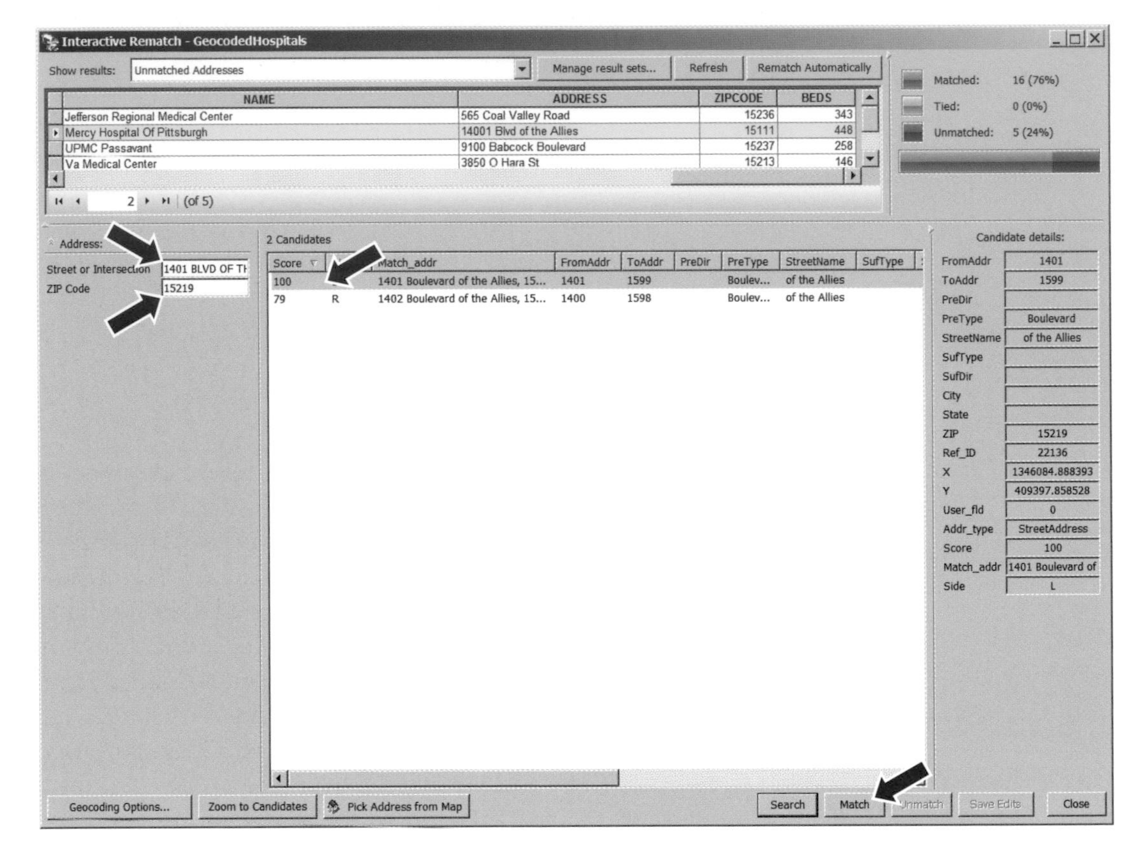

8 Select the candidate that has a score of 100 and click the Match button. ArcMap changes the status of the record to M (matched) and the score to 100 and adds the x,y coordinates of the address location.

Interactively rematch another address

1 In the Interactive Rematch - GeocodedHospitals dialog box, select the unmatched record for the "Va Medical Center" with an address of 3850 O Hara St. ArcMap shows a 79 percent match score, which is good enough for your purposes. (See facing page.)

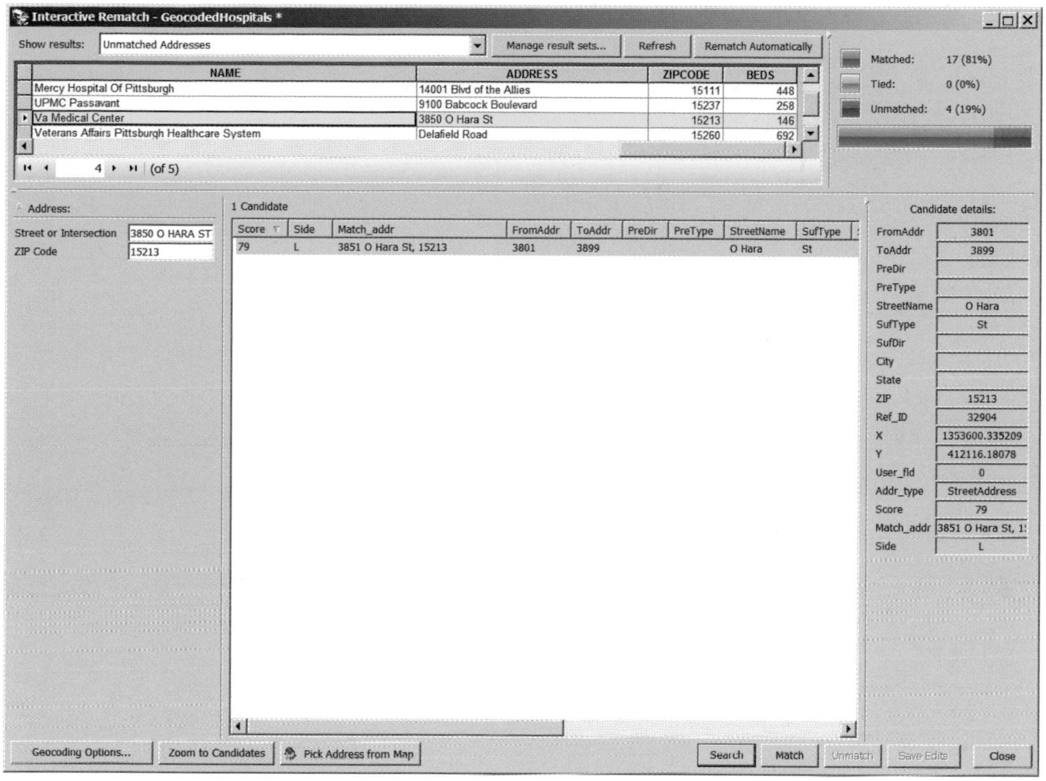

2 Click Match. ArcMap places a point on the map at O Hara Street and the address status changes to M (matched) in the attribute table.

The next address for another VA hospital is a bit more challenging. For this address, you will look at the map in the next exercise to see the problems and find solutions.

3 Close the Interactive Rematch dialog box.

Use street TIGER/Line maps to find addresses

In the previous exercise, you rematched a record that had an error in the input table (hospitals database). Sometimes errors are in the reference table (street centerlines). For example, TIGER/Line files may be missing values in the address range fields. If you don't see an obvious solution when rematching or if you are unfamiliar with the geographic region, you may need to look at the street map to help figure out what changes are needed. In this section, you will learn more about the unmatched address in question by looking at the Streets table.

1 On the Selection menu, click Select By Attributes.

2 **In the Select By Attributes dialog box, click the Layer arrow and click Streets. For Method, click "Create a new selection."**

3 **In the list of fields, double-click "FENAME", click the = button, press the SPACEBAR, and type** 'Delafield', **using single quotation marks. Click OK.** You will see Delafield selected on the map. ▶

4 **On the Selection menu, click Zoom To Selected Features.**

5 **Label Streets using the FENAME field.**

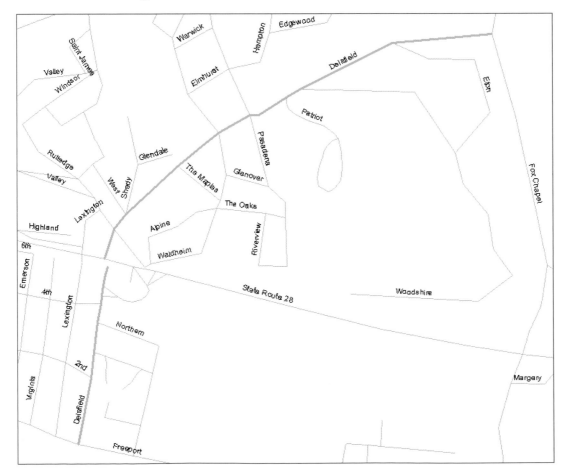

6 **In the table of contents, right-click Streets and click Open Attribute Table.**

7 **At the bottom of the Streets table, click the "Show selected records" button.**

8 **Scroll to the right in the table and notice the street ranges for Delafield Road, and the ZIP Code.** Notice that some of the "from" and "to" ranges for streets are missing, and the ZIP Code for the street segments is 15215.

OBJECTID *	Shape *	TLID	FNODE	TNODE	LENGTH	FEDIRP	FENAME	FETYPE	FEDIRS	CFCC	FRADDL	TOADDL	FRADDR	TOADDR	ZIPL	ZIPR	CENSUS1	CENSUS2	CFCC1	CFCC2	SOURCE	Shape_Length
30374	Polyline	51645813	44700	45464	0.18496		Delafield	Rd		A41	1051	1099	0	0	15215		0	0	A	A4	A	979.471217
31673	Polyline	51647389	42681	42730	0.05745		Delafield	Rd		A41	601	699	608	698	15215	15215	0	0	A	A4	A	303.150684
31675	Polyline	51647393	42680	42694	0.02137		Delafield	Ave		A41	601	699	600	698	15215	15215	0	0	A	A4	A	112.773958
31676	Polyline	51647394	42730	42793	0.0347		Delafield	Rd		A41	701	799	700	750	15215	15215	0	0	A	A4	A	183.332804
31680	Polyline	51647398	42793	43112	0.13036		Delafield	Rd		A41	801	805	752	798	15215	15215	0	0	A	A4	A	689.133289
31685	Polyline	51647404	43112	43350	0.09627		Delafield	Rd		A41	807	899	800	898	15215	15215	0	0	A	A4	A	509.020289
31689	Polyline	51647408	43350	43568	0.0673		Delafield	Rd		A41	901	999	900	998	15215	15215	0	0	A	A4	A	356.044463
31691	Polyline	51647410	43568	43632	0.01575		Delafield	Rd		A4	0	0	0	0			0	0	A	A4	A	83.433162
31706	Polyline	51647431	43632	43867	0.06		Delafield	Rd		A41	1001	1007	0	0	15215		0	0	A	A4	A	317.391385
31709	Polyline	51647435	43972	44700	0.19052		Delafield	Rd		A41	1009	1049	0	0	15215		0	0	A	A4	A	1008.10514
57493	Polyline	51683295	43867	43972	0.02708		Delafield	Rd		A41	0	0	0	0			0	0	A	A4	A	148.039922
71186	Polyline	51811463	42671	42680	0.01514		Delafield	Rd		A41	501	599	500	598	15215	15215	0	0	A	A4	A	79.884614
71187	Polyline	51811464	42670	42671	0.01945		Delafield	Rd		A41	401	499	400	498	15215	15215	0	0	A	A4	A	102.60969
71188	Polyline	51811465	42663	42670	0.01403		Delafield	Rd		A41	301	399	0	0	15215		0	0	A	A4	A	74.029779
71189	Polyline	51811466	42640	42663	0.03493		Delafield	Rd		A41	231	299	274	298	15215	15215	0	0	A	A4	A	184.26248
71190	Polyline	51811467	42610	42648	0.05574		Delafield	Rd		A41	225	229	236	272	15215	15215	0	0	A	A4	A	294.04477
71191	Polyline	51811468	42597	42610	0.04838		Delafield	Rd		A41	201	223	200	234	15215	15215	0	0	A	A4	A	255.232855
71192	Polyline	51811469	42507	42597	0.12607		Delafield	Rd		A41	101	199	100	198	15215	15215	0	0	A	A4	A	665.115461

(18 out of 81646 Selected)

9 **Close the Streets attribute table.** The street segment shown in the figure (between Patriot and Woodshire) is the segment that contains the VA hospital address (1010 Delafield Road).

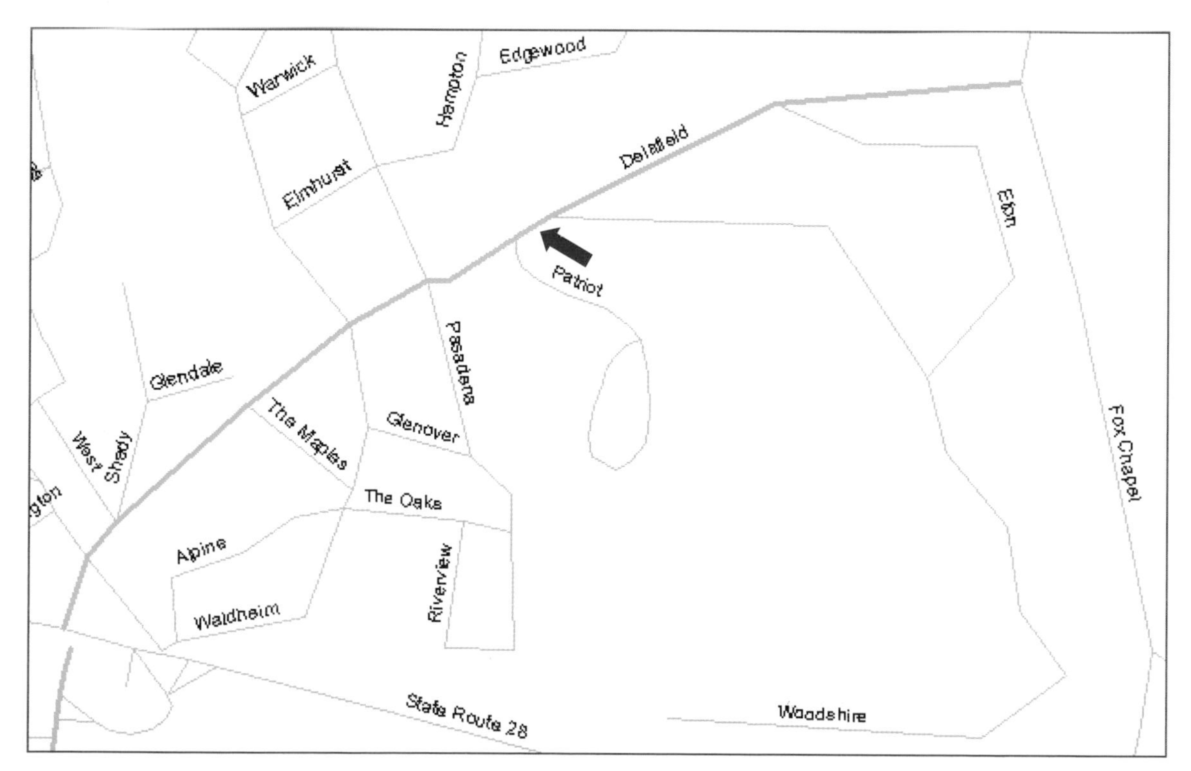

T 6-5

10 **Use the Identify tool to identify the records of this street segment. Close the Identify window when you are finished.** ▶

Identify

Identify from: <Top-most layer>

Streets selection
Delafield

Location: 1,373,229.807 431,314.645 Feet

Field	Value
OBJECTID	57493
Shape	Polyline
TLID	51683295
FNODE	43867
TNODE	43972
LENGTH	0.02799
FEDIRP	
FENAME	Delafield
FETYPE	Rd
FEDIRS	
CFCC	A41
FRADDL	0
TOADDL	0
FRADDR	0
TOADDR	0
ZIPL	
ZIPR	
CENSUS1	0
CENSUS2	0
CFCC1	A
CFCC2	A4
SOURCE	A

Identified 1 feature

Edit the street table

The “from” and “to” address fields are missing, so next, you will edit the attribute table to enter the missing segment information.

1 **Use the Clear Selected Features button to clear the selected features and use the Select Features tool on the Tools toolbar to select only the Delafield Road street segment between Patriot and Woodshire.**

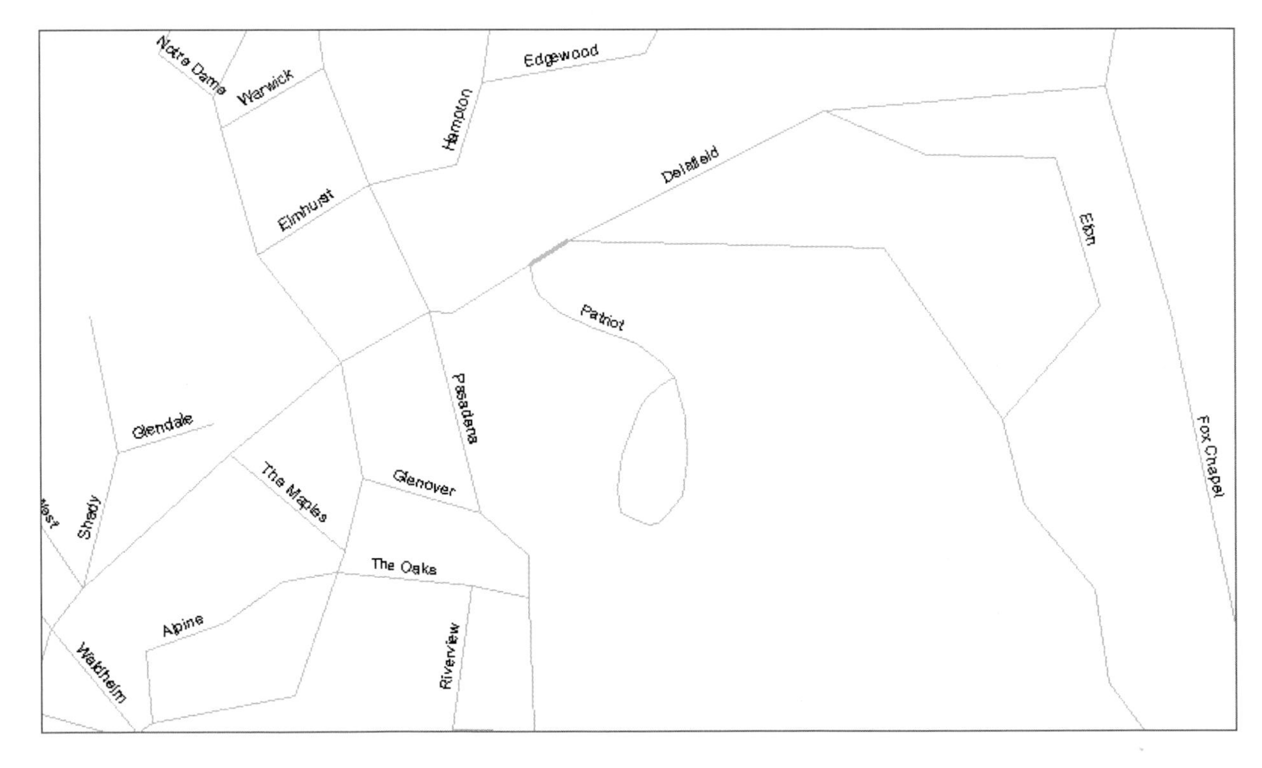

2 **In the table of contents, right-click Streets and click Open Attribute Table.**

3 **On the Customize menu, click Toolbars > Editor.**

4 **On the Editor toolbar, click Editor > Start Editing.**

5 **In the Start Editing window, click Streets and click OK.** ▶

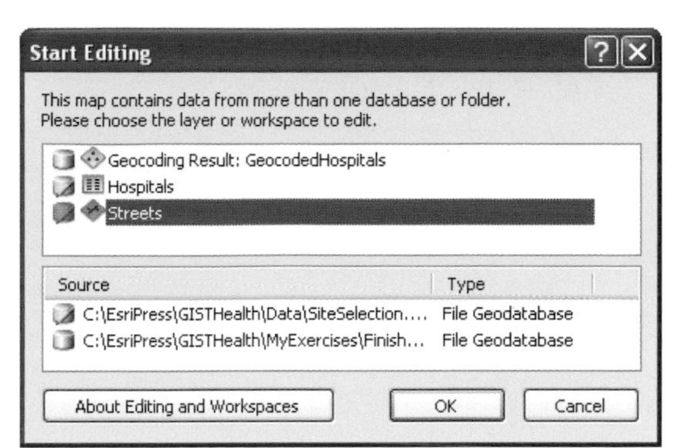

6 **In the FRADDR field of the attribute table, type** 1006, **in the TOADDR field, type** 1012, **and in the ZIPL and ZIPR fields, type** 15215. When rematched, the VA hospital will be placed in the middle of this street segment.

OBJECTID *	Shape *	TLID	FNODE	TNODE	LENGTH	FEDIRP	FENAME	FETYPE	FEDIRS	CFCC	FRADDL	TOADDL	FRADDR	TOADDR	ZIPL	ZIPR
57493	Polyline	51683295	43867	43972	0.02799		Delafield	Rd		A41	0	0	1006	1012	15215	15215

7 **On the Editor toolbar, click Editor > Stop Editing and click Yes to save your edits.**

8 **Close the table and the Editor toolbar.** The features should be automatically cleared from selection. If they are not, clear the selected features.

Rebuild the address locator

Because you edited the street centerline file, you now need to rebuild the address locator so the new segment will be recognized when rematching addresses.

1 **On the Menu bar, click the Catalog window button, browse to Chapter6.gdb, right-click AlleghenyCountyStreets, and click Rebuild.** ▶

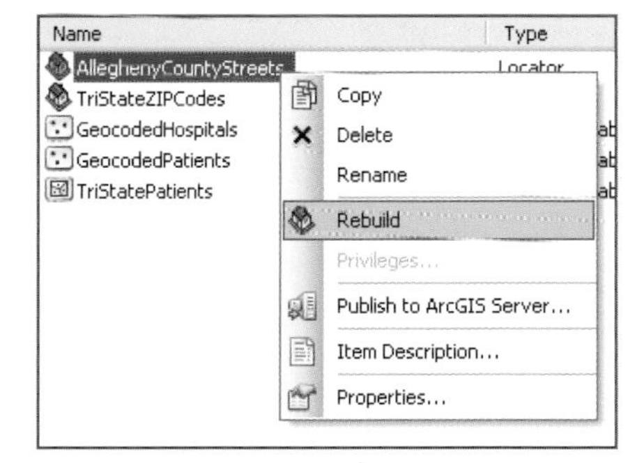

2 **Click OK to rebuild the locator.** Wait while the address locator is rebuilt.

Rematch addresses

1 **In the table of contents, click the Geocoding Result: Geocoded Hospitals layer to select it.**

2 **On the Geocoding toolbar, click Review/Rematch Addresses.**

3 **In the Interactive Rematch - GeocodedHospitals dialog box, select the unmatched record for DELAFIELD ROAD.**

4 In the Street or Intersection box, type 1010 **before the existing street address, then type** 15215 **in the ZIP Code box, and press ENTER twice.**

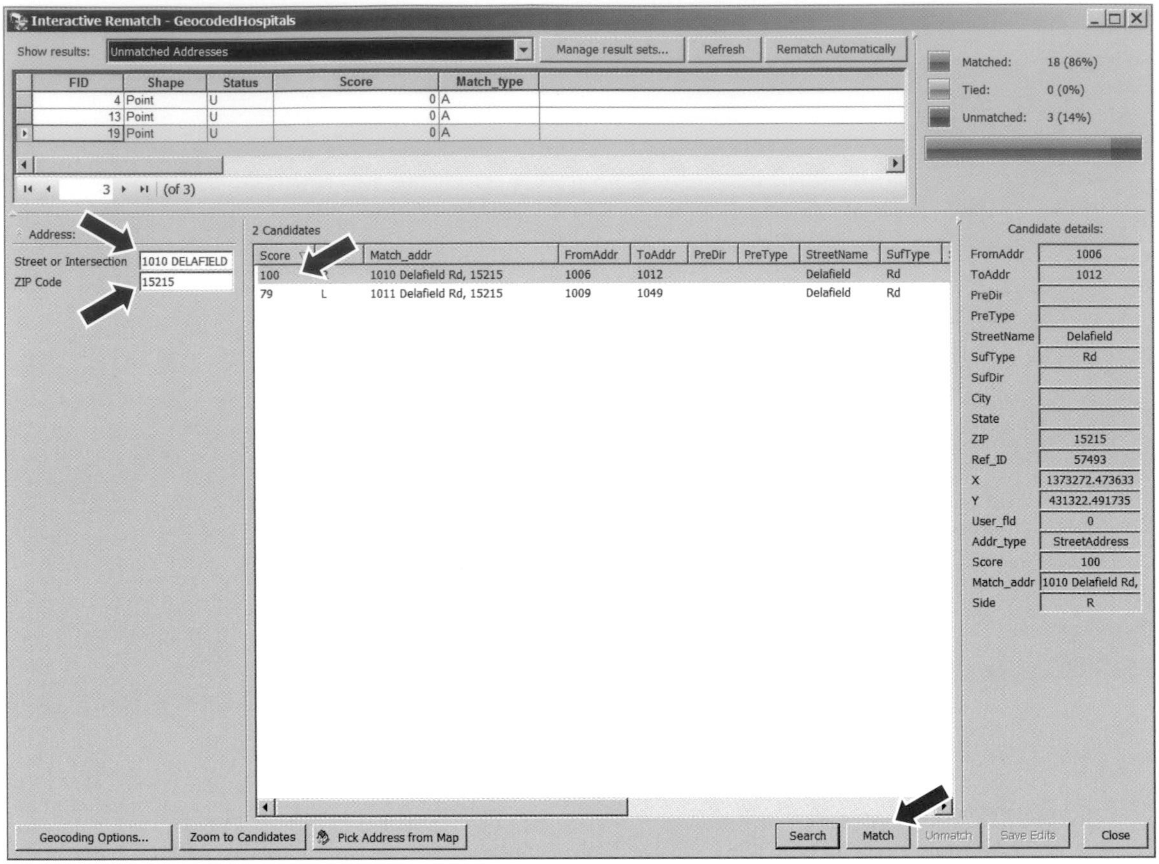

5 Click in the Candidate details box to bring up candidates. Select the candidate that has a score of 100 and click Match and then Close. A point is placed approximately halfway along the line segment you edited. (See facing page.)

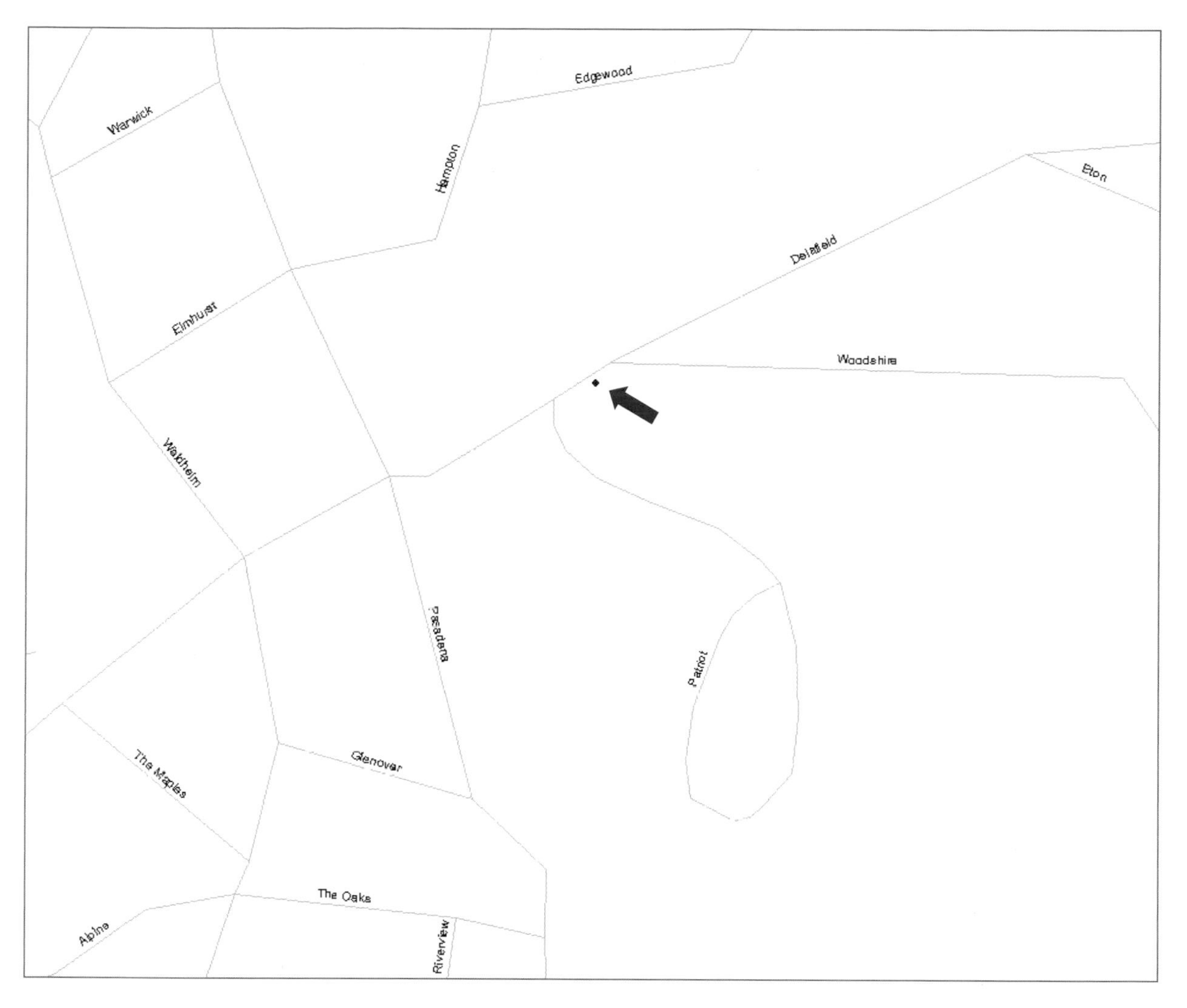

T 6-5

6 **Zoom to the full extent of the data.** Congratulations! You successfully geocoded three hospitals in your study.

Save the map document

1 **On the File menu, click Save As.**

2 **Save your map document as** Tutorial6-5YourName.mxd **to your Chapter6 folder in MyExercises.** Do not close ArcMap.

Tutorial 6-6
Creating a final comparison map

Now that you have patients and hospitals geocoded, you can create a map that compares both layers. An interesting map might compare the hospital locations and the number of beds for each hospital (an attribute in the hospital table) to the location of existing patients.

1 **Open Tutorial6-3YourName.mxd from your Chapter6 folder in MyExercises.** A copy of this map document is available in the Chapter6 folder in FinishedExercises if you need it.

2 **On the Standard toolbar, click Add Data, browse to Chapter6.gdb, and add GeocodedHospitals.**

3 **In the table of contents, right-click GeocodedHospitals and click Zoom To Layer.**

4 **Click Add Data, browse through the Data folder to SiteSelection.gdb, add Rivers, and symbolize to your liking.**

YOUR TURN

Create a graduated-point map showing the number of beds for the existing hospitals compared to a choropleth map of patient locations.

Can you tell from this map what areas are underserving patients and where a health-care organization might want to open a clinic? What other map layers would be good to include in an analysis?

Save the map document

1 **On the File menu, click Save As.**

2 **Save your map document as** Tutorial6-6YourName.mxd **to your Chapter6 folder in MyExercises.** Close ArcMap.

Summary

GIS is useful to the hospital now that you have placed your own patient data and competitor hospitals on the map. Already you can see some promising areas for locating a satellite clinic, either in the northwestern or eastern portion of the county.

You have just performed some remarkable feats in GIS by using powerful ArcGIS programs along with some of the US national map infrastructure—TIGER/Line street maps and ZIP Code maps. ArcGIS geocoding programs provide built-in expertise for analyzing location data to accomplish something akin to what your postal delivery person does when interpreting street-mail address data relative to actual locations. ArcGIS spatial joins have the unique capability to assign area identifiers to individual points. It then becomes a simple task to aggregate data by spatial identifiers to produce useful statistics such as counts and percentages. Geocoding and spatial aggregation are two of the main functions that can spatially enable an organization's data and make it ready for spatial analysis.

Assignment 6-1
Map mammography clinics by ZIP Code compared with female population

Many health-care organizations are concerned that high malpractice costs, inadequate government and private insurance payments for mammography services, aging screening equipment, a shortage of mammography technicians and radiologists, and the closure of money-losing radiology clinics are all contributing to high breast cancer rates.

In this assignment, you will geocode mammography clinics in Pennsylvania to ZIP Codes, and then compare this data with the number of females by ZIP Code between the ages of 40 and 74, the age range for recommended yearly breast screening, to see if there are areas in the state that are inadequately covered. Although there is an ongoing debate about the recommended age for annual mammography screening, it is typically agreed that annual screening should be done for women in this age range, especially if there is a history of family breast cancer.

Start with this data

- *\EsriPress\GISTHealth\Data\SiteSelection.gdb\PAClinics:* table of mammography clinic locations in Pennsylvania. Clinic locations used in this assignment are ones inspected by the federal government, with data downloaded in 2005 from the US Food and Drug Administration (FDA) website.
- *\EsriPress\GISTHealth\Data\UnitedStates.gdb\PACounties:* polygon feature class of Pennsylvania counties.
- *\EsriPress\GISTHealth\Data\UnitedStates.gdb\PAZIPCodes:* polygon feature class of Pennsylvania ZIP Codes. Includes US Census female population (2000) age 40–74.

Create a file geodatabase

Create a file geodatabase called **Assignment6-1YourName.gdb** and save it to your Chapter6 folder in MyAssignments. Import the preceding feature classes and table into it.

Create a new address locator

Create an address locator called **PAZIPCodeLocator** and save it to Assignment6-1YourName.gdb. Use the style US Address ZIP (5-Digit), and PAZIPCodes as the reference table.

Create a map comparing geocoded state mammography clinics to female population

Create a map document called **Assignment6-1YourName.mxd** and save it to your Chapter6 folder in MyAssignments, using relative paths. Include a map layout comparing a count of mammography clinics as graduated points and a choropleth map showing the number of females age 40–74 in Pennsylvania ZIP Codes. Add PACounties as a Hollow fill and an outline width of 2, but do not label the counties.

Save the geocoded mammography clinics to your file geodatabase as a point feature class called **GeocodedPAClinics.** You should match approximately 98 percent of the clinics. For this assignment, this is sufficient, and there is no need to rematch additional clinics.

Save your spatially joined GeocodedPAClinics and PAZIPCodes locator called **PAClinicZIPJoin** to your file geodatabase.

Export your map layout as a JPEG image file called **Assignment6-1YourName.jpg** to your Chapter6 folder in MyAssignments.

Create a Word document

Create a Microsoft Word document called Assignment6-1YourName.docx and save it to your Chapter6 folder in MyAssignments. Insert your map layout image including general observations about the number of clinics by ZIP Code and the female population age 40–74.

Are there obvious areas of the state where clinics are needed? Using the attribute table of spatially joined clinics and female population, list the number of clinics for the top five ZIP Codes by highest female population age 40–74. Does it seem that there are enough clinics to serve this population?

WHAT TO TURN IN

If your work is to be graded, turn in the following files:

- ***File geodatabase:*** \EsriPress\GISTHealth\MyAssignments\Chapter6\Assignment6-1YourName.gdb
- ***ArcMap document:*** \EsriPress\GISTHealth\MyAssignments\Chapter6\Assignment6-1YourName.mxd
- ***Microsoft Word document:*** \EsriPress\GISTHealth\MyAssignments\Chapter6\Assignment6-1YourName.docx

If instructed to do so, instead of individual files, turn in a compressed file, **Assignment6-1YourName.zip**, that includes all the preceding files. Do not include path information in the compressed file.

Assignment 6-2
Map mammography clinics in a county by street address

In assignment 6-1, you geocoded mammography clinics in Pennsylvania by ZIP Code to investigate the overall supply and demand for mammography clinics in the state. When the map is zoomed in closer to a relatively small area within the state, you can see detailed spatial information, including clinics located on the street network. Then, through additional analysis on the population of women, you can use detailed US Census tracts to start identifying possible relocation areas for existing clinics or locations for new clinics. In this assignment, you will geocode mammography clinics in Allegheny County by street address and compare the resulting spatial distribution of clinics to the population by census tract of women age 40–74, the age range for recommended yearly breast screening.

Start with this data

- ***\EsriPress\GISTHealth\Data\SiteSelection.gdb\AlleghenyCountyClinics:*** table of mammography clinic locations in Allegheny County
- ***\EsriPress\GISTHealth\Data\SiteSelection.gdb\Municipalities:*** polygon features of Allegheny County municipalities
- ***\EsriPress\GISTHealth\Data\SiteSelection.gdb\Rivers:*** polygon features of Allegheny County rivers
- ***\EsriPress\GISTHealth\Data\SiteSelection.gdb\Streets:*** polyline features of Allegheny County streets
- ***\EsriPress\GISTHealth\Data\SiteSelection.gdb\Tracts:*** polygon features of Allegheny County census tracts (2000), including US Census female population age 40–74

Create a file geodatabase

Create a file geodatabase called **Assignment6-2YourName.gdb** and save it to your Chapter6 folder in MyAssignments. Import the preceding feature classes and table into it.

Create a new address locator

Create an address locator called **AlleghenyCountyStreetsLocator** and save it to Assignment6-2YourName.gdb. Use the style US Addresses - Dual Range, and Streets as the reference table.

Create a map comparing geocoded mammography clinics to female population

Create a map document called **Assignment6-2YourName.mxd** and save it to your Chapter6 folder in MyAssignments, using relative paths. Include a map layout showing mammography clinics in Allegheny County geocoded to streets compared to a choropleth map of the density of female population age 40–74. Add Municipalities as a Hollow fill and an outline width of 1.15, but do not label the municipalities.

Save the new geocoded clinics to your file geodatabase as a point feature class called **GeocodedAlleghenyCountyClinics.** Add x,y coordinates to the output file. You should get a match percentage of 71 percent matched (36) and 29 percent unmatched (15). Your results might vary depending on the software version used. See "Hints" for rematching.

Export your map layout as a JPEG image file called **Assignment6-2YourName.jpg** and save it to your Chapter6 folder in MyAssignments.

Create a Word document

Create a Microsoft Word document called **Assignment6-2YourName.docx** and save it to your Chapter6 folder in MyAssignments. Include your map image. Based on the density of female population per square mile, name a municipality where you think a clinic should open and justify why you picked this municipality. Also include a log of the steps you used to rematch clinic addresses. For each address investigated, list the original address, the address matching problem, the source, and the correction.

Hints

- *For a variety of reasons, some of the mammography clinics will not geocode; for example, addresses may have missing street numbers, wrong ZIP Codes, misspellings, or simply be outside the county. Try using map layers from this assignment or online mapping programs to find reasons why addresses did not match. Rematch as many unmatched clinics as possible by using interactive rematching.*
- *In the Symbology dialog box, normalize female population age 40–74 by square miles to get the population density per square mile.*

WHAT TO TURN IN

If your work is to be graded, turn in the following files:

- **File geodatabase:** \EsriPress\GISTHealth\MyAssignments\Chapter6\Assignment6-2YourName.gdb
- **ArcMap document:** \EsriPress\GISTHealth\MyAssignments\Chapter6\Assignment6-2YourName.mxd
- **Microsoft Word document:** \EsriPress\GISTHealth\MyAssignments\Chapter6\Assignment6-2YourName.docx

If instructed to do so, instead of individual files, turn in a compressed file, **Assignment6-2YourName.zip**, that includes all the preceding files. Do not include path information in the compressed file.

Chapter 7

Processing and analyzing spatial data

Objectives

- Extract features to build a study area
- Dissolve polygons to create neighborhood population counts
- Append map layers
- Use spatial joins to aggregate data
- Create buffers to conduct proximity analysis

Health-care scenario

Doctors and researchers at a pediatric hospital in Pittsburgh want to explore the possibilities for a prevention program to reduce youth-pedestrian injuries from cars. They have two hypotheses. One is that poverty contributes to youth-pedestrian injuries because of congested and low-quality public spaces for play, resulting in children playing in or near streets. Poverty also leads to a tendency for low parental guardianship, especially in female-headed households. A second hypothesis is that proximity to parks reduces child-pedestrian injuries because play areas in parks tend to be away from vehicular traffic, and adults often accompany children to parks and their supervision can prevent accidents. Contrary to the second hypothesis is the possibility of *increased* risks of pedestrian injuries to children walking to and from parks, but researchers believe that the net effect is lowered risks of injury for children living near parks.

One policy-related restriction, peculiar to Pittsburgh, is that an injury prevention program should be designed at the neighborhood level. Pittsburgh has strong neighborhood organizations that would be instrumental to successfully implementing these programs. Note that Pittsburgh's neighborhoods are made up of one or more census tracts each, so it should be easy to aggregate census data at the neighborhood level to investigate pedestrian injuries using census data on poverty.

The primary dataset you will use in this study is a collection of 94 cases of severe pedestrian injuries of children up to age 14, drawn from a recent five-year period. The data has several limitations. Among them is that a sample size of 94 is too few cases to draw strong conclusions. For example, Pittsburgh has 90 neighborhoods, so the average is slightly less than one injury per neighborhood, suggesting that there may not be enough data to perceive a pattern. In this case, however, youth-pedestrian injuries are concentrated in relatively few neighborhoods, so there are patterns to observe and attempt to explain. It is true, however, that additional observations would make the patterns more reliable.

A second and perhaps more serious limitation is that the data does not include accident addresses, but only the residence addresses of the accident victims. Most youth-pedestrian injuries do occur near home, so the residence address is a rough approximation of an injury location, for the most part. Of course, some accidents occur away from home—for example, near schools. Analysis at the neighborhood level helps reduce the location problem of this data, because Pittsburgh neighborhoods are relatively large and self-contained communities that have their own primary schools. So, a residence address can be an acceptable substitute for the address of injuries that occur near schools. To study the effect of parks on reducing youth-pedestrian accidents, it is still more important to have the actual accident location. A child living near a park, for example, may be injured near school or someplace relatively distant from home, and the residence data will give incorrect information by associating the accident with the park. Although this error introduces some noise into the study of parks' effect on reducing accidents in their vicinity, it does not produce any specific patterns or biases. If you find any patterns, such as reduced injuries near parks per 10,000 youths, you can assume that the patterns would only be stronger with better, more precise location data.

The last limitation is that the injury data is from the only pediatric hospital in Pittsburgh. Serious pediatric injuries may have been treated at other hospitals, but these injuries should be relatively few because of the special competencies of the pediatric hospital. Mitigating the problem further is the fact that the pediatric hospital is centrally located in Pittsburgh, and no part of Pittsburgh is more than 6 miles from the hospital. Although the data may be somewhat incomplete, it should not be a serious problem. In any event, it is clear from all the data limitations that this study is highly exploratory.

Solution approach

In this chapter, you will build an analysis from basemap layers and several data sources, and then use GIS to conduct a sophisticated spatial analysis. The tasks for building the analysis are many and are fairly comprehensive, covering the kinds of GIS preparation work you are likely to encounter as a GIS analyst. You carried out some of this work in earlier tutorials—there is a lot to remember and some repetition here in new circumstances helps.

The GIS data you will use includes the following:

- Several TIGER/Line map layers in latitude–longitude coordinates for Allegheny County, which includes the city of Pittsburgh, downloaded from the US Census Bureau website
- Two injury datasets that were address matched using TIGER/Line streets by the methods outlined in chapter 6
- A data table of poverty variables of interest downloaded and prepared from the US Census Bureau website
- Two map layers from the Pittsburgh City Planning Department in state plane coordinates for Parks and Neighborhoods
- A data table from City Planning defining each city neighborhood in terms of the census tracts that make up neighborhoods

You will use this data to study youth pedestrian injuries in Pittsburgh. Along the way, you will use many GIS tasks and functions: extracting by attribute value; clipping, selecting, and extracting features by location; editing polygons; appending map layers; setting the data frame and map layer projections; and dissolving polygons.

Your first step is to select and extract a boundary map layer that has the single polygon consisting of Pittsburgh's boundary. This layer will serve as a "cookie cutter" for extracting Pittsburgh streets, water polygons, and census tracts from the TIGER/Line county maps. Carrying out extractions raises some interesting issues and problems. You will need to clip river polygons at the boundary of Pittsburgh to give them the same extent as the rest of Pittsburgh—otherwise, they extend too far beyond Pittsburgh's boundary. When you use the clip function in ArcToolbox, you will create new river polygon lines coinciding with Pittsburgh's boundary. Unfortunately, some portions of the river polygons are on Pittsburgh's boundary, and Pittsburgh extends out only to the center of the rivers. In these cases, you will edit the rivers after clipping them to give them their full width. While brief, this work will give you a taste of editing and creating features.

To aid in the process of appending map layers to make a single output map layer, the work of address matching the residences of injury victims was carried out by two individuals, Mary Smith and Bill Jones. This will break up the intense work of interactively rematching unmatched addresses and other work needed to prepare the injury points layer. As you gain practice in appending map layers, you will have to append Smith's and Jones's layers.

The next task is to start accommodating the various projections and coordinate systems of the input map layers—a mixture of latitude and longitude geographic and state plane rectilinear coordinates. As done in chapter 4, you will create projection files for the City Planning map layers, and then assign a projection to the data frame for your map document. All layers will then overlay one another as part of the same system.

Last, you will dissolve TIGER/Line census tracts to create a new version of the Pittsburgh neighborhoods map layer, keeping your data TIGER-based. The version of neighborhoods obtained from City Planning was derived from tract boundaries that a City Planning GIS analyst edited to align them with physical features in aerial photographs. When overlaying the original TIGER tracts and the City Planning neighborhoods, the result is "sliver polygons," or very narrow polygons that lie between slightly different boundaries. To eliminate these slivers, you will replace the City Planning neighborhoods layer with a new one you create.

The analysis in this chapter uses two spatial analysis functions: intersection and buffers. You will use intersection as the basis for aggregating point and polygon data to neighborhood polygons. You will use multiple-ring buffers to study injury rates as a function of distance from park polygons. Not much more needs to be said about these GIS analyses in this introduction, but rest assured that the work you will do is a powerful demonstration of some of the unique capabilities of GIS.

The PedestrianInjuries geodatabase in the Data folder has several feature classes and a data table that the authors downloaded from the US Census Bureau website for Allegheny County, Pennsylvania:

- tgr42003ccd00: polygons for cities, boroughs, towns, and townships
- tgr42003lkA: lines for street centerlines
- tgr42003trt00: polygons for Census 2000 tracts
- tgr42003wat: polygons for water bodies and rivers

The geodatabase also includes two point feature classes that Smith and Jones address matched from the injury data table obtained from the pediatric hospital. The data is completely address matched and the resulting points are edited and moved to centers of street segments to protect privacy. These map layers are

- InjuriesJones: half of the address-matched injury points
- InjuriesSmith: the other half of the address-matched injury points

The PedestrianInjuries geodatabase also includes two data tables: PopPov and PghCrosswalk. PopPov was prepared from SF 3 data downloaded from the US Census Bureau website. The PopPov table includes the following attributes:

- STFID: census tract identifier
- POP: total population
- POP5TO17: population 5 to 17 years old
- PCINC: per capita income
- POVTOT: total population below the poverty line
- POV5TO17: population 5 to 17 years old below the poverty line
- FPOVTOT (POVTOT/POP): fraction of population below the poverty line
- FPOV5TO17 (POV5TO17/POP5TO17): fraction of population 5 to 17 years old below the poverty line

The PghCrosswalk table cross-references every census tract identification number (STFID) with its neighborhood name.

Finally, the Pittsburgh geodatabase includes map layers and a data table from the Pittsburgh City Planning Department. These layers include the following:

- BlockCentroids: census block centroids made from census block polygons in Pittsburgh
- Neighborhoods: polygons for Pittsburgh neighborhoods, each made up of one or more census tracts
- Parks: polygons for Pittsburgh parks that have playgrounds, playing fields, or other facilities for youth activities

Tutorial 7-1
Preparing a study region

The first set of tasks concerns extracting an outline of the Pittsburgh municipality from the larger Allegheny County feature class downloaded from the US Census Bureau website. You will start by extracting a boundary for Pittsburgh that you will use as a "cookie cutter" for extracting Pittsburgh layers.

Create a new study file geodatabase

1 **Start ArcCatalog and browse to your Chapter7 folder.**

2 **Right-click Chapter7 and click New > File Geodatabase.**

3 **Rename the file geodatabase** Chapter7.gdb.

4 **Close ArcCatalog.**

Extract the Pittsburgh municipality

1 **Start ArcMap and open Tutorial7-1.mxd.** This is an empty map that has the data frame already assigned as NAD_1983_State Plane_ Pennsylvania_South_FIPS_3702_Feet.

2 **Add all the feature classes and tables from PedestrianInjuries.gdb in the Data folder to the map.** Although the coordinate systems of the layers vary, the layers will overlay each other nicely because they all have assigned projection (.prj) files.

3 **In the table of contents, click List By Drawing Order and turn off all layers except tgr42003ccd00.**

4 **In the table of contents, right-click tgr42003ccd00 and click Open Attribute Table.**

5 In the table, scroll down and locate the row that has an ObjectID value of 89 and a Name value of Pittsburgh. Select this record by clicking the row-selector button at the left end of the row, and then close the table. The Pittsburgh polygon is now selected.

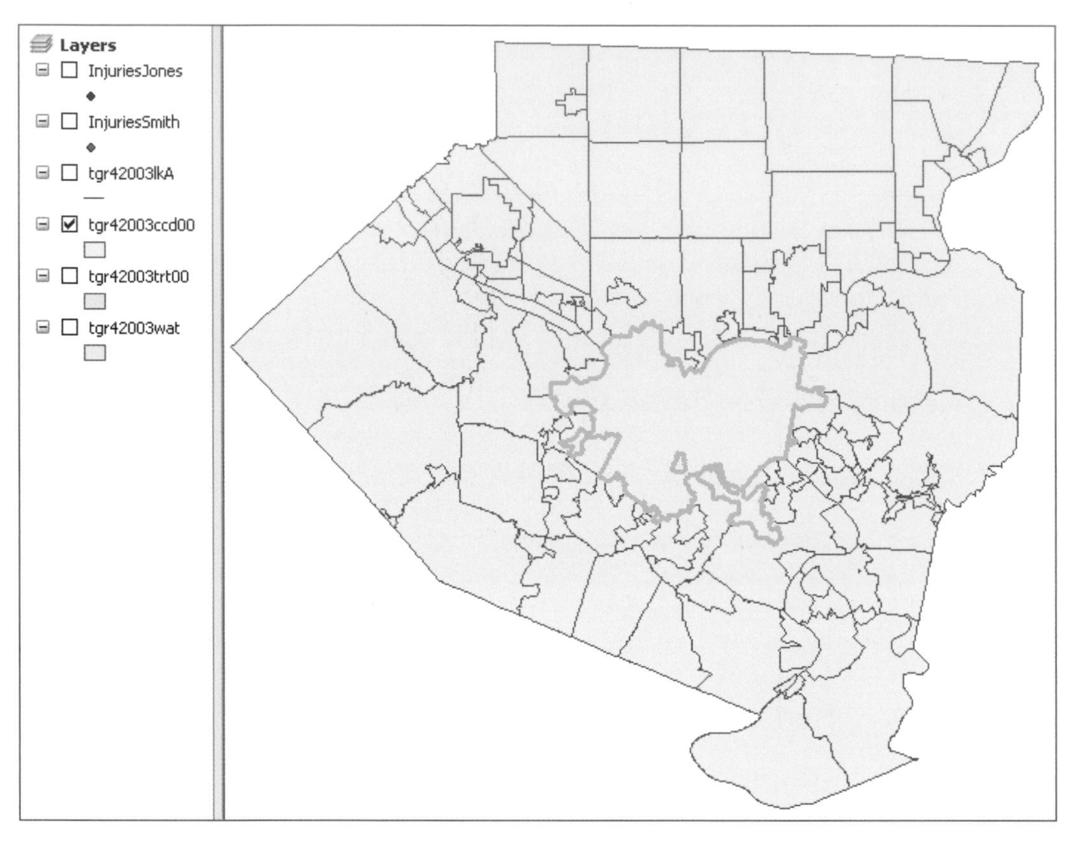

6 In the table of contents, right-click tgr42003ccd00 and click Data > Export Data.

7 In the Export Data dialog box, name the output feature class Pittsburgh**, use the same coordinate system as the data frame, and save it to Chapter7.gdb in your Chapter7 folder in MyExercises. Click OK and then Yes to add the layer to your map.**

8 In the table of contents, right-click tgr42003ccd00 and click Remove.

9 In the table of contents, right-click Pittsburgh and click Zoom To Layer. The Pittsburgh municipality is the only layer currently displayed in your map. (See facing page.) In the upcoming steps, you will use this layer to clip the water features that lie within Pittsburgh.

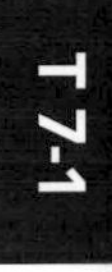

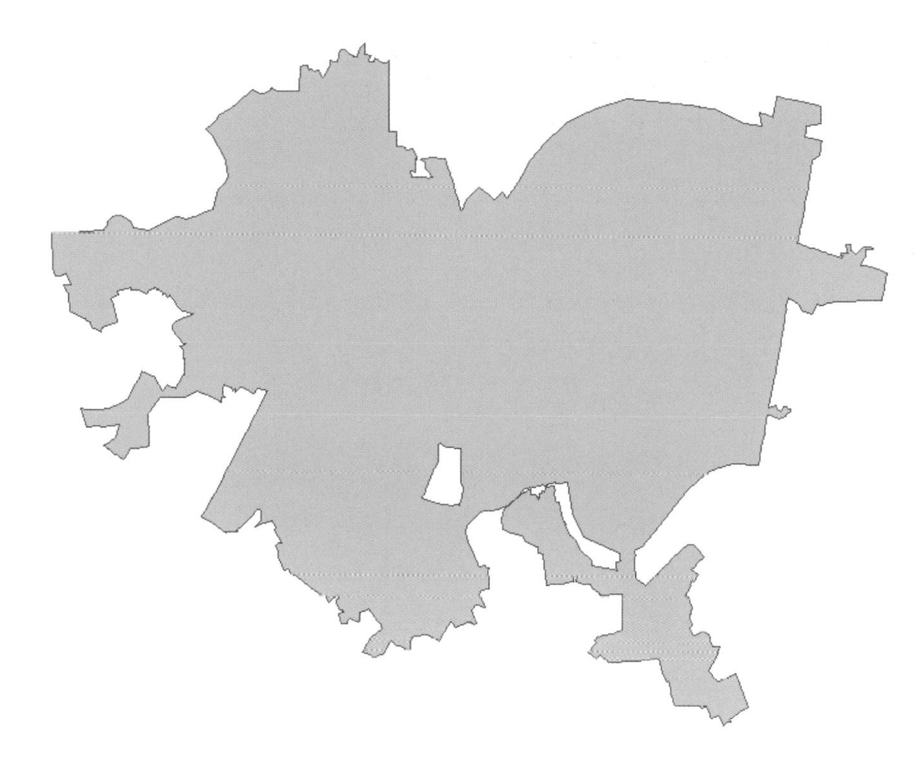

10 On the Bookmarks menu, click Create Bookmark, name the bookmark Pittsburgh**, and click OK.**

Clip water polygons

In this exercise, you will clip the water polygons using the Pittsburgh polygon. The polygons for Pittsburgh's three major rivers extend beyond Pittsburgh's boundary, so the Clip tool will truncate these polygons at Pittsburgh's boundary.

1 In the table of contents, press and drag the tgr42003wat layer just above Pittsburgh so that the rivers and other water polygons overlay the Pittsburgh boundary polygon.

2 Turn the tgr42003wat layer on.

3 On the Geoprocessing menu, click Clip.

4 In the Clip dialog box, in the Input Features list, click tgr42003wat. In the Clip Features list, click Pittsburgh. Name the output feature class Rivers **and save it to Chapter7.gdb. After these settings are made, click OK, and wait for the Clip tool to finish processing.** ▶

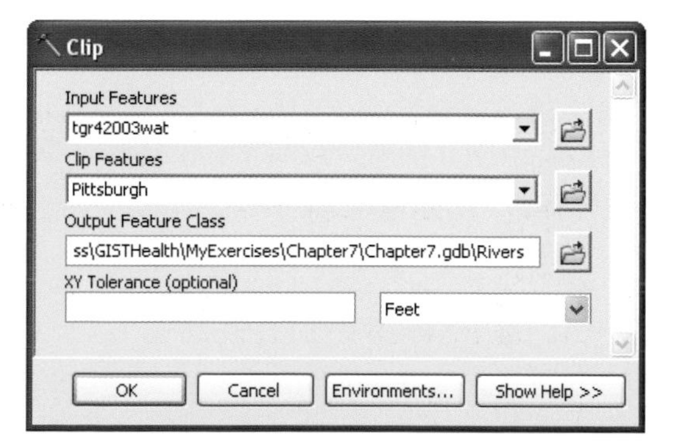

5 **Symbolize Pittsburgh using a Hollow fill and an outline of width** 1.5.

6 **Symbolize Rivers using a light-blue fill color.**

7 **Symbolize tgr42003wat using a light-orange fill color (or any color other than blue).**

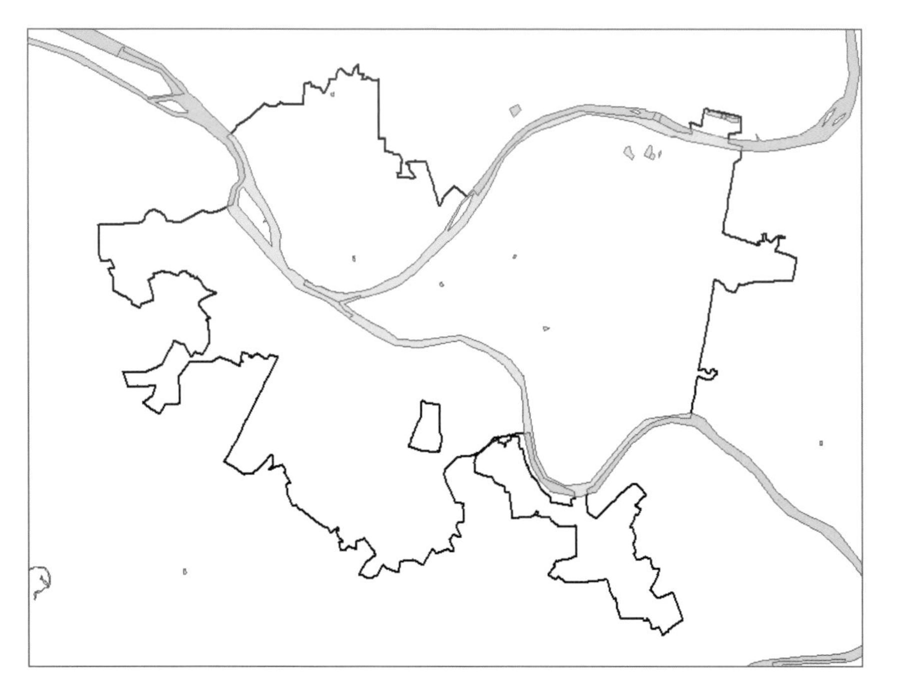

Edit Rivers features

The Clip tool did a nice job of producing the Rivers map layer, except for one problem: In places where a river is on the boundary of Pittsburgh, the boundary goes through the center of the river. In such locations, the river has half its width clipped off—the part of the river that extends past the Pittsburgh boundary. You can easily remedy this problem by editing Rivers using the heads-up digitizing tool in ArcMap. While digitizing, you will use tgr42003wat as a guide and move the vertices (points) on Rivers to match the points of the former Rivers layer.

1 **On the Tools toolbar, use the Zoom In button and zoom to the Rivers layer where it intersects the western boundary of Pittsburgh, as shown in the figure.** (See facing page.)

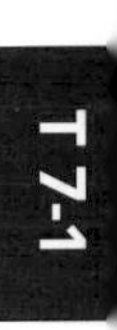

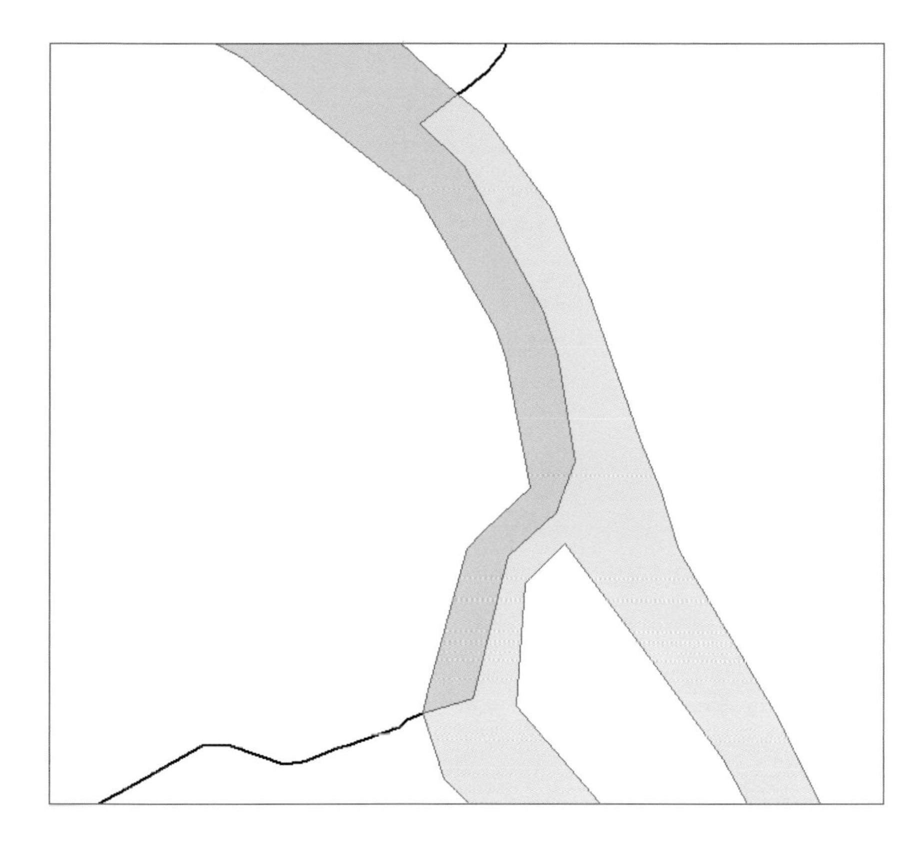

2 On the Customize menu, click Toolbars > Editor.

3 On the Editor toolbar, click the Editor arrow and click Start Editing.

4 In the Start Editing dialog box, click Rivers and click OK. ▶

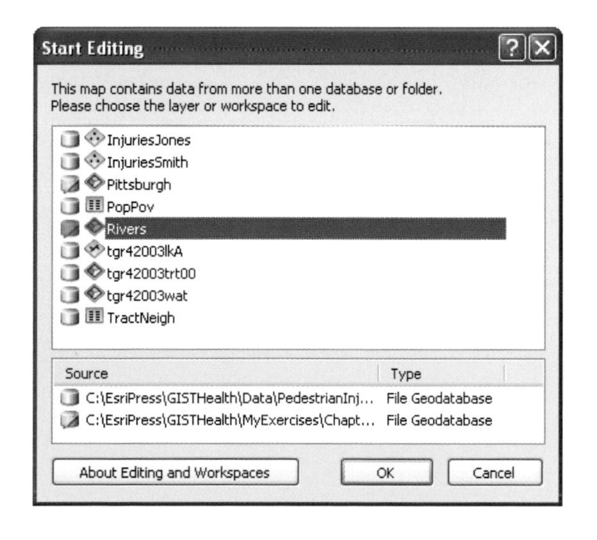

5 Click Continue to accept the warning that one or more layers do not match the projection of the data frame.

6 Click the Create Features button to open the Create Features panel. In the Create Features panel, click Rivers. ▶

7 On the Editor toolbar, click Editor > Snapping > Snapping Toolbar.

8 On the Snapping toolbar, click the Vertex Snapping and Edge Snapping buttons to turn them on, and click the Point Snapping and End Snapping buttons to turn them off. ▶

9 On the Editor toolbar, click the Edit tool button and in the map display, double-click anywhere on the Rivers layer.

Create Features
<Search>
Pittsburgh
Pittsburgh
Rivers
Rivers
Construction Tools
Polygon
Rectangle
Circle
Ellipse
Freehand
Auto Complete Polygon

Snapping
Snapping ▾

Now you can see all the vertices making up the Rivers polygon. Next, you will edit these vertices to align them with their bounding features in tgr42003wat.

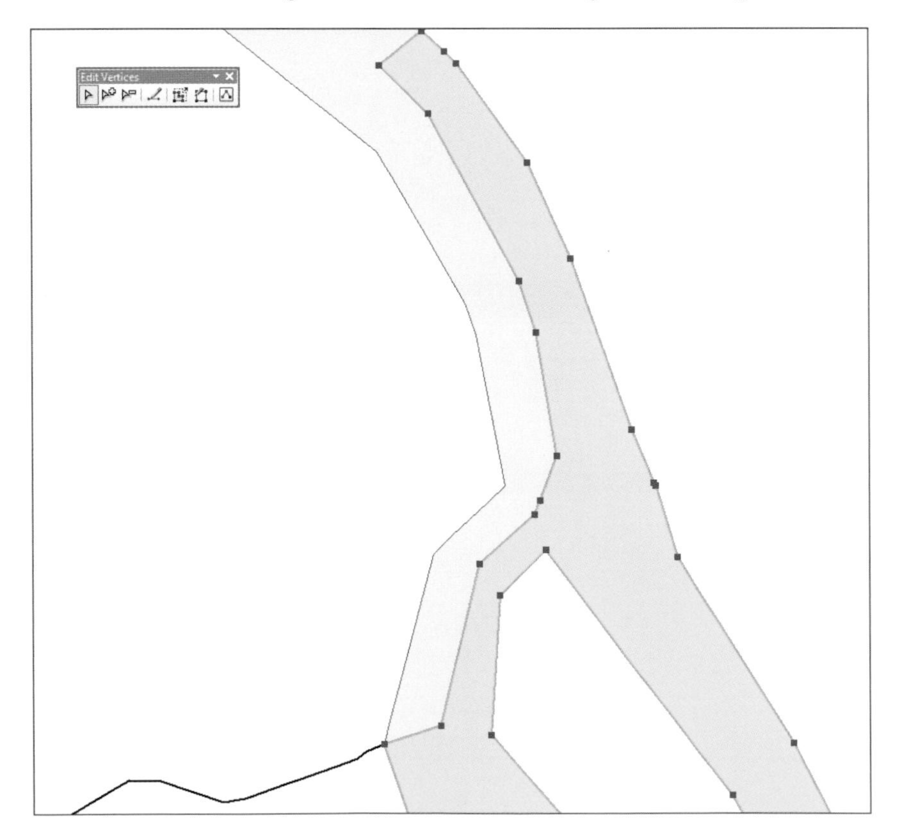

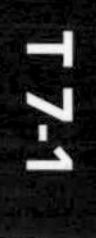

10 **Move the pointer over the leftmost vertex of Rivers, and when the pointer icon changes to the vertex selection icon, drag the vertex parallel to the existing Rivers line segment and drop it on top of the tgr42003wat boundary as shown in the figure.**

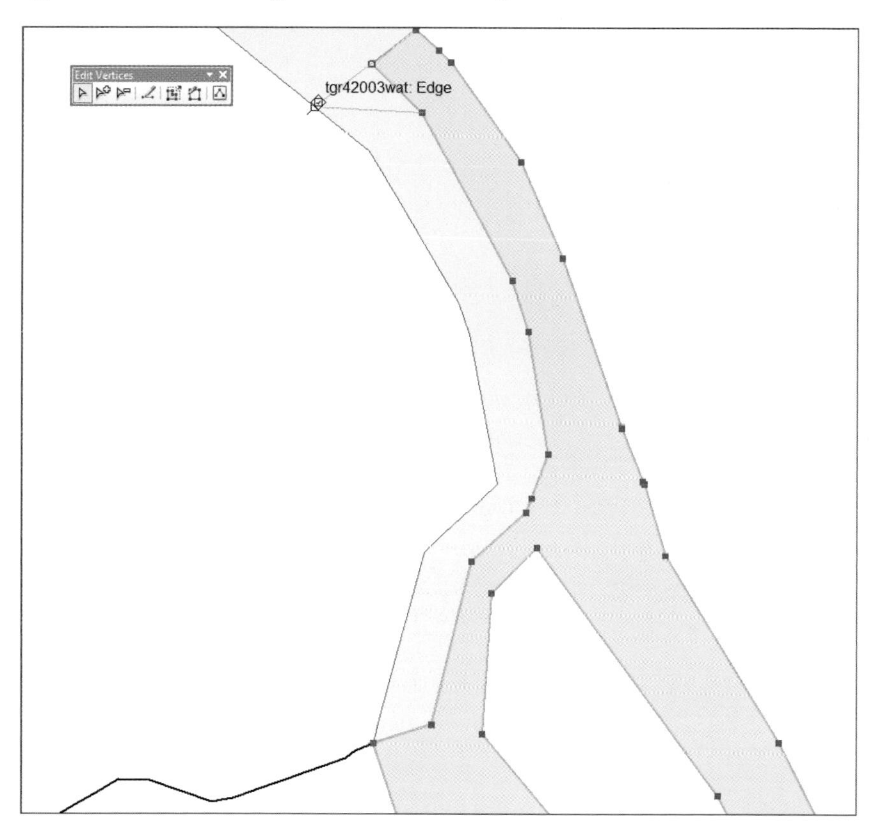

11 Continue to move the vertices in Rivers so they are coincident with the outer boundary of tgr42003wat, which is just outside of and following along the contour of the Pittsburgh boundary.

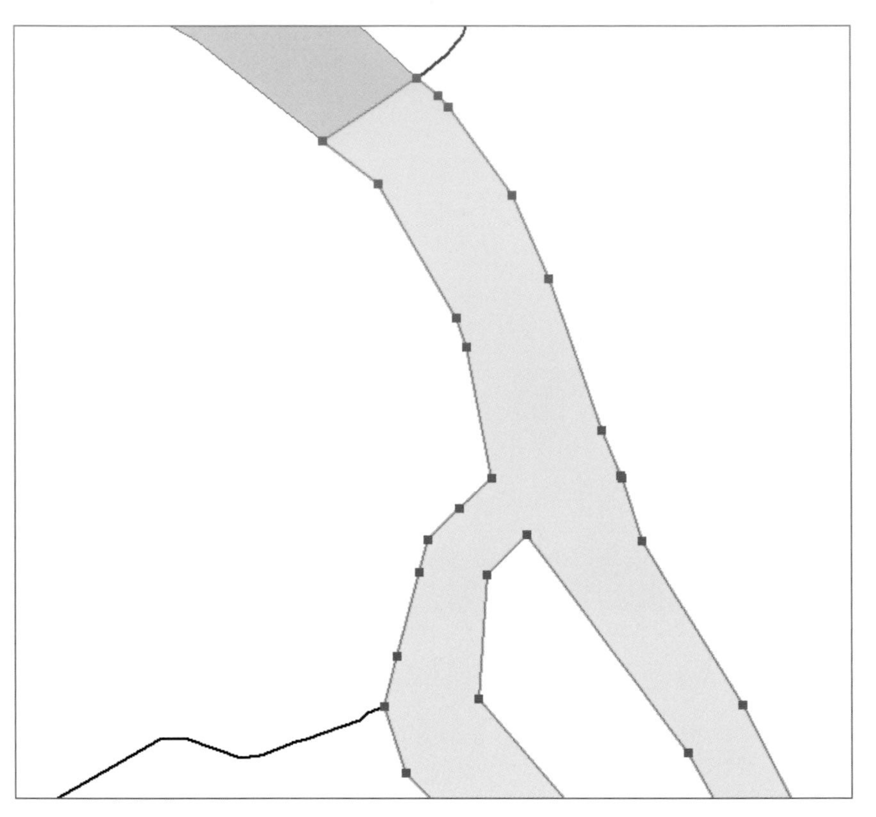

Hints

- *If you run into any problems and want to start over, on the Editor toolbar, click Editor > Stop Editing and do not save changes. Then start over.*
- *Be sure to allow time for the vertex selection icon to appear before trying to move a vertex.*
- *If a layer other than Rivers has its vertices activated, click a white area outside of Pittsburgh, and then click the blue-fill area of Rivers to reactivate its vertices.*
- *If you want to add a new vertex to Rivers, right-click the Rivers boundary where you would like to add the vertex and click Insert Vertex.*

12 When you have finished editing this portion of Rivers, on the Editor toolbar click Editor > Stop Editing. Click Yes to save your edits.

13 Use your Pittsburgh bookmark to zoom out to see all of Pittsburgh.

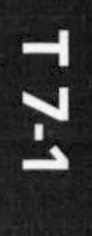

YOUR TURN

Rivers has two more polygons to edit, one on the northern side of Pittsburgh and the other on the southern side. Time permitting, edit both. If time is limited, edit just one. When you are finished, stop editing and save your edits.

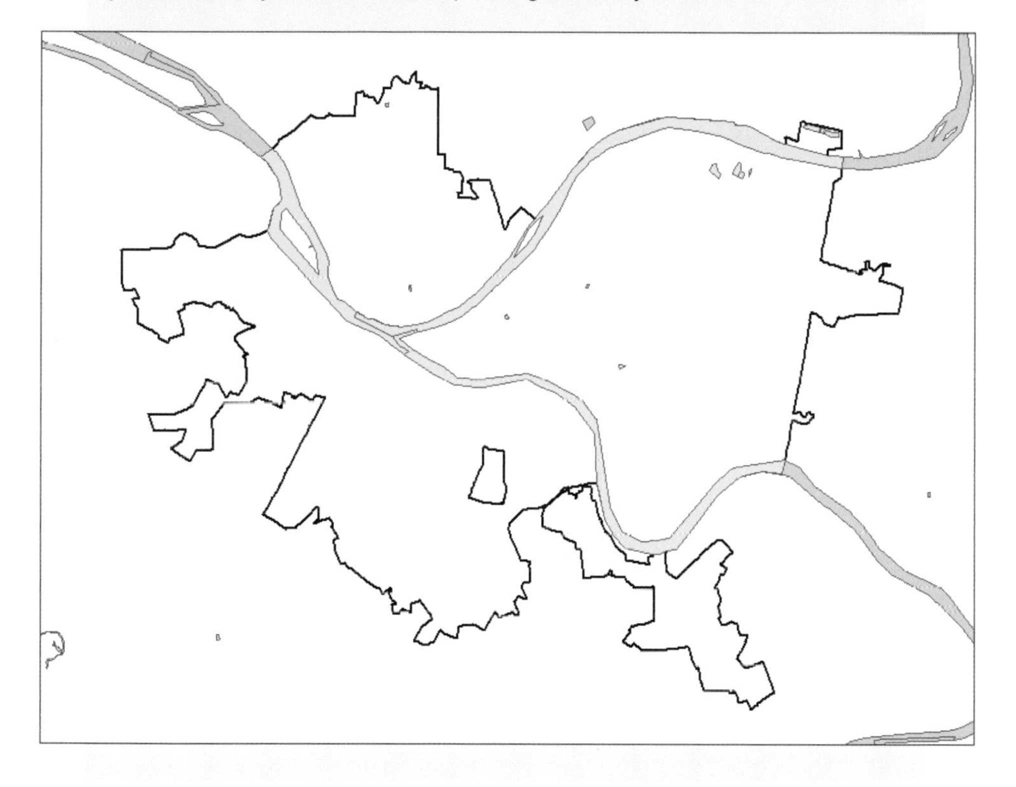

Extract streets and tracts for Pittsburgh

You should never clip street centerline segments because that would lead to location errors in address matching. If a street segment were located half in Pittsburgh and half outside the city, the resulting street segment clipped to be inside of Pittsburgh (and half as long as the original), would still have its original attribute record and street number range covering the whole segment. Address matching for the clipped segment would place points for the entire range of original street numbers all inside of Pittsburgh, including the half of the segment actually outside of Pittsburgh. Thus, to extract Pittsburgh streets in this exercise, you will include the original length of all street segments that intersect or are within Pittsburgh's boundary.

1 In the table of contents, turn on the tgr42003lkA layer in your map.

2 On the Selection menu, click Select By Location. Set the options in the Select By Location dialog box so that they match the figure. ▶

Select By Location

Select features from one or more target layers based on their location in relation to the features in the source layer.

Selection method:

select features from

Target layer(s):

- ☐ InjuriesJones
- ☐ InjuriesSmith
- ☑ tgr42003lkA
- ☐ Rivers
- ☐ Export_Output
- ☐ tgr42003wat
- ☐ Pittsburgh
- ☐ tgr42003trt00

☐ Only show selectable layers in this list

Source layer:

Pittsburgh

☐ Use selected features (0 features selected)

Spatial selection method for target layer feature(s):

intersect the source layer feature

☐ Apply a search distance

7000.000000 Feet

About select by location OK Apply Close

3 Click Apply and then OK.

4 In the table of contents, right-click tgr42003lkA, click Data > Export Data, name the output feature class Streets**, and save it to Chapter7.gdb.**

5 Click OK and then Yes.

6 Turn tgr42003lkA off and symbolize Streets using a light-medium-gray fill color.

7 Move the Pittsburgh layer to the top of the table of contents and turn off trg42003wat. Notice that some street segments extend outside of Pittsburgh's boundary, as anticipated.

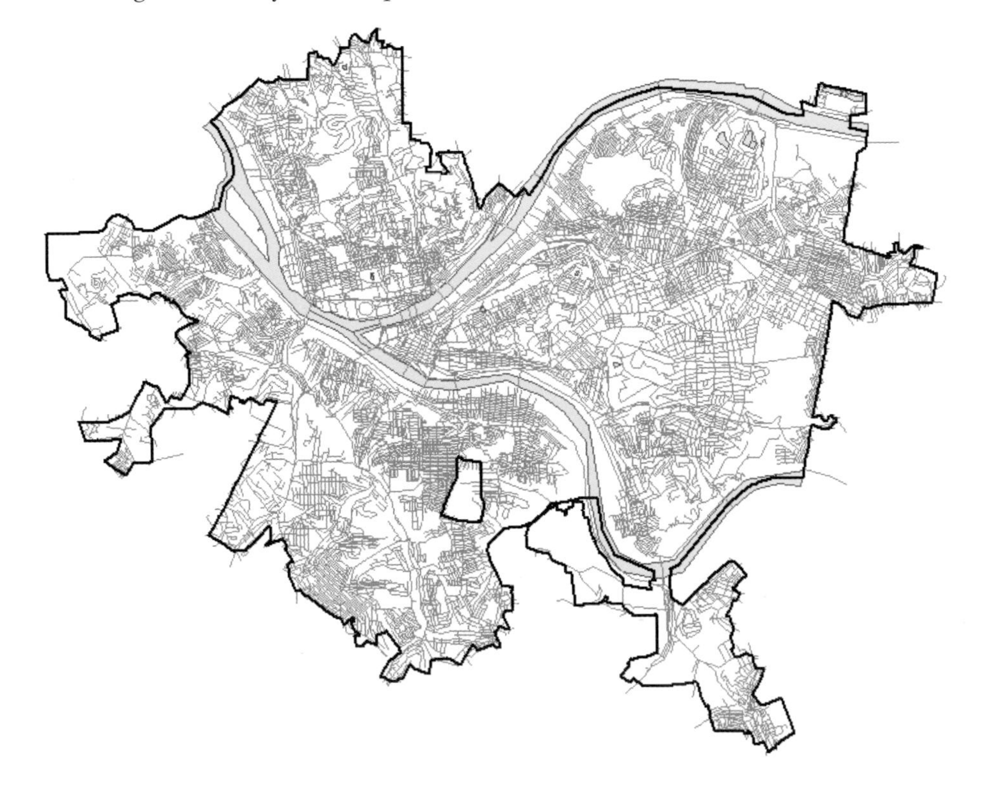

YOUR TURN

Using a procedure similar to that described in the preceding steps for extracting rivers and streets, extract the census tracts that are within Pittsburgh. In this case, though, select the features from tgr42003trt00, and in the Select By Location query, use the have their centroid in the source layer feature" function instead of intersect the source layer feature." If you were to use Intersect, you'd also be selecting tracts just outside of and touching Pittsburgh, which you don't want in this case. Name the output feature class **Tracts** and save it to Chapter7.gdb.

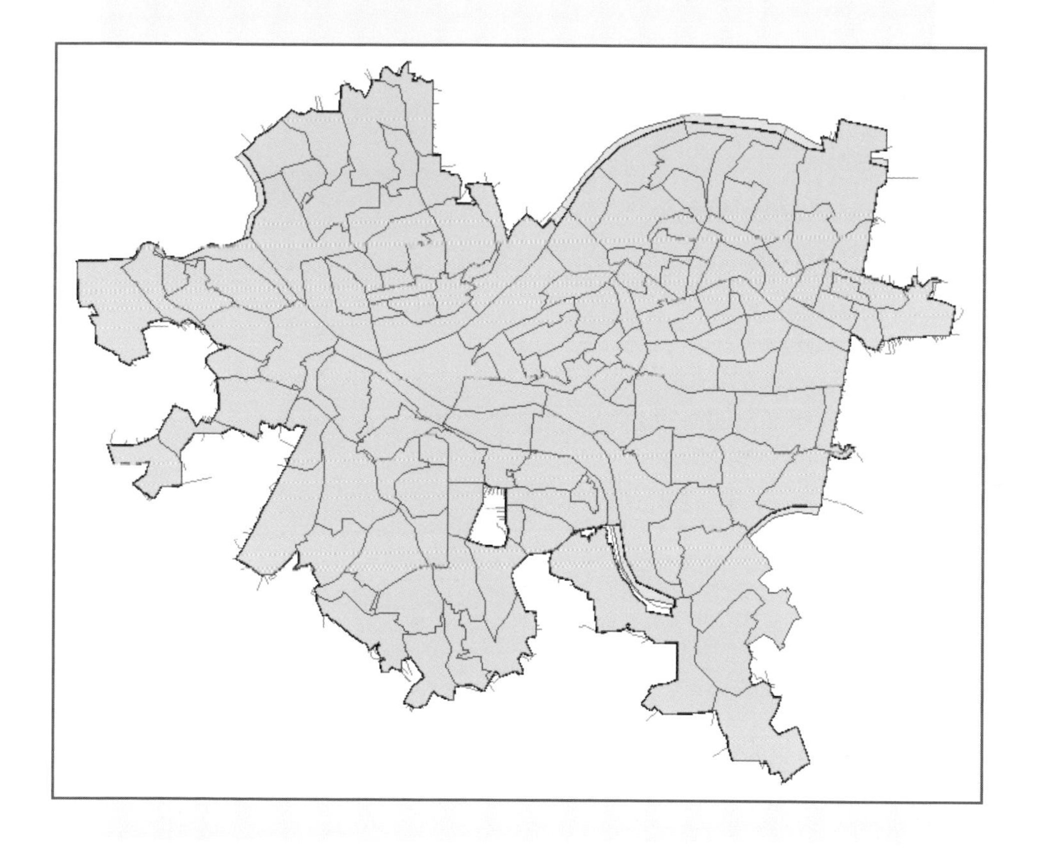

Save the map document

1 **On the File menu, click Save As.**

2 **Save your map document as** Tutorial7-1YourName.mxd **to your Chapter7 folder in MyExercises.** Do not close ArcMap.

Tutorial 7-2
Making additional table and map preparations

The Tracts feature class, as downloaded and prepared in the previous tutorial, has no census data attached to it. The authors downloaded and prepared a table of desirable census poverty variables, PopPov, which you will now join to Tracts.

Join Tracts and the census data table

1 In the table of contents, right-click Tracts and click Joins and Relates > Join.

2 In the Join Data dialog box, match the settings in the figure and click OK. If the OK button is not highlighted, click STFID in step 3 on the dialog box. ▶

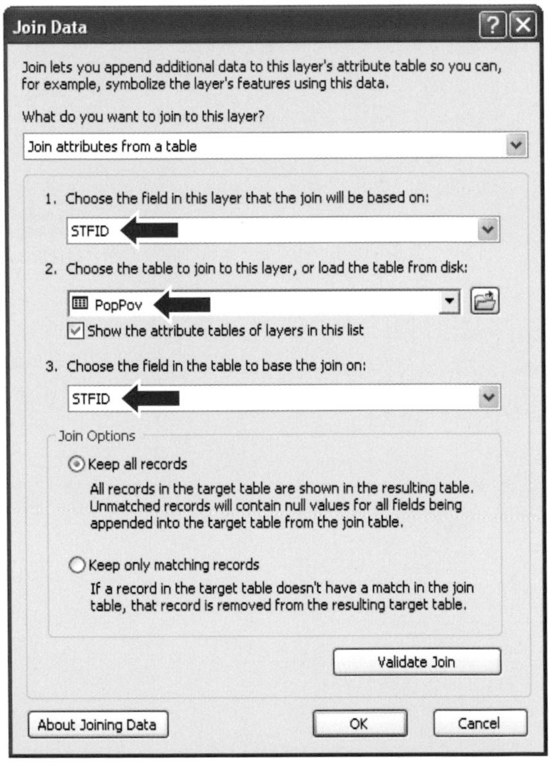

Join Data

Join lets you append additional data to this layer's attribute table so you can, for example, symbolize the layer's features using this data.

What do you want to join to this layer?

Join attributes from a table

1. Choose the field in this layer that the join will be based on:

STFID

2. Choose the table to join to this layer, or load the table from disk:

PopPov

Show the attribute tables of layers in this list

3. Choose the field in the table to base the join on:

STFID

Join Options

Keep all records

All records in the target table are shown in the resulting table. Unmatched records will contain null values for all fields being appended into the target table from the join table.

Keep only matching records

If a record in the target table doesn't have a match in the join table, that record is removed from the resulting target table.

Validate Join

About Joining Data OK Cancel

3 In the table of contents, right-click Tracts and click Open Attribute Table.

4 Scroll to the right in the table to confirm that the attributes from the PopPov table were joined to the Tracts table.

Tracts

STFID	TRACTID	Shape_Length	Shape_Area	OBJECTID *	POP	POP5TO17	PCINC	POVTOT	FPOVTOT	FPOV5TO17	POV5TO17	STFID *
42003010300	103	0.057203	0.000124	1	4221	44	5190	635	0.15044	0.5	22	42003010300
42003020100	201	0.082042	0.000223	2	4874	64	23081	704	0.14444	0	0	42003020100
42003020300	203	0.079702	0.0002	3	315	59	18456	115	0.36508	0.49153	29	42003020300
42003030500	305	0.049469	0.000071	4	2693	480	11643	897	0.33309	0.35208	169	42003030500
42003040200	402	0.056167	0.000062	5	2242	243	8623	386	0.17217	0.25103	61	42003040200

(0 out of 141 Selected)

5 Close the Tracts table.

Append injury features

In this exercise, you will append the feature class address matched by Smith to the feature class address matched by Jones. For two feature classes to be appended, they must be the same vector data type (point, line, or polygon) and have identical attribute names and field types in their feature attribute tables. This is true of the two injury feature classes being used. The Smith feature class has 46 records and the Jones feature class has 48.

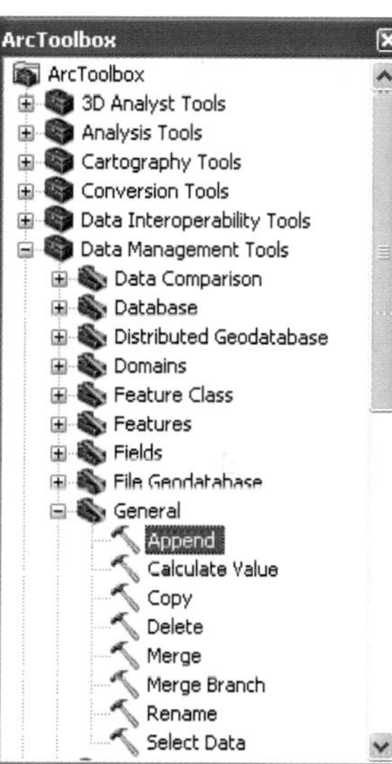

1. **In the table of contents, right-click InjuriesJones, click Data > Export Data, and save the feature class as** InjuriesJones **to Chapter7.gdb. Then add it to your map document.** This step is necessary so that you don't modify the original InjuriesJones database.

2. **Remove the original InjuriesJones layer from the table of contents.**

3. **On the Standard toolbar, click ArcToolbox.**

4. **In the ArcToolbox window, expand the Data Management toolbox and then the General toolset. In the General toolset, double-click the Append tool.** ▶

5. **In the Append dialog box, for Input Datasets, click InjuriesSmith.**

6. **For Target Dataset, click InjuriesJones. Click OK, and then wait until the process is completed.** ▶

7. **Close ArcToolbox.**

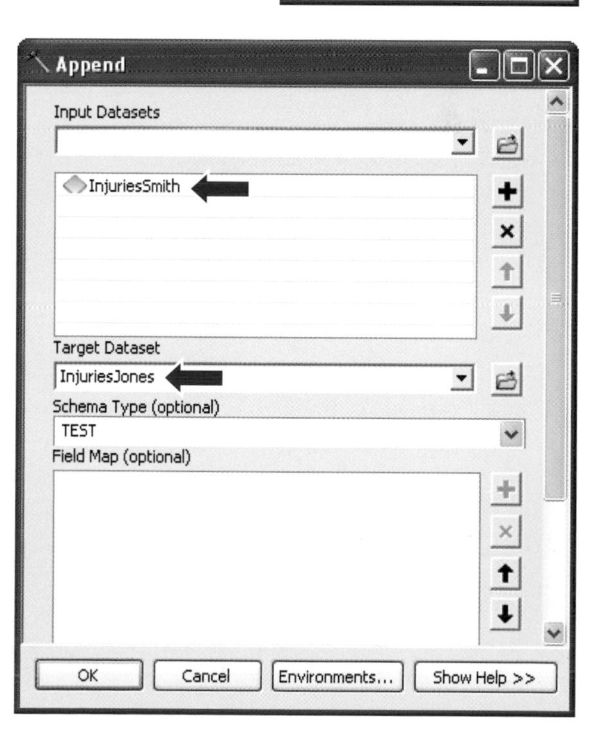

8 Open the InjuriesJones attribute table.

Originally, InjuriesJones had only 48 rows of data. Now you can see that it has 94 rows, because you appended Smith's 46 records (and points) to it. Next, you will use ArcCatalog to rename InjuriesJones to InjuryResidences. But first you'll have to remove InjuriesJones from your current ArcMap session so that you have write permission to rename the feature class in ArcCatalog. ▶

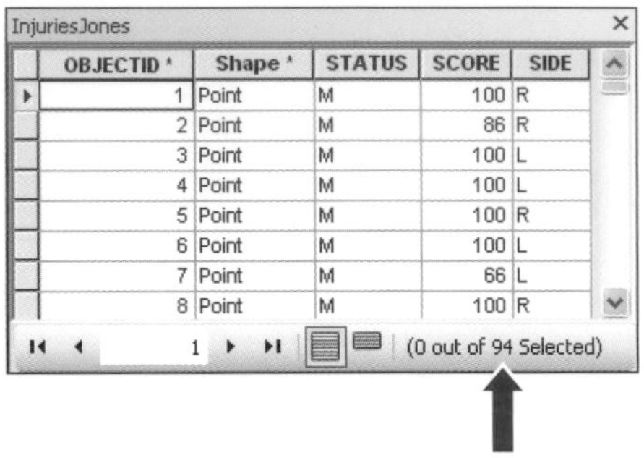

InjuriesJones

OBJECTID *	Shape *	STATUS	SCORE	SIDE
1	Point	M	100	R
2	Point	M	86	R
3	Point	M	100	L
4	Point	M	100	L
5	Point	M	100	R
6	Point	M	100	L
7	Point	M	66	L
8	Point	M	100	R

1 (0 out of 94 Selected)

9 Close the InjuriesJones table.

Clean up the map and rename a feature class

1 In the table of contents, right-click InjuriesJones and click Remove. Then do the same for InjuriesSmith, tgr42003lkA, tgr4003wat, and tgr42003trt00 (the latter four layers are no longer needed).

2 On the Standard toolbar, click Catalog.

3 In the Catalog tree, browse to Chapter7.gdb.

4 Right-click InjuriesJones, click Rename, and type InjuryResidences.

5 Close Catalog.

6 In ArcMap, on the Standard toolbar, click Add Data and add InjuryResidences to the map.

7 Turn on all the layers in your map except Tracts and Streets.

8 Symbolize InjuryResidences using a Circle 2 point symbol set to a size 7 **and a red fill color.**

Add Pittsburgh City Planning map layers

Now you will add two layers from the Pittsburgh City Planning Department: Neighborhoods and Parks.

1 On the Standard toolbar, click Add Data, browse through the Data folder to Pittsburgh.gdb, and add Neighborhoods and Parks to the map document.

2 **Symbolize Neighborhoods using a Hollow fill and an orange outline of width 1.15. Symbolize the Parks layer using a medium-green fill and no outline. Symbolize Tracts using a Hollow fill and an outline of width 1.15.**

3 **Turn Streets off and Tracts on.**

4 **Zoom to the northern portion of Pittsburgh above the rivers and compare the Tracts polygons with those of Neighborhoods.** Although Neighborhoods and Tracts should be coterminous, you can see that the tracts used to build neighborhoods were slightly different from the TIGER/Line tracts in your map document. The image in the figure clearly shows that the boundaries do not match perfectly: The overlay of the two polygon layers creates small sliver polygons, which should not be there. To remedy this problem, you will simply build new neighborhood polygons using the PghCrosswalk table supplied by City Planning. The table includes tract ID numbers and neighborhood names.

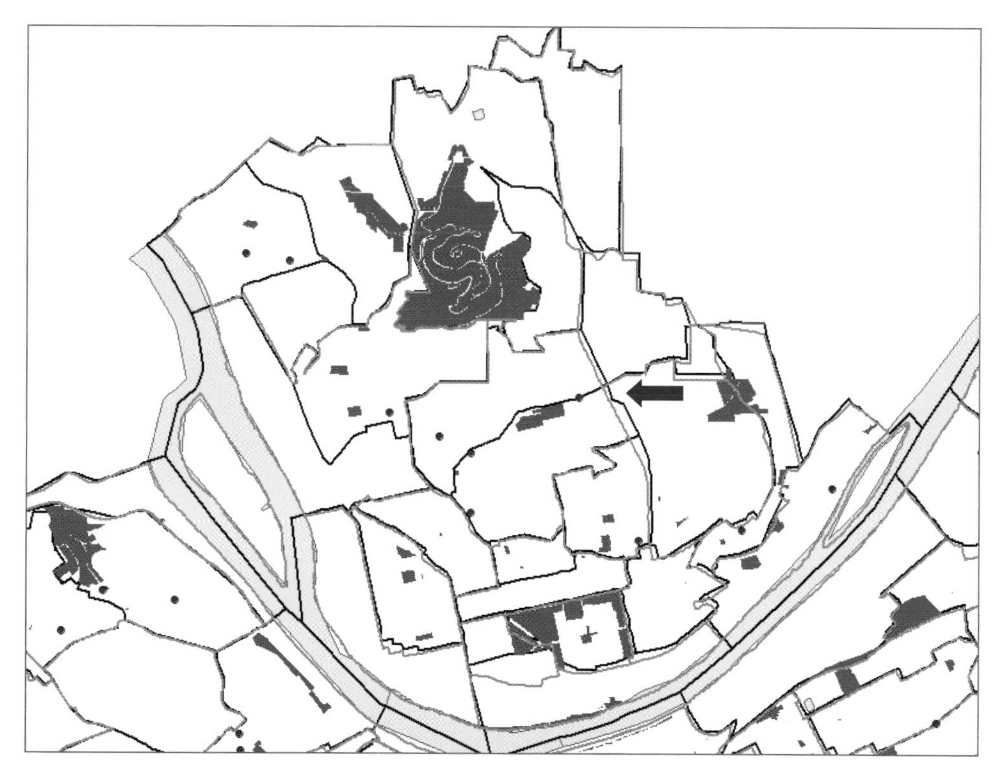

Dissolve tracts to build the Neighborhoods map layer

In this exercise, you will use the dissolve function and the inputs of the TIGER/Line Tracts feature class you extracted, as well as the PghCrosswalk table that lists each tract of a neighborhood. The dissolve function removes boundaries between adjacent polygons that have the same value for a specified value of a specified attribute.

T 7-2

1 In the table of contents, click List By Source, right-click PghCrosswalk, and click Open. You can see that this file has the information needed to dissolve tracts into neighborhoods. STFID is the tract identifier and HOOD is the neighborhood name. ▶

PghCrosswalk

OBJECTID *	STFID *	HOOD
1	42003220400	Allegheny Center
2	42003220100	Allegheny West
3	42003180300	Allentown
4	42003160300	Arlington
5	42003160400	Arlington Heights
6	42003202300	Banksville

(0 out of 140 Selected)

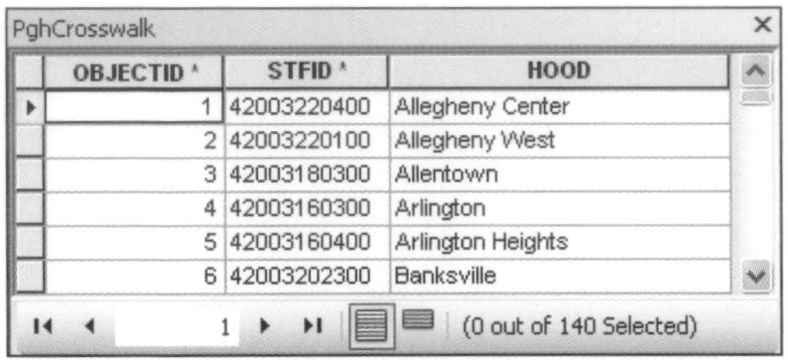

2 Close the table and in the table of contents, click List By Drawing Order.

Next, you will join the PghCrosswalk table to the Tracts feature attribute table. Then the Dissolve tool will have the inputs it needs in the desired form.

3 In the table of contents, right-click Tracts, click Joins and Relates > Join, and in the Join Data dialog box, match the settings in the figure. ▶

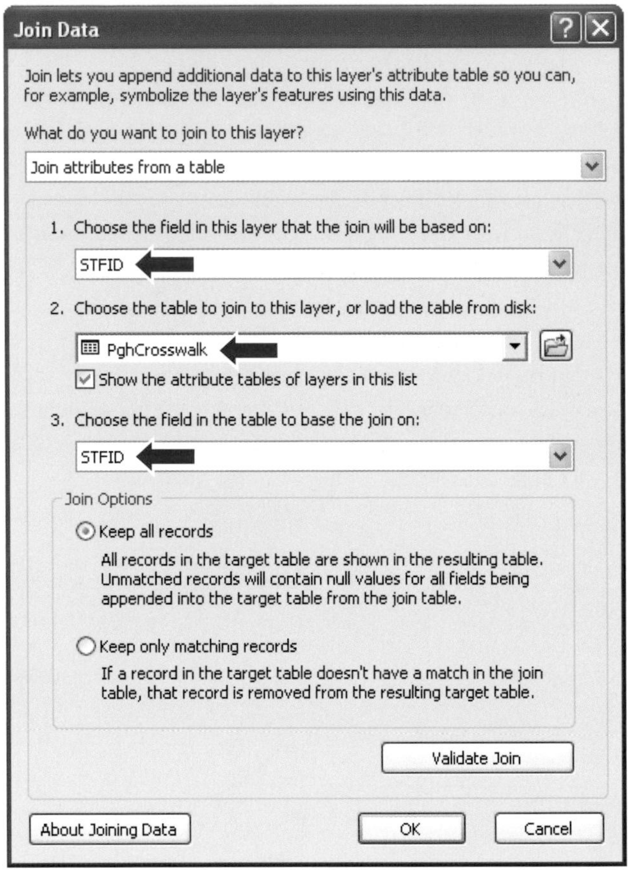

Join Data

Join lets you append additional data to this layer's attribute table so you can, for example, symbolize the layer's features using this data.

What do you want to join to this layer?

Join attributes from a table

1. Choose the field in this layer that the join will be based on:

STFID

2. Choose the table to join to this layer, or load the table from disk:

PghCrosswalk

Show the attribute tables of layers in this list

3. Choose the field in the table to base the join on:

STFID

Join Options

Keep all records

All records in the target table are shown in the resulting table. Unmatched records will contain null values for all fields being appended into the target table from the join table.

Keep only matching records

If a record in the target table doesn't have a match in the join table, that record is removed from the resulting target table.

Validate Join

About Joining Data OK Cancel

4 Click OK. The join adds the neighborhood name to the Tracts table in the HOOD field.

5 On the Geoprocessing menu, click Dissolve.

6 In the Dissolve dialog box, for Input Features, click Tracts. Name the output feature class NeighborhoodsTracts **and save it to Chapter7.gdb.**

7 **In the "Dissolve_Field(s) (optional)" list, scroll to the bottom of the list of fields and select the PghCrosswalk.HOOD check box.** ▶

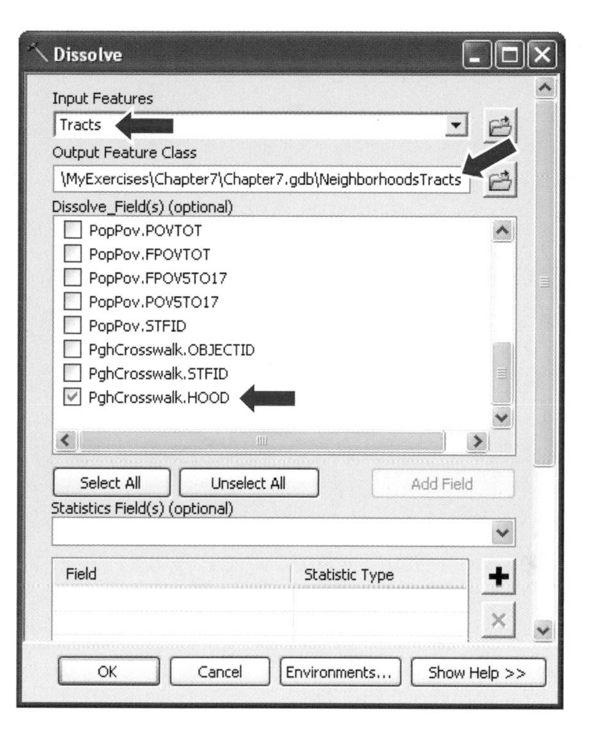

8 **Click OK and wait until the dissolve process is completed.** If you have trouble dissolving Tracts, use a finished copy of NeighborhoodsTracts in \FinishedExercises\Chapter7\Chapter7.gdb

9 **In the table of contents, remove the original Neighborhoods layer and symbolize the new NeighborhoodsTracts layer using a Hollow fill and an orange outline of width** 1.15. Now you can see that the tracts and the new neighborhoods are coterminous. In neighborhoods made up of more than one census tract, you can see the interior black lines of Tracts that were dissolved to make the new neighborhoods layer.

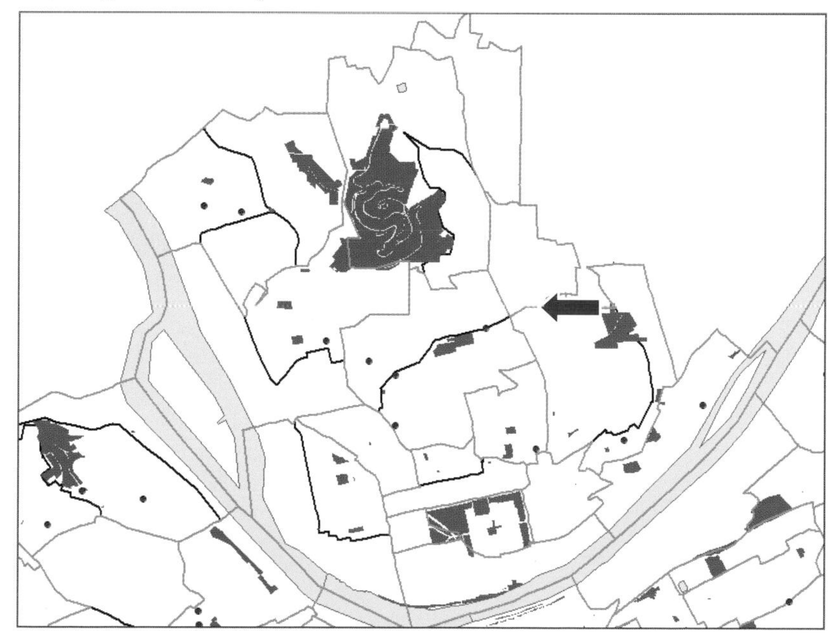

Save the map document

1 **On the File menu, click Save As.**

2 **Save your map document as** Tutorial7-2YourName.mxd **to your Chapter7 folder in MyExercises.** Do not close ArcMap.

Tutorial 7-3
Investigating the correlation between poverty and injuries

The objective of this tutorial is to aggregate poverty and injury data to neighborhoods, produce a map that displays these variables at the neighborhood level, and produce a correlation coefficient for the relationship between the two variables. Aggregation of each variable requires two steps: (1) intersect NeighborhoodsTracts with InjuryResidences or Tracts to assign neighborhood identifiers to injury points or tract polygons, and (2) count injuries by neighborhood identifier and sum a poverty variable by neighborhood. The result is two aggregate datasets by neighborhood, which you will then join to produce the final dataset for plotting and analysis.

Intersect map layers

First, you will intersect NeighborhoodsTracts polygons and InjuryResidences points to create a new point feature class that has NeighborhoodsTracts data attached to each point.

1 **Turn off Parks, Streets (should already be off), and Tracts and turn on all other layers.**

2 Zoom to the Pittsburgh bookmark.

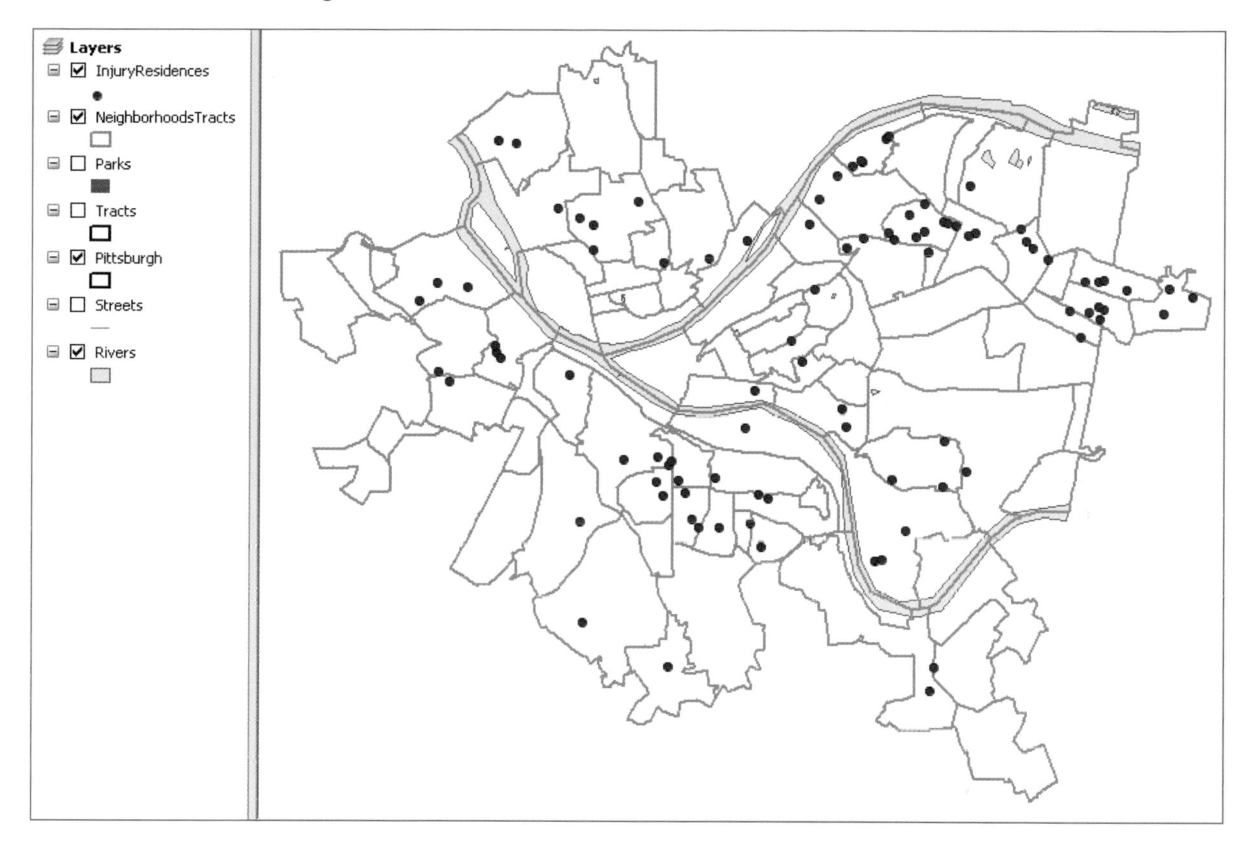

3 On the Geoprocessing menu, click Intersect.

4 In the Intersect dialog box, for Input Features, click NeighborhoodsTracts, and then go back and click InjuryResidences. Name the output feature class NeighborhoodsTractsInjuries and save it to Chapter7.gdb. Finally, scroll to the bottom of the Intersect dialog box and for Output Type, click POINT. ▶

5 Click OK and wait for the intersect layer to be created.

6 Right-click NeighborhoodsTractsInjuries and click Open Attribute Table.

Intersect
Input Features
Features Ra...
NeighborhoodsTracts
InjuryResidences
Output Feature Class
rcises\Chapter7\Chapter7.gdb\NeighborhoodsTractsInjuries
JoinAttributes (optional)
ALL
XY Tolerance (optional)
Feet
Output Type (optional)
POINT
OK Cancel Environments... Show Help >>

7 Examine the table to see that every injury record now has a neighborhood name attached as a result of the intersection.

NeighborhoodTractsInjuries

OBJECTID *	Shape *	FID_NeighborhoodsTracts	HOOD	FID_InjuryResidences	STATUS	SCORE	SIDE
1	Point	37	Hays	84	M	100	L
2	Point	59	Overbrook	51	M	92	L
3	Point	54	New Homestead	10	M	100	L
4	Point	15	Brookline	45	M	100	L
5	Point	38	Hazelwood	40	M	100	R
6	Point	38	Hazelwood	60	M	100	R

80 (0 out of 93 Selected)

8 Close the NeighborhoodsTractsInjuries table.

YOUR TURN

Use similar steps to intersect NeighborhoodsTracts and Tracts. For Output Type, click INPUT and name the output feature class **NeighborhoodsTractsIntersect**. Save the new feature class to Chapter7.gdb. Examine the resulting intersected feature class to see that each of the 140 tracts in Pittsburgh has a neighborhood name attached. You will notice that there are 141 records in the attribute table and that one of them has no data. This is because it is a polygon outside the city of Pittsburgh boundary and can be ignored. When you are finished, close the table.

Count injuries by neighborhood

In this exercise, you will use the NeighborhoodsTractsInjuries point feature class you just created to count the number of injuries in each neighborhood.

1 In the table of contents, right-click NeighborhoodsTractsInjuries, click Open Attribute Table, right-click the field name HOOD, and click Summarize.

2 In the Summarize dialog box, name the output table CountInjuries **and save it to Chapter7.gdb.** ▶

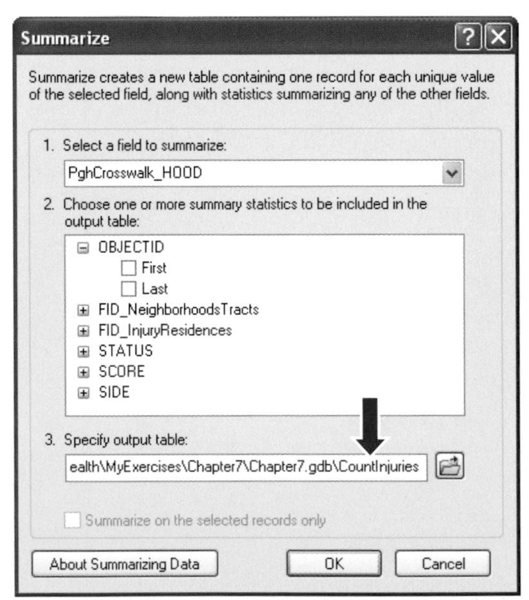

3 Click OK and then Yes.

4 Close the NeighborhoodsTractsInjuries table.

5 In the table of contents, right-click CountInjuries and click Open.

6 **Right-click the Count_PghCrosswalk_HOOD column and click Sort Descending.** Examine this table to see that it has the number of injuries by neighborhood.

CountInjuries

OBJECTID *	PghCrosswalk_HOOD	Count_PghCrosswalk_HOOD
17	Garfield	9
22	Homewood North	4
23	Homewood South	4
25	Larimer	4
28	Mount Washington	4
32	Perry South	4

0 (0 out of 48 Selected)

7 **Close the table and in the table of contents, click List By Drawing Order.**

T 7-3

Summarize poverty data by neighborhood

In this exercise, you will use census tract data to summarize poverty data by neighborhood. You will sum the HOOD field in the NeighborhoodsTractsIntersect layer to produce a table called SumPopPov that has the number of youths age 5 to 17 who live in poverty summed by neighborhood.

1 **In the table of contents, right-click NeighborhoodsTractsIntersect, click Open Attribute Table, right-click the field name HOOD, and click Summarize.**

2 **In the Summarize dialog box, match the settings in the figure.**

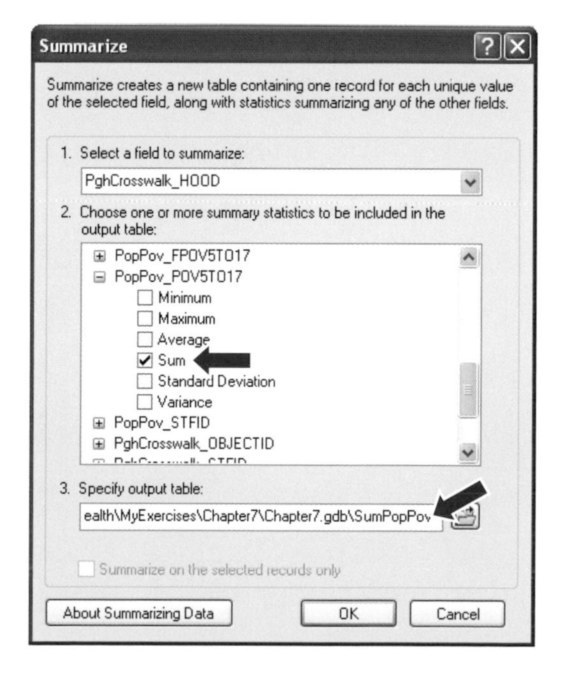

3 **Save the table as** SumPopPov **to Chapter7.gdb.**

4 Click Yes to add the table to the map document. The SumPopPov table has the population age 5 to 17 in poverty for each neighborhood.

SumPopPov

OBJECTID *	PghCrosswalk_HOOD	Count_PghCrosswalk_HOOD	Sum_PopPov_POV5TO17
1		0	59
2	Allegheny Center	1	11
3	Allegheny West	1	0
4	Allentown	1	197
5	Arlington	1	112
6	Arlington Heights	1	0

(0 out of 88 Selected)

Join tables

In this exercise, you will join the number of injuries in each neighborhood (CountInjuries) to the summary table you created in the previous exercise, which shows the population age 5 to 17 in poverty for each neighborhood (SumPopPov), and then join this table to the feature class of neighborhoods and census tracts.

1 In the table of contents, click List By Source, right-click SumPopPov, and click Joins and Relates > Join.

2 In the Join Data dialog box, match the settings in the figure and click OK. ▶

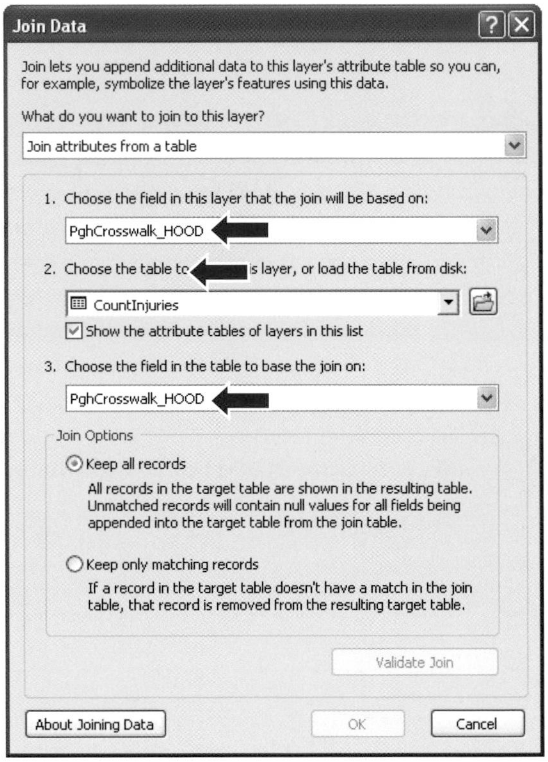

Join Data

Join lets you append additional data to this layer's attribute table so you can, for example, symbolize the layer's features using this data.

What do you want to join to this layer?

Join attributes from a table

1. Choose the field in this layer that the join will be based on:

PghCrosswalk_HOOD

2. Choose the table to join to this layer, or load the table from disk:

CountInjuries

Show the attribute tables of layers in this list

3. Choose the field in the table to base the join on:

PghCrosswalk_HOOD

Join Options

Keep all records

All records in the target table are shown in the resulting table. Unmatched records will contain null values for all fields being appended into the target table from the join table.

Keep only matching records

If a record in the target table doesn't have a match in the join table, that record is removed from the resulting target table.

Validate Join

About Joining Data | OK | Cancel

3 Right-click SumPopPov, click Open, right-click the PghCrosswalk_HOOD column, and click Sort Ascending. You now have a record for each neighborhood that has neighborhood-level data for injuries and the youth-poverty population. The null values indicated in the table are expected: They are for neighborhoods that do not have injuries.

SumPopPov

OBJECTID *	PghCrosswalk_HOOD	Cnt_PghCrosswalk_HOOD	Sum_PopPov_POV5TO17	OBJECTID *	PghCrosswalk_HOOD *	Cnt_PghCrosswalk_HOOD
1		0	59	<Null>	<Null>	<Null>
2	Allegheny Center	1	11	<Null>	<Null>	<Null>
3	Allegheny West	1	0	<Null>	<Null>	<Null>
4	Allentown	1	197	1	Allentown	1
5	Arlington	1	112	2	Arlington	2
6	Arlington Heights	1	0	<Null>	<Null>	<Null>

(0 out of 88 Selected)

4 Close the SumPopPov table.

5 Remove the NeighborhoodsTractsInjuries and NeighborhoodsTractsIntersect layers from the table of contents.

6 **Right-click NeighborhoodsTracts click Joins and Relates > Join, and match the settings in the figure. Click OK.** In item 3, click the first of the two PghCrosswalk_HOOD fields. ▶

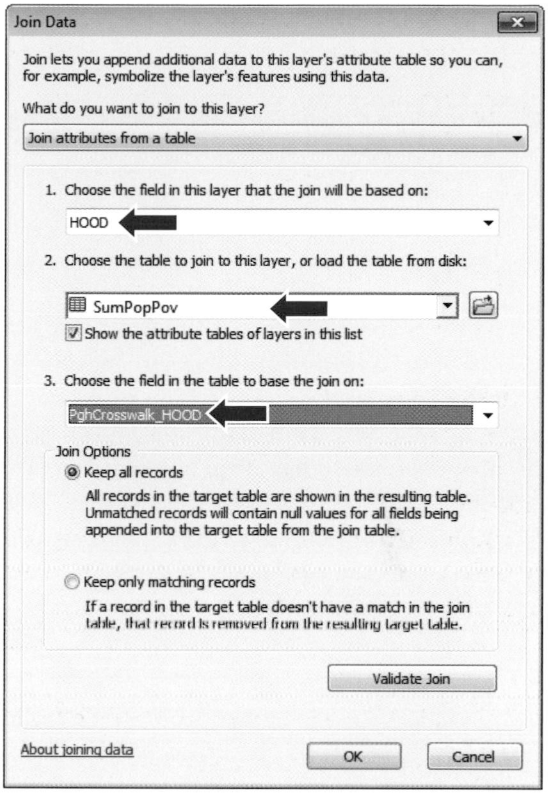

Join Data

Join lets you append additional data to this layer's attribute table so you can, for example, symbolize the layer's features using this data.

What do you want to join to this layer?

Join attributes from a table

1. Choose the field in this layer that the join will be based on:

HOOD

2. Choose the table to join to this layer, or load the table from disk:

SumPopPov

☑ Show the attribute tables of layers in this list

3. Choose the field in the table to base the join on:

PghCrosswalk_HOOD

Join Options

◉ Keep all records

All records in the target table are shown in the resulting table. Unmatched records will contain null values for all fields being appended into the target table from the join table.

○ Keep only matching records

If a record in the target table doesn't have a match in the join table, that record is removed from the resulting target table.

Validate Join

About joining data

OK Cancel

7 **In the table of contents, right-click Neighborhoods Tracts and click Open Attribute Table.** The resulting table contains records for each neighborhood/tract that include a count of injuries and the youth-poverty population for each one.

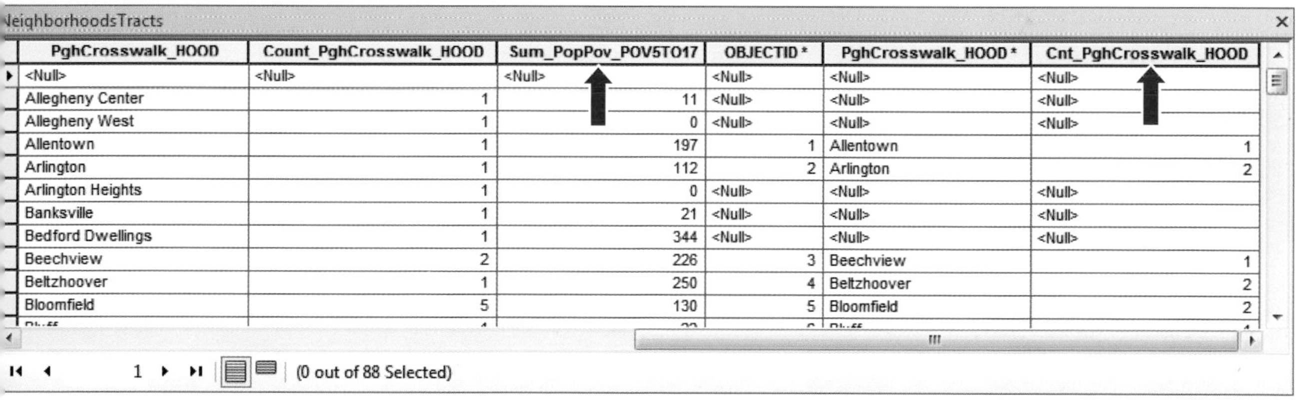

NeighborhoodsTracts

PghCrosswalk_HOOD	Count_PghCrosswalk_HOOD	Sum_PopPov_POV5TO17	OBJECTID *	PghCrosswalk_HOOD *	Cnt_PghCrosswalk_HOOD
<Null>	<Null>	<Null>	<Null>	<Null>	<Null>
Allegheny Center	1	11	<Null>	<Null>	<Null>
Allegheny West	1	0	<Null>	<Null>	<Null>
Allentown	1	197	1	Allentown	1
Arlington	1	112	2	Arlington	2
Arlington Heights	1	0	<Null>	<Null>	<Null>
Banksville	1	21	<Null>	<Null>	<Null>
Bedford Dwellings	1	344	<Null>	<Null>	<Null>
Beechview	2	226	3	Beechview	1
Beltzhoover	1	250	4	Beltzhoover	2
Bloomfield	5	130	5	Bloomfield	2

(0 out of 88 Selected)

8 **Close the table.**

Symbolize map layers

In this exercise, you will symbolize the layers to show the number of children living in poverty by neighborhood compared with the injury locations.

1 **In the table of contents, click List By Drawing Order.**

2 Right-click NeighborhoodsTracts, click Properties, and click the Symbology tab.

3 In the Show panel, click Quantities > Graduated colors. Under Fields, for Value, click Sum_PopPov_POV5TO17.

4 Under Classification, click the Classify button. In the Classification dialog box, for Method, click Quantile and click OK.

5 In the Symbol column on the Symbology tab, double-click the symbol associated with the 0–22 range and change the fill color to a bright light blue (such as Yogo Blue). Then click OK twice.

6 Continue down the list of symbols by making the following symbol color selections for each value range: 23–69, Sugilite Sky; 70–137, Arctic White; 138–225, Topaz Sand; and 226–838, Seville Orange. Once the colors are set for all the symbols, click OK to close Layer Properties.

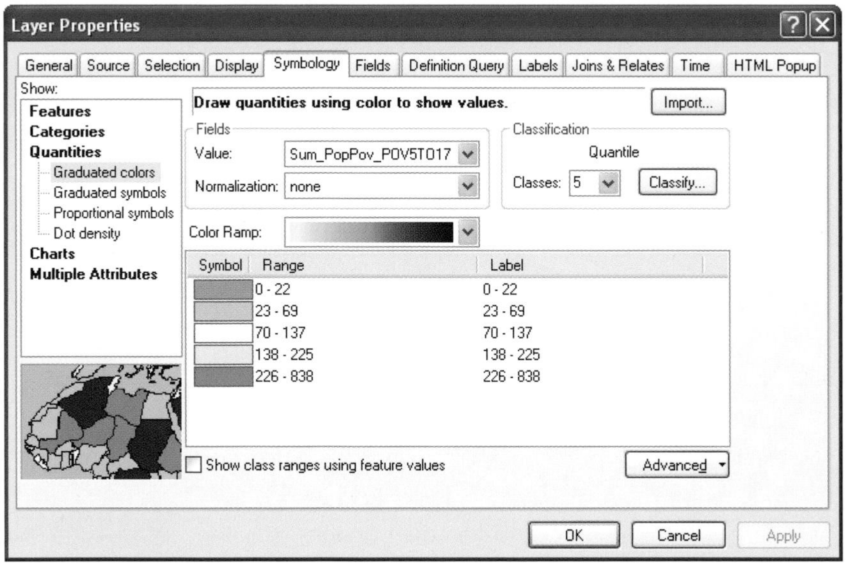

7 Turn on InjuryResidences.

Now you can see the neighborhoods that have children living in poverty. (See facing page.) The top 40 percent of these neighborhoods, seen in shades of orange, clearly have more injuries than the lowest 40 percent of neighborhoods, seen in shades of blue. Next, you will start to quantify this relationship.

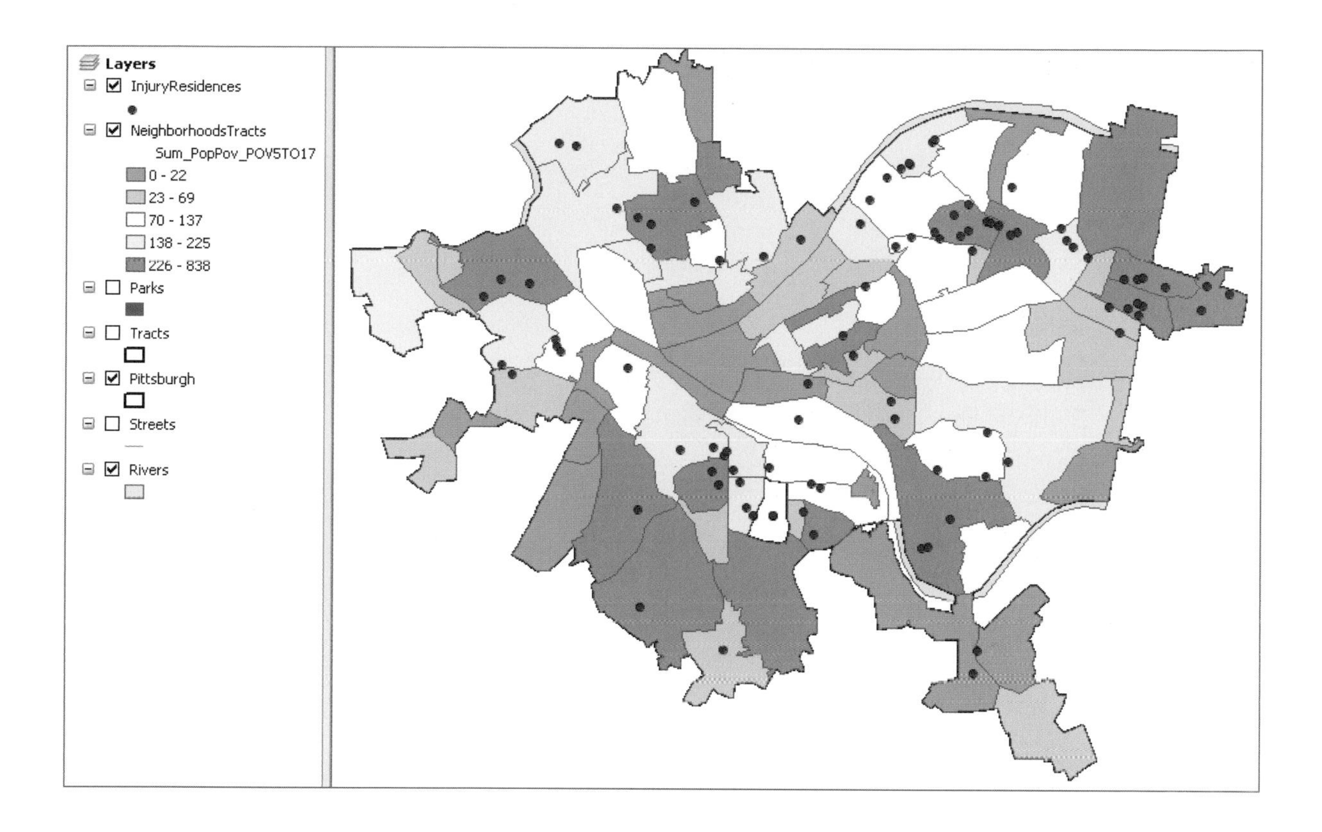

Count injuries by the top and bottom 40 percent quantiles

Now that you have map layers showing the locations of injuries and poverty, it is easy to calculate whether neighborhoods that have high poverty are the ones where injuries are occurring.

1 **On the Selection menu, click Select By Attributes.**

2 **In the Select By Attributes dialog box, for Layer, click NeighborhoodsTracts; in the list of fields, double-click "SumPopPov.Sum_PopPov_POV5T017"; click the >= button; and type** 138 **in the lower expression panel.** This step builds an attribute query to select all neighborhoods in the top 40 percent of youth population living in poverty. ▶

Select By Attributes
Layer: NeighborhoodsTracts
Only show selectable layers in this list
Method: Create a new selection
"SumPopPov.PghCrosswalk_HOOD"
"SumPopPov.Cnt_PghCrosswalk_HOOD"
"SumPopPov.Sum_PopPov_POV5T017"
"CountInjuries.OBJECTID"
"CountInjuries.PghCrosswalk_HOOD"
"CountInjuries.Cnt_PghCrosswalk_HOOD"
= <> Like
> >= And
< <= Or
_ % () Not
Is
Get Unique Values Go To:
SELECT * FROM NeighborhoodsTracts_SumPopPov_CountInjuries
"SumPopPov.Sum_PopPov_POV5T017" >= 138
Clear Verify Help Load... Save...
OK Apply Close

3 **Click OK.** The resulting map shows neighborhoods that have high poverty selected.

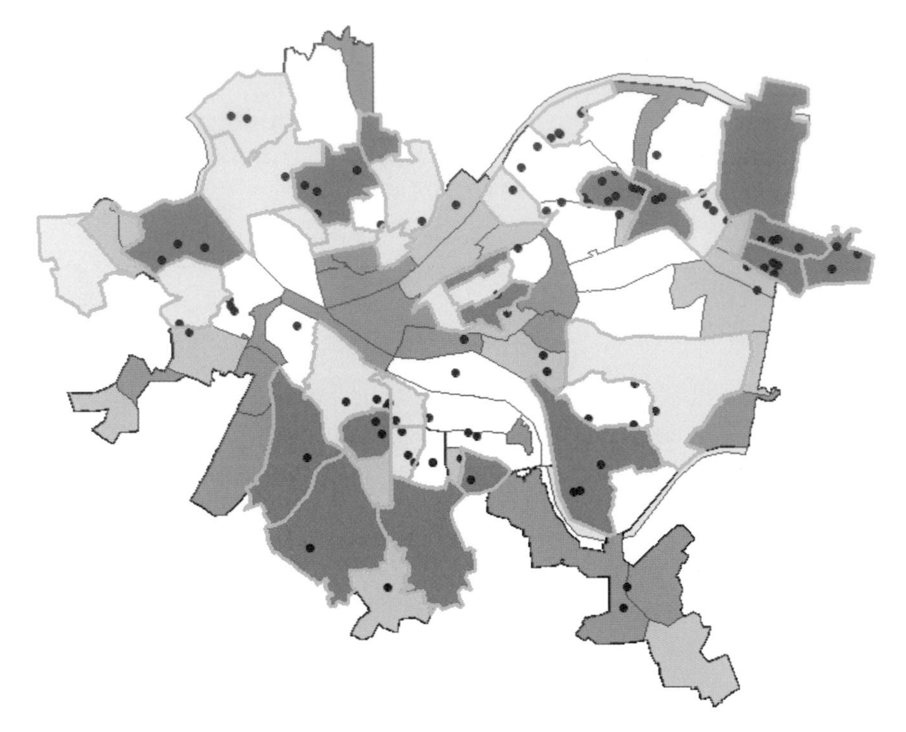

4 **On the Selection menu, click Select By Location. In the Select By Location dialog box, match the settings in the figure.** ▶

5 **Click Apply and then OK.**

Select By Location

Select features from one or more target layers based on their location in relation to the features in the source layer.

Selection method:

select features from

Target layer(s):

☑ InjuryResidences
☐ NeighborhoodsTracts
☐ Parks
☐ Tracts
☐ Pittsburgh
☐ Streets
☐ Rivers
☐ Export_Output

☐ Only show selectable layers in this list

Source layer:

NeighborhoodsTracts

☑ Use selected features (34 features selected)

Spatial selection method for target layer feature(s):

intersect the source layer feature

☐ Apply a search distance

7000.000000 Feet

About select by location OK Apply Close

6 **Open the InjuryResidences attribute table.** In the resulting selection statistics of InjuryResidences, you will find that 61 of 94 injuries (65 percent) fall into the top 40 percent of neighborhoods by youth population living in poverty. This is a good indication that poverty is a factor in serious youth-pedestrian injuries.

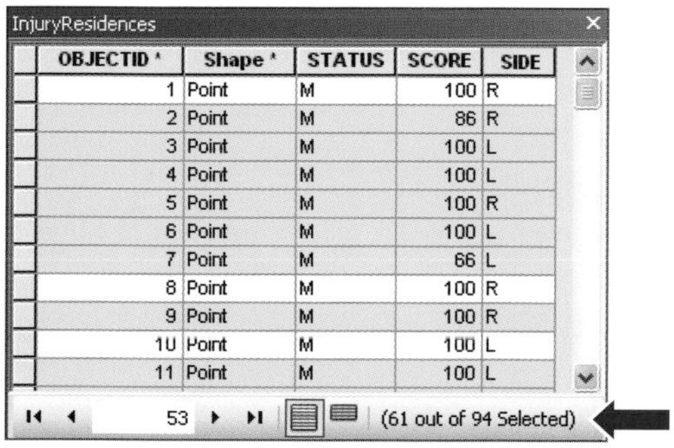

InjuryResidences

OBJECTID *	Shape *	STATUS	SCORE	SIDE
1	Point	M	100	R
2	Point	M	86	R
3	Point	M	100	L
4	Point	M	100	L
5	Point	M	100	R
6	Point	M	100	L
7	Point	M	66	L
8	Point	M	100	R
9	Point	M	100	R
10	Point	M	100	L
11	Point	M	100	L

53 (61 out of 94 Selected)

7 **If necessary, close any open tables.**

8 **On the Selection menu, click Clear Selected Features.**

YOUR TURN

Determine the number of injuries in the lowest 40 percent of neighborhoods by youth poverty population. ***Hint:*** *The attribute selection criterion needed is "SumPopPov.Sum_PopPov_POV5T017" <= 69 and the result is that only 13 of 94 injuries (14 percent) are in neighborhoods that have the lowest youth-poverty population.* Clear the selection.

If you were to calculate the correlation coefficient for Sum_PopPov_POV5TO17 (the youth population in poverty by neighborhood) and Count_PghCrosswalk_HOOD (the number of injuries by neighborhood), you would find a rather high correlation between these variables.

Save the map document

1 **On the File menu, click Save As.**

2 **Save your map document as** Tutorial7-3YourName.mxd **to your Chapter7 folder in MyExercises.** Do not close ArcMap.

Tutorial 7-4
Investigating injuries near parks

In this tutorial, your last task is to conduct a proximity analysis of parks and serious youth-pedestrian injuries. You will use ArcToolbox to construct 600 ft and 1,200 ft buffers around parks, and then analyze injury rates per 10,000 youths in the 0-to-600 ft and 600-to-1,200 ft rings around parks. Injury rates are expected to be higher for youths living in the 600-to-1,200 ft ring.

Build multiple-ring buffers

1 Turn off NeighborhoodsTracts, Streets, and Tracts in your map and turn on all other layers.

2 On the Standard toolbar, click ArcToolbox, expand the Analysis toolbox and then the Proximity toolset, and double-click the Multiple Ring Buffer tool. ▶

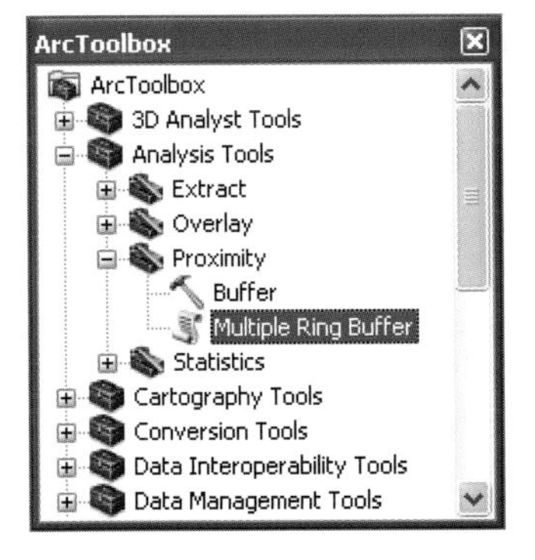

3 In the Multiple Ring Buffer dialog box, for Input Features, click Parks; name the output feature class ParksBuffers**; and save the feature class to Chapter7.gdb. In the Distances box, type** 0.5 **and click the Plus (+) button.** This step enters the distance of the first buffer and amounts to a trick. You need the ring that is 0 to 600 ft, but the multiple-ring buffer cannot use the value 0 as an input. Instead, you have to use a small value, near 0, so you used 0.5 ft.

4 In the Distances box, type 600 **and click the Plus button. Then enter a distance value of** 1200**.**

5 For Buffer Unit, click Feet. ▶

6 **Click OK and wait for the buffers to be created.** Be patient. This process could take time. If you have trouble creating the multi-ring buffers, use \FinishedExercises\Chapter7\Chapter7.gdb\ParksBuffer.

7 **Close ArcToolbox.**

8 **Right-click ParksBuffers, click Properties, and click the Symbology tab.**

9 **In the Show panel, click Quantities > Graduated colors. Under Fields, for Value, click "distance."**

10 **In the Symbol column, double-click the symbol associated with the 0.5 range value and set the symbology to a Hollow fill and a medium-gray outline. For the other two symbols in this column, use light- and medium-gray fill colors. Once the symbology is defined, click OK.**

11 **Format the labels using two decimal places and click OK.**

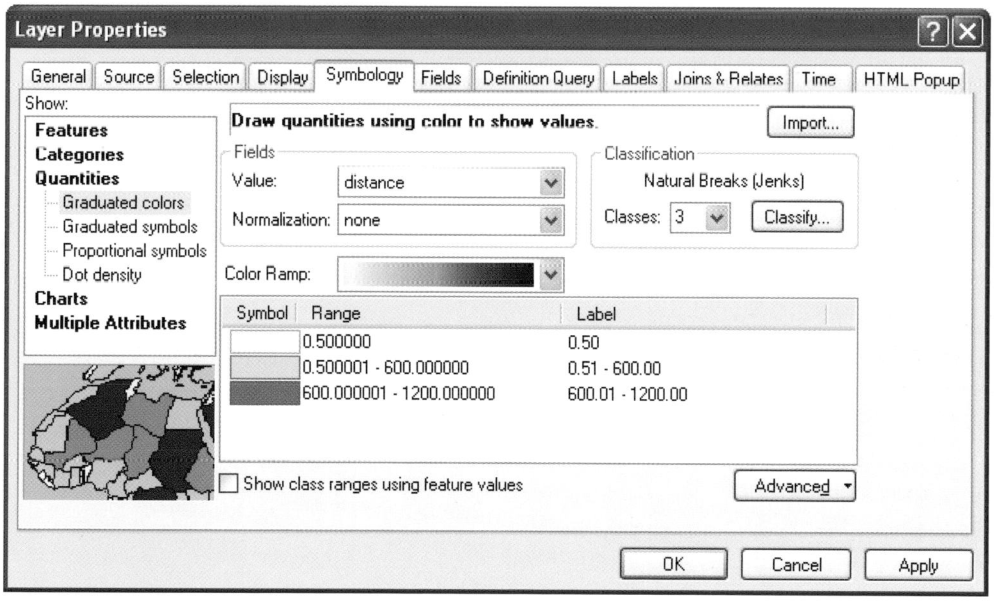

The resulting map shows the Parks proximity buffers.

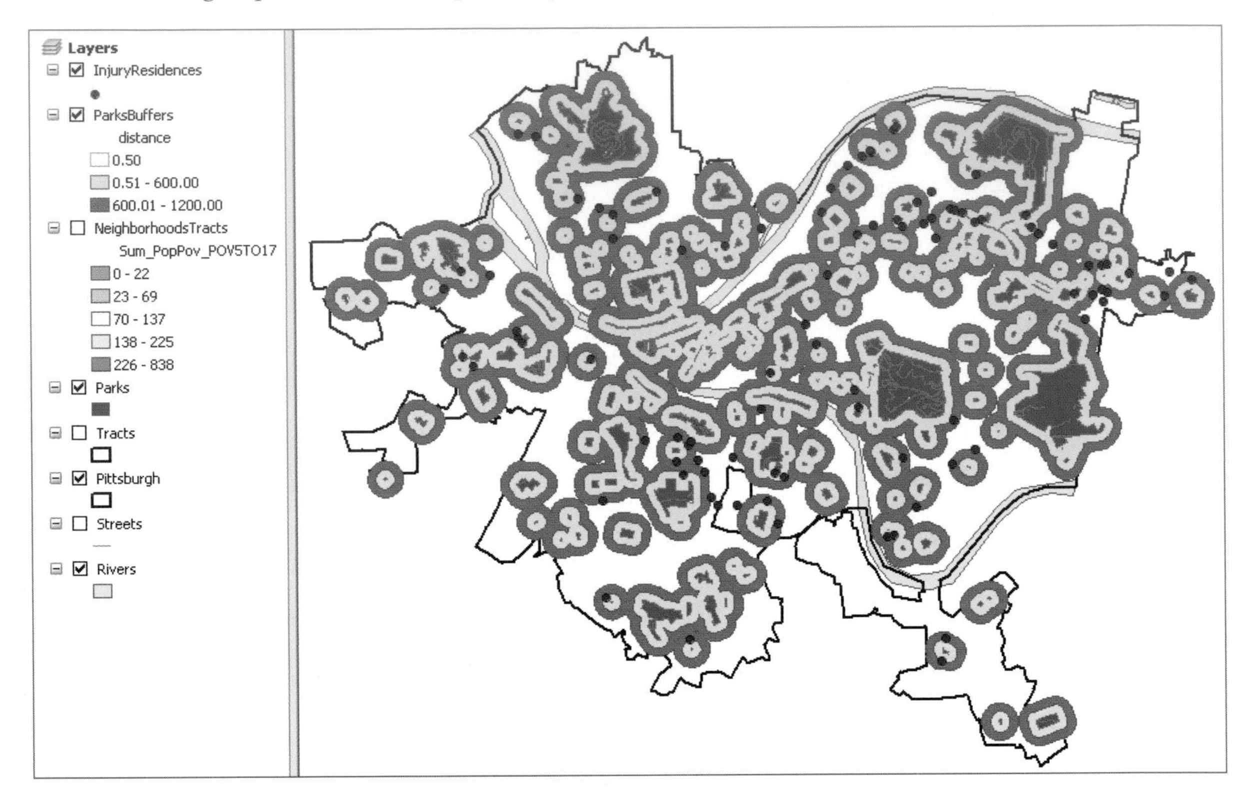

Analyze injuries and population using buffers

In this exercise, you will select injury and block centroid points within the park buffers to determine injury rates within the 600 ft and 1,200 ft buffers.

1 **Add BlockCentroids to your map from Pittsburgh.gdb in the Data folder.**

2 **Symbolize the layer using a Circle 1 point symbol set to a size 2 and a dark-gray fill color.**

3 **In the table of contents, right-click ParksBuffers and click Open Attribute Table. In the table, click the row selector button for the second row, which has a distance value of 600.**

ParksBuffers

Shape *	distance	OBJECTID *	Shape_Length	Shape_Area
Polygon	0.5	1	852186.882709	115164760.740708
Polygon	600	2	1745718.565342	462562090.93932
Polygon	1200	3	1641637.918078	507991430.327739

2 (1 out of 3 Selected)

4 **Close the table.**

5 On the Selection menu, click Select By Location and match the settings in the figure. Click Apply and then Close. ▶

6 Right-click InjuryResidences, click Open Attribute Table, and note that there are 31 injuries in the 600 ft buffer. Close the table.

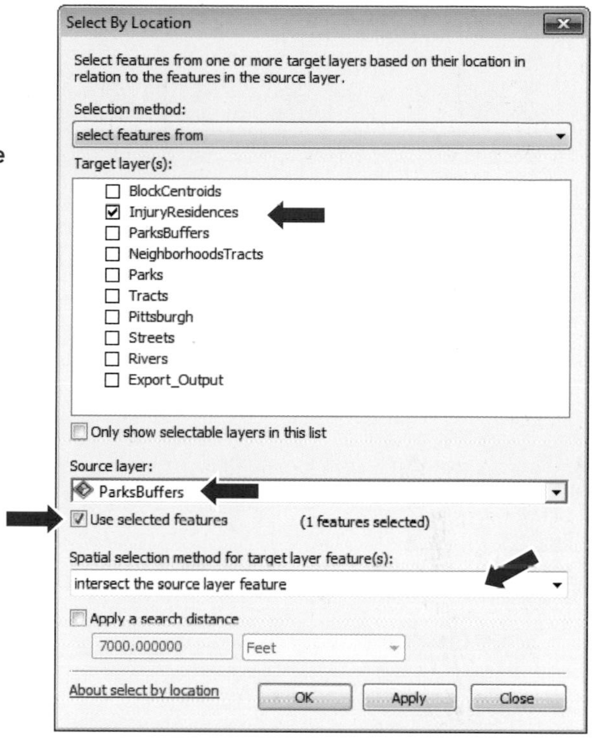

Select By Location

Select features from one or more target layers based on their location in relation to the features in the source layer.

Selection method:

select features from

Target layer(s):

☐ BlockCentroids
☑ InjuryResidences
☐ ParksBuffers
☐ NeighborhoodsTracts
☐ Parks
☐ Tracts
☐ Pittsburgh
☐ Streets
☐ Rivers
☐ Export_Output

☐ Only show selectable layers in this list

Source layer:

ParksBuffers

☑ Use selected features (1 features selected)

Spatial selection method for target layer feature(s):

intersect the source layer feature

☐ Apply a search distance

7000.000000 Feet

About select by location OK Apply Close

7 On the Selection menu, click Select By Location and match the settings in the figure. Click Apply and then Close. ▶

Select By Location

Select features from one or more target layers based on their location in relation to the features in the source layer.

Selection method:

select features from

Target layer(s):

☑ BlockCentroids
☐ InjuryResidences
☐ ParksBuffers
☐ NeighborhoodsTracts
☐ Parks
☐ Tracts
☐ Pittsburgh
☐ Streets
☐ Rivers
☐ Export_Output

☐ Only show selectable layers in this list

Source layer:

ParksBuffers

☑ Use selected features (1 features selected)

Spatial selection method for target layer feature(s):

intersect the source layer feature

☐ Apply a search distance

7000.000000 Feet

About select by location OK Apply Close

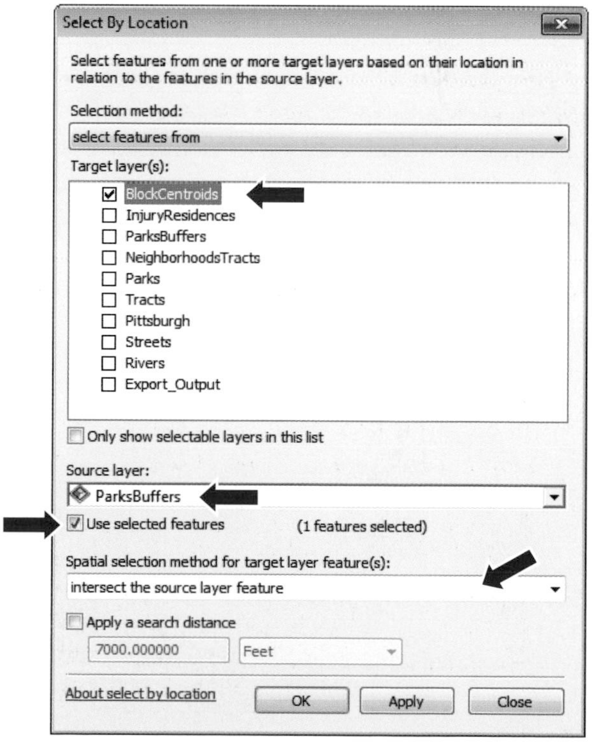

8 **Right-click BlockCentroids, click Open Attribute Table, right-click the AGE_5_17 field name, and click Statistics.** Note that there is a sum of 17,479 youths in the 600 ft buffer.

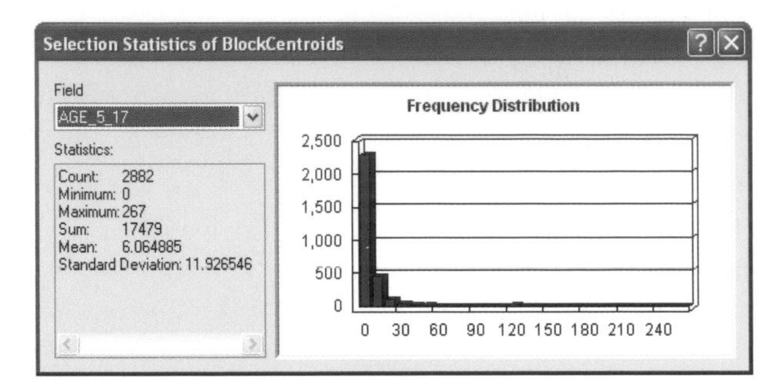

9 **Close the Selection Statistics of BlockCentroids window and close the table.**

10 **On the Selection menu, click Clear Selected Features.**

YOUR TURN

Repeat the preceding analysis to get the number of injuries and sum of youths in the 600-to-1,200 ft buffer. You will find that there are 45 injuries and 17,492 youths in the 600-to-1,200 ft buffer ring.

The table that follows summarizes the results you have found. Injuries per 10,000 youths are 45 percent higher in the 600-to-1,200 ft buffer ring than in the 0-to-600 ft buffer ring, suggesting that youths living in the 600 ft buffer ring have relatively fewer serious injuries. It can be speculated that this is because the latter youths play more in parks, which are safer environments that are removed from vehicular traffic. The ratio of 1.45 is derived by dividing 25.73 by 17.74.

Parks buffer ring	Injuries	Youth population	Injuries per 10,000 youths	Ratio
0–600	31	17,479	17.74	1.00
600–1,200	45	17,492	25.73	1.45

Save the map document

1 **On the File menu, click Save As.**

2 **Save your map document as** Tutorial7-4YourName.mxd **to your Chapter7 folder in MyExercises.** Close ArcMap.

Summary

You have investigated hypothesized relationships between serious youth-pedestrian injuries in Pittsburgh and two explanatory variables: poverty and access to parks. It was expected that injury rates would increase with poverty levels and decrease with proximity to parks. The basis for this work was a sample of 94 injuries collected over a five-year period by a pediatric hospital—a relatively small number of cases considering the population of 90 Pittsburgh neighborhoods. For this reason and others, this study was highly exploratory.

Nevertheless, you found some evidence to support both hypotheses. A total of 65 percent of serious-youth-injury residences are in the top 40 percent of neighborhoods by number of youths living in poverty, whereas only 14 percent of such injuries are in the lowest 40 percent of neighborhoods by youth-poverty population. The simple correlation between the number of injuries by neighborhood and the total youth population living in poverty by neighborhood is nearly 0.6. You also found that the serious-injury rate per 10,000 youths is 45 percent higher in the 600-to-1,200 ft buffer ring of parks, compared with the 0-to-600 ft buffer ring. This supports the hypothesis that living near parks reduces youth-pedestrian injuries.

In future work, the authors hope to use a larger sample of injury data—for example, one that includes moderate injuries from all Pittsburgh hospitals. The study could be improved if accident-location addresses were obtained in addition to the residence addresses of victims. It also seems relevant to start including additional physical features as explanatory variables, such as natural surroundings and the actual locations of play facilities.

This chapter provides a recap and extension of many of the GIS skills you learned in chapters 1 through 6. If you have successfully completed the tutorials in these chapters, you have acquired nearly every skill needed to use GIS to study a region of interest that is not a county or state.

The work accomplished in this chapter illustrates the unique and powerful spatial analysis capabilities of GIS. Spatial joins are key to data aggregation—transforming individual events into aggregate measures to use in modeling. Buffers provide a way to study the impact of proximity of populations to facilities. The next chapter takes spatial analysis to the next level, asking you to spatially interpolate data—a common task that faces analysts studying spatial phenomena.

Assignment 7-1

Conduct proximity analysis for playgrounds

In the last tutorial in chapter 7, you conducted a proximity analysis of parks and serious youth-pedestrian injuries using 600 ft and 1,200 ft buffers. In this assignment, you will run the same buffer analysis on playgrounds.

Start with this data

- *\EsriPress\GISTHealth\Data\Pittsburgh.gdb\BlockCentroids:* point centroids for the youth population in the city of Pittsburgh.
- *\EsriPress\GISTHealth\Data\Pittsburgh.gdb\Neighborhoods:* polygon features for neighborhoods in the city of Pittsburgh.
- *\EsriPress\GISTHealth\Data\Pittsburgh.gdb\Playgrounds:* polygon features of playgrounds in the city of Pittsburgh. ***Note:*** *Playgrounds is missing a projection (.prj) file. The correct projection (NAD_1983_StatePlane_Pennsylvania_South_FIPS_3702_Feet) must be assigned for buffers in this assignment to work properly.*
- *\EsriPress\GISTHealth\MyExercises\Chapter7\Chapter7.gdb\InjuryResidences:* point features of pedestrian injuries joined from InjuriesSmith and InjuriesJones earlier in this chapter. ***Note:*** *also available in FinishedExercises.*
- \EsriPress\GISTHealth\MyExercises\Chapter7\Chapter7.gdb\Rivers: polygon features of rivers created earlier in this chapter. ***Note:*** *also available in FinishedExercises.*

Create a file geodatabase

Create a file geodatabase called **Assignment7-1.gdb** and save it to your Chapter7 folder in MyAssignments. Import the preceding features and add them to your map document, symbolized to your liking.

Conduct additional sensitivity analysis for buffers around playgrounds

Create a map document called **Assignment7-1YourName.mxd** and save it to your Chapter7 folder in MyAssignments, using relative paths. Include a map layout that contains a buffer analysis of playgrounds and the number of injuries, sum of youths, and a ratio using buffers of 0.5, 600, and 1,200 ft.

Save new buffer features to Assignment7-1.gdb.

Create a Word document

Create a Microsoft Word document called **Assignment7-1YourName.docx** that includes a table of your analysis results similar to the table you created earlier in this chapter comparing the number of youth injuries with the number of youths in the 600 ft and 1,200 ft buffers. Insert an image of your map of playground buffers below the table. Save it to your Chapter7 folder in MyAssignments

Hints

- *Assign the projection NAD_1983_StatePlane_Pennsylvania_South_FIPS_3702_Feet to playgrounds—otherwise, the buffers will not work*
- *Use FEET as the buffer unit.*

Export your map as a JPEG image file called **Assignment7-1YourName.jpg** and save it to your Chapter7 folder in MyAssignments.

WHAT TO TURN IN

If your work is to be graded, turn in the following files:

- ***File geodatabase:*** \EsriPress\GISTHealth\MyAssignments\Chapter7\Assignment7-1YourName.gdb
- ***ArcMap document:*** \EsriPress\GISTHealth\MyAssignments\Chapter7\Assignment7-1YourName.mxd
- ***Microsoft Word document:*** \EsriPress\GISTHealth\MyAssignments\Chapter7\Assignment7-1YourName.docx

If instructed to do so, instead of individual files, turn in a compressed file, **Assignment7-1YourName.zip**, that includes all the preceding files. Do not include path information in the compressed file.

Assignment 7-2
Map injuries near schools and convenience stores

Youth-pedestrian injuries may also occur near swimming pools, convenience stores, and other likely kids' destinations in the neighborhood. Children are sometimes injured near schools on weekends, holidays, or even on school days when they return to play on school grounds after crossing guards have gone for the day and school zone lights are no longer flashing.

In this assignment, you will run a buffer analysis similar to the one you did for parks and playgrounds but this time for schools and convenience stores in the city of Pittsburgh.

Start with this data

- *\EsriPress\GISTHealth\Data\Pittsburgh.gdb\Neighborhoods:* polygon feature class of Pittsburgh neighborhoods
- *\EsriPress\GISTHealth\Data\Pittsburgh.gdb\BlockCentroids:* point features of the youth population in the city of Pittsburgh
- *\EsriPress\GISTHealth\Data\Pittsburgh.gdb\ConvenienceStores:* point features of convenience stores in the city of Pittsburgh
- *\EsriPress\GISTHealth\Data\UnitedStates.gdb\PASchools:* XY table of Pennsylvania schools
- *EsriPress\GISTHealth\MyExercises\Chapter7\Chapter7.gdb\InjuryResidences:* point feature class of pedestrian injuries joined from InjuriesSmith and InjuriesJones earlier in this chapter

Create a file geodatabase

Create a file geodatabase called **Assignment7-2YourName.gdb** and save it to your Chapter7 folder in MyAssignments. Import the preceding feature classes and table and add them to your map document.

Conduct a sensitivity analysis of injuries for buffers around schools and convenience stores

Create a map document called **Assignment7-2YourName.mxd** and save it to your Chapter7 folder in MyAssignments, using relative paths. Include a 600 ft and 1,200 ft buffer analysis around schools. Repeat the buffer analysis for convenience stores and serious pedestrian injuries. See "Hints."

Create a Word document

Create a Microsoft Word document called **Assignment7-2YourName.docx** that includes a table showing the number of serious pedestrian injuries, sum of youth, injuries per 10,000 youths, and ratio in the 600 ft and 1,200 ft buffers around schools. Repeat for convenience stores. Insert images of each buffer analysis of schools and convenience stores. Save it to your Chapter7 folder in MyAssignments.

Hints

- *You will need the skills learned in tutorial 4-8 for creating school points from an XY event table. Select only schools within Pittsburgh neighborhoods and create a new point feature class of these schools. When exporting the selected points for Pittsburgh, use the same coordinate system as the data frame (NAD_1983_StatePlane_Pennsylvania_South_FIPS_3702_Feet)—otherwise, the schools buffer might not be created properly.*
- *There is no need for the 0.5 ft buffer in this assignment because the input features are points.*
- *Use FEET for the buffer units.*
- *For the youth population, use AGE_5_17, the school-age youth population.*

WHAT TO TURN IN

If your work is to be graded, turn in the following files:

- ***File geodatabase:*** \EsriPress\GISTHealth\MyAssignments\Chapter7\Assignment7-2YourName.gdb
- ***ArcMap document:*** \EsriPress\GISTHealth\MyAssignments\Chapter7\Assignment7-2YourName.mxd
- ***Microsoft Word document:*** \EsriPress\GISTHealth\MyAssignments\Chapter7\Assignment7-2YourName.docx

If instructed to do so, instead of individual files, turn in a compressed file, **Assignment7-2YourName.zip**, that includes all the preceding files. Do not include path information in the compressed file.

Assignment 7-3
Study injury rates by neighborhood

In this assignment, researchers at the Pittsburgh pediatric hospital where the pedestrian-injury data was collected would like to explore the possibilities of a prevention program to reduce vehicular injuries to child pedestrians to identify which neighborhoods have the highest injury rates.

Pittsburgh has 90 neighborhoods, so unless child-pedestrian injuries are highly concentrated in relatively few neighborhoods, there will be too few data points for strong evidence, either way, to support the hypothesis. So this study is highly exploratory and would be strengthened by injury data from multiple sources (such as other hospitals, the police department, ambulance companies, etc.).

Start with this data

- ***\EsriPress\GISTHealth\MyExercises\Chapter7\Chapter7.gdb\Rivers:*** polygon features of rivers created earlier in this chapter. *Note: also available in FinishedExercises.*
- ***\EsriPress\GISTHealth\Data\Pittsburgh.gdb\Neighborhoods:*** polygon feature class of Pittsburgh neighborhoods.
- ***\EsriPress\GISTHealth\Data\Pittsburgh.gdb\BlockCentroids:*** point centroids for the youth population in Pittsburgh (US Census 2000).
- ***\EsriPress\GISTHealth\MyExercises\Chapter7\Chapter7.gdb\InjuryResidences:*** point feature class of pedestrian injuries joined from InjuriesSmith and InjuriesJones earlier in this chapter.

Create a file geodatabase

Create a file geodatabase called **Assignment7-3YourName.gdb** and save it to your Chapter7 folder in MyAssignments. Import the preceding features and add them to your map document. Import the rivers as polygons to use as a visual reference.

Create a map analyzing injury rates per neighborhood

Create a map document called **Assignment7-3YourName.mxd** and save it to your Chapter7 folder in MyAssignments, using relative paths. Include a map layout that contains a choropleth map of neighborhoods showing the pedestrian-injury rate per 1,000 kids using four rates: **3.00 and under, 3.01-6.00, 6.01-9.00, 9.01 and over**. See "Hints." Label your map using the neighborhood name and the count of injuries by neighborhood for neighborhoods that have injuries. Add rivers for visual reference.

Export your map as a JPEG image file called **Assignment7-3YourName.jpg** and save it to your Chapter7 folder in MyAssignments.

Hints

- *Spatially join point centroids to the neighborhoods, creating a new polygon feature class called* ***PopulationByNeighborhood*** *and save it to Assignment7-3YourName.gdb. Use the Sum option to summarize the population fields for neighborhoods.*
- *Spatially join injuries point features to PopulationByNeighborhood, creating a new polygon feature class called* ***InjuriesByNeighborhood*** *and save it to Assignment7-3YourName.gdb.*
- *Create a new field called* ***AGE_18_UNDER*** *that adds columns Sum_AGE_UNDER5 and Sum_AGE_5_17.*
- *To get the rate of injuries, create a new field called* ***INJRATE*** *with type FLOAT that calculates the count of injuries by neighborhood (Count_1) divided by the population under 18 (AGE_18_UNDER) multiplied by 1,000.*
- *Some neighborhoods will have no injuries. Add these neighborhoods as a Hollow fill and medium-dark-gray outline to display them.*

Create a Word document

Create a Microsoft Word document called **Assignment7-3YourName.docx** that includes an image of your map layout. Include a few bullets or sentences about what neighborhood(s) you would recommend for an injury prevention program based on the injury rate and the number of injuries. Save it to your Chapter7 folder in MyAssignments

WHAT TO TURN IN

If your work is to be graded, turn in the following files:

- ***File geodatabase:*** \EsriPress\GISTHealth\MyAssignments\Chapter7\Assignment7-3YourName.gdb
- ***ArcMap document:*** \EsriPress\GISTHealth\MyAssignments\Chapter7\Assignment7-3YourName.mxd
- ***Microsoft Word document:*** \EsriPress\GISTHealth\MyAssignments\Chapter7\Assignment7-3YourName.docx

If instructed to do so, instead of individual files, turn in a compressed file, **Assignment7-3YourName.zip**, that includes all the preceding files. Do not include path information in the compressed file.

Chapter 8

Transforming data using approximate methods

Objectives

- Use geoprocessing functions to aggregate data
- Use indicator variables and spatial joins to apportion data
- Build a model to automate data aggregation

Health-care scenarios

Analysis of health policy issues generally depends on area data, such as the number of infected persons per health referral region or the number of uninsured persons per census tract. It is data that is obtained from multiple sources and for different types of polygon boundary layers. It is often necessary to transform this data into a common set of polygons to use in mapping and modeling—for example, from census tracts to health administrative territories or from census block groups to administrative zones. But although it is generally reasonable to transform data from smaller areas into larger ones, the reverse is not recommended. Some cases may yield no errors in data transformation, but many others require approximations that could result in errors.

In the first scenario, the Dartmouth Atlas of Health Care Project, which is part of the Center for the Evaluative Clinical Sciences at Dartmouth Medical School in Hanover, New Hampshire, has brought together researchers in diversified disciplines—including epidemiology, economics, and statistics—to examine how medical resources are distributed and used in the United States. Using very large health-care claims databases—including Medicare, Blue Cross organizations, and other sources of data—this project makes it possible to address fundamental issues that affect the US health-care system, including undesirable variations in the quality of health care across the country.

Analysts working on the Dartmouth project have defined hospital service areas (local health-care markets for hospital care) and hospital referral regions (regional markets for tertiary medical care) as the working geography for health-care analysis. Unfortunately, these areas are not coterminous with census area boundaries; that is, they were not constructed by dissolving census block groups or census tracts. Thus, the census areas overlap research regions, and it is not possible to simply aggregate the census data to these regions. If analyses are to include demographic and economic data, some spatial processing is necessary to transform and, in some cases, split or apportion the census data across health service areas and health referral regions.

In another scenario, local health officials define the boundaries of emergency medical services (EMS) zones and need to know the vulnerable populations in these areas. These populations are defined using census variables such as poverty, but the spatial boundaries for the census data are not coterminous with EMS zones.

Solution approach

The GIS analyst faces three scenarios in transforming aggregate data spatially. If the source polygons of the variable being transformed are smaller than and coterminous with the target polygons, the solution is a simple data aggregation of source polygon variables—for example, transforming census tract data so it can be aggregated to county polygons (figure 8.1). A simple data query sums the tract data by county, and the resulting county-level data can then be joined to a county polygon map layer.

The second case is when the source polygons are much smaller than the target polygons and not coterminous. The example used in this chapter is extremely safe and accurate, containing over 10,000 source polygons per target polygon. The approach to this scenario is still simple, with its accuracy depending on error cancellation. The source polygons are converted into centroid points, and the centroid points are spatially joined to the target polygons to associate a source polygon with a single target polygon. Then the centroid data is summed by target polygons to complete the aggregation process. In the final data, some source

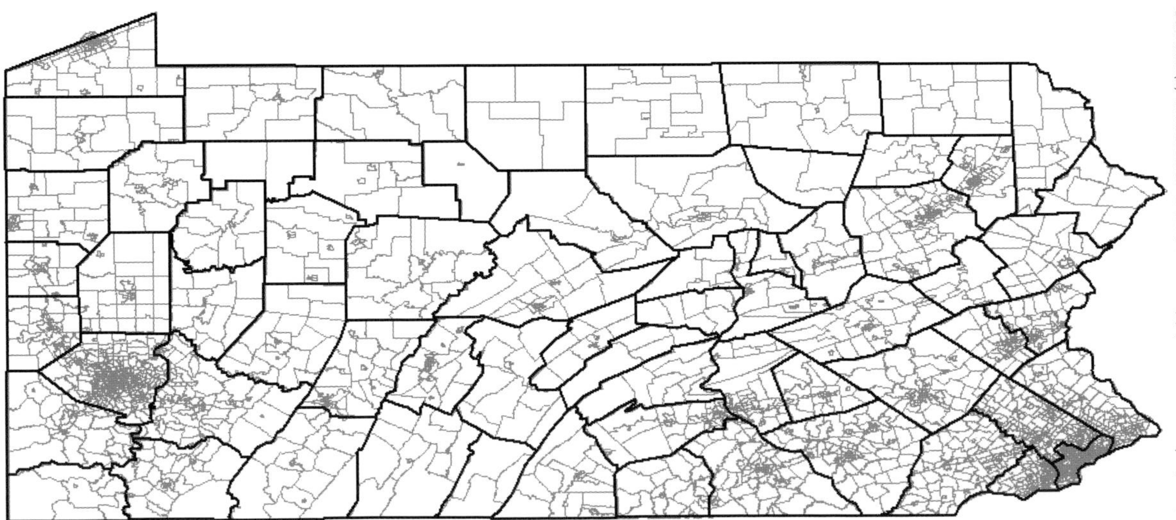

Figure 8.1 County and coterminous census tract boundaries in Pennsylvania

Sources: (a) Census 2000 TIGER/Line Data; (b) Esri Data & Maps (2005).

polygons cross target polygons, which results in errors because each source polygon's data is allocated to only a single target polygon. This is the target polygon in which the source polygons' centroids lie, where the data should be split between two or more polygons. Having a much smaller source polygon than the target polygons means that there will be many such errors per target polygon, but the errors tend to cancel each other out. You will use this version of simple data aggregation in tutorial 8-1.

The third approach is used when source and target polygons are comparable in size, and the source polygons are at least somewhat smaller. The cancellation of errors associated with allocating all a source polygon's data to a single target polygon doesn't work because there are too few source polygons per target polygon. An example is census block groups as source polygons and EMS zones as target polygons when there are not many block groups per EMS zone. In this case, it is necessary to split up the attribute variable of interest for a source polygon that crosses two or more target polygons and allocate this variable to each target polygon.

An example is shown in figure 8.2, which displays all the block groups within or intersected by an EMS zone. The figure shows block groups that cross the EMS boundary so that you can easily see them. If you were to allocate census block group data to EMS zone 9 using census block group centroids and spatial overlay, the EMS zone would have none of the data from tracts 420030103001, 420030305002, 420030305001, and 420030605001, but it would have all the data from the other block groups. Very likely, there would be a sizable error in the resulting EMS zone estimate of the census variable of interest.

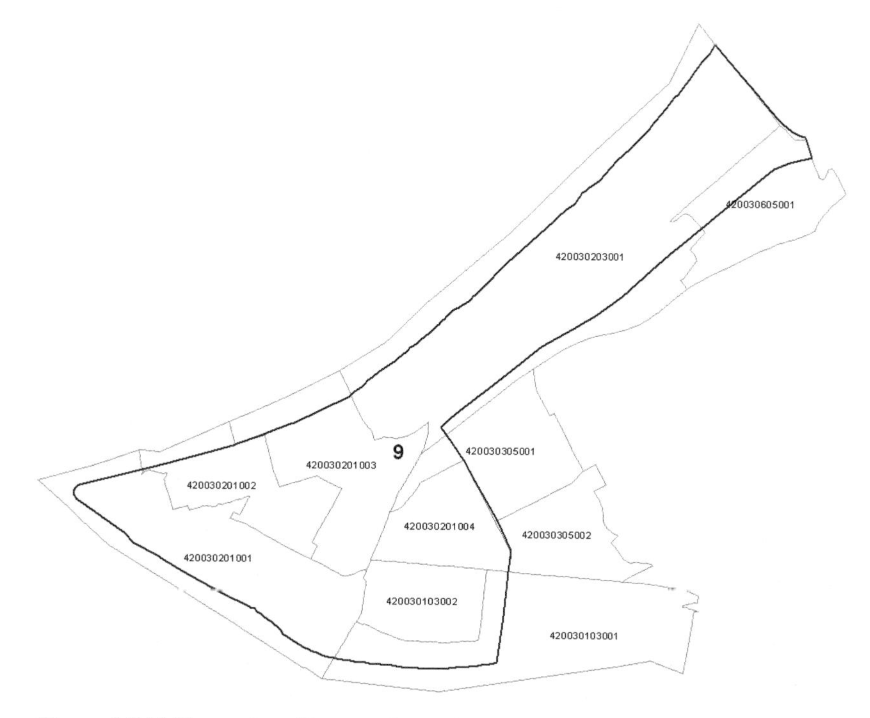

Figure 8.2 EMS zone 9 and intersecting or interior census block groups

Thus, you need an approximate means for splitting the source polygon's data. Suppose that a source polygon is split into two parts, one part in target polygon A and the other part in target polygon B. A simple approach is to assume that the actual split of the source polygon variable is proportional to the source polygon's area in target polygons A and B. Then the analyst can approximately split, or apportion, the attribute to A and B using the proportions of the source polygon in A and B as weights as in a weighted average. The weights are positive and must sum to 1, and thus can be used to distribute all parts from a source to two or more target polygons.

People and other entities, however, are often not distributed uniformly across areas, as is assumed for this approach, and this can lead to potentially sizable errors if proper apportionment is not used. For example, no people, or very few, live in parks, lakes, or agricultural fields, all of which have area. A better approximation is to use short-form SF 1 census variables, such as total population, which is available at the census block level as an indicator variable of apportionment. You would assume that the SF 3 variable of interest is proportional in its spatial distribution to the SF 1 indicator variable.

In this case, the indicator data is joined to block centroid points and the centroids are assigned to source and target polygons. The proportion of the source indicator variable in A and B is the basis of apportionment. The assumption here is that the attribute of interest is uniformly distributed over the indicator population of the source polygon, which is often a reasonable assumption for small locales. The attractiveness of this approach, relative to using area as the apportionment variable, is that it accounts for uninhabitable areas such as lakes, cemeteries, and so forth. You will use the block-population-based apportionment in this chapter's tutorials.

Tutorial 8-1

Aggregating block data for the elderly population to health referral regions

Census block polygons in Nebraska are not coterminous with health referral region polygons: Some census blocks overlap the much larger boundaries of health referral regions. In this tutorial, for example, a selected block is split between two health referral regions.

In this example, aggregating US Census data at the block level to health referral regions fits the situation where the source polygons are much smaller than the target polygons and are noncoterminous. So you will use simple aggregation from block-polygon centroids and aggregate a census attribute to health referral polygons, using a spatial join. Blocks and block centroids for Nebraska are already downloaded for your use, and the census attribute of interest, AGE_65_UP for the population age 65 and older, is permanently joined. The block centroids were created using steps similar to those in tutorial 5-8.

Open an existing map

1 **Start ArcMap and open Tutorial8-1.mxd.** A choropleth map of Dartmouth Health Atlas health referral regions in Nebraska shows Medicare enrollees using data from Continuous Medicare History Sample (CMHS) 5% from the Centers for Medicare and Medicaid Services. The data is for a random 5 percent sample of Medicare enrollees selected on the basis of the terminal digits in their Social Security numbers.

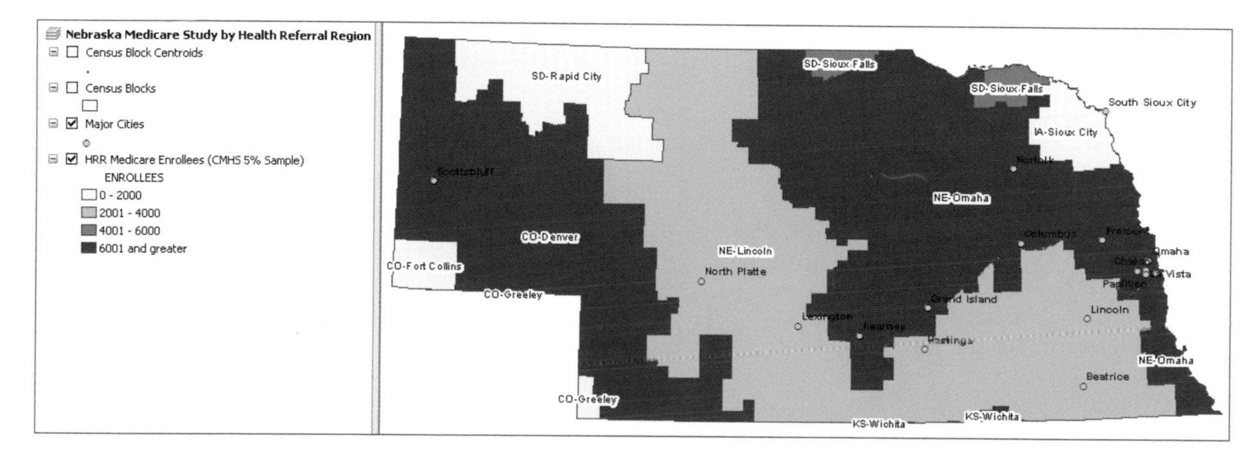

T 8-1

YOUR TURN

Turn on the Census Blocks layer in your map to see that there are many blocks per referral region. Then use the half-dozen bookmarks that are provided to see overlaps of blocks across referral areas. Some are small and others large. Turn on the Census Block Centroids layer and use the bookmarks again. Turn off blocks and block centroids and zoom out to the full extent.

Create a file geodatabase

1 Open the Catalog window and browse to your Chapter8 folder.

2 Right-click Chapter8 and click New > File Geodatabase.

3 Rename the file geodatabase Chapter8.gdb.

4 Close Catalog.

Intersect health referral regions and block centroids

Census block centroids contain the same data as census block polygons and are better for aggregating data to polygons. Using block centroids assumes that the centroid of the census block polygon falls within the polygon to which it is being aggregated. In previous chapters, you used the spatial join process to aggregate data. In this exercise, you will use the geoprocessing Intersect tool, which will be the first step in a model to automate this process.

1 On the Geoprocessing menu, click Intersect.

2 In the Intersect dialog box, match the settings in the figure. Name the output feature class BlockCentroidsHRRIntersect **and click OK.** ▶

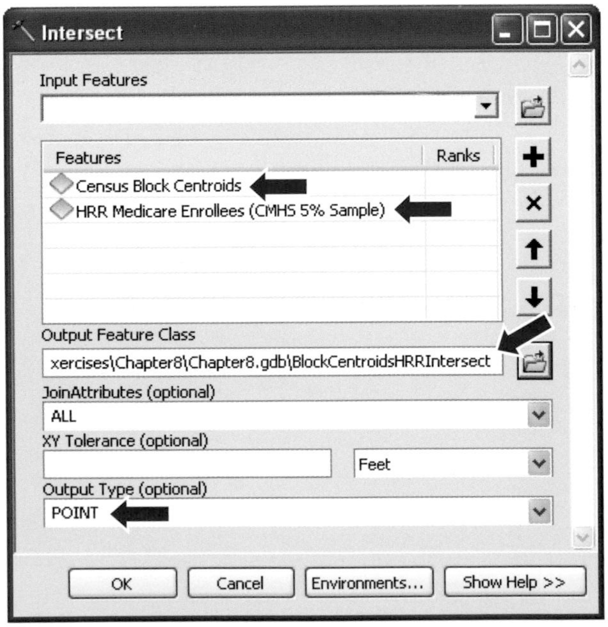

Intersect

Input Features

Features	Ranks
Census Block Centroids	
HRR Medicare Enrollees (CMHS 5% Sample)	

Output Feature Class

xercises\Chapter8\Chapter8.gdb\BlockCentroidsHRRIntersect

JoinAttributes (optional)

ALL

XY Tolerance (optional)

Feet

Output Type (optional)

POINT

OK Cancel Environments... Show Help >>

3 **Open the BlockCentroidsHRRIntersect attribute table to see that each block has the HRR_LABEL field.**

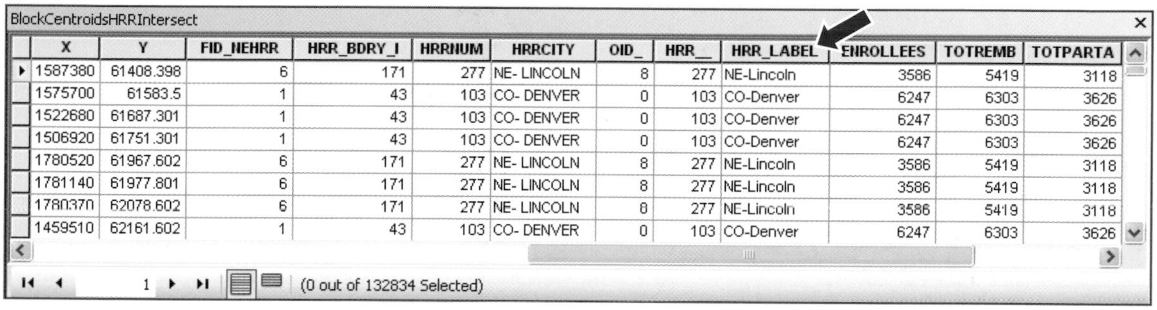

BlockCentroidsHRRIntersect

X	Y	FID_NEHRR	HRR_BDRY_I	HRRNUM	HRRCITY	OID_	HRR_	HRR_LABEL	ENROLLEES	TOTREMB	TOTPARTA
1587380	61408.398	6	171	277	NE- LINCOLN	8	277	NE-Lincoln	3586	5419	3118
1575700	61583.5	1	43	103	CO- DENVER	0	103	CO-Denver	6247	6303	3626
1522680	61687.301	1	43	103	CO- DENVER	0	103	CO-Denver	6247	6303	3626
1506920	61751.301	1	43	103	CO- DENVER	0	103	CO-Denver	6247	6303	3626
1780520	61967.602	6	171	277	NE- LINCOLN	8	277	NE-Lincoln	3586	5419	3118
1781140	61977.801	6	171	277	NE- LINCOLN	8	277	NE-Lincoln	3586	5419	3118
1780370	62078.602	6	171	277	NE- LINCOLN	8	277	NE-Lincoln	3586	5419	3118
1459510	62161.602	1	43	103	CO- DENVER	0	103	CO-Denver	6247	6303	3626

(0 out of 132834 Selected)

4 **Close the table.**

Use the Dissolve tool to aggregate data

You could use the table Summarize option to aggregate the population field to a summary table, but in this exercise you will use the geoprocessing Dissolve tool to aggregate block data to the health referral region level. This is a tool that could be used in a later model to automate this process, which you will learn more about in tutorial 8-3.

1 **On the Geoprocessing menu, click Dissolve.**

2 **In the Dissolve dialog box, for Input Features, click BlockCentroidsHRRIntersect and match the settings in the figure. Name the output feature class** HRRAge65Plus **and save it to Chapter8.gdb.** ▶

3 **Click OK.** The resulting layer is added to the map.

4 **Remove the BlockCentroidsHRRIntersect, Census Block Centroids, and Census Blocks layers from your map.**

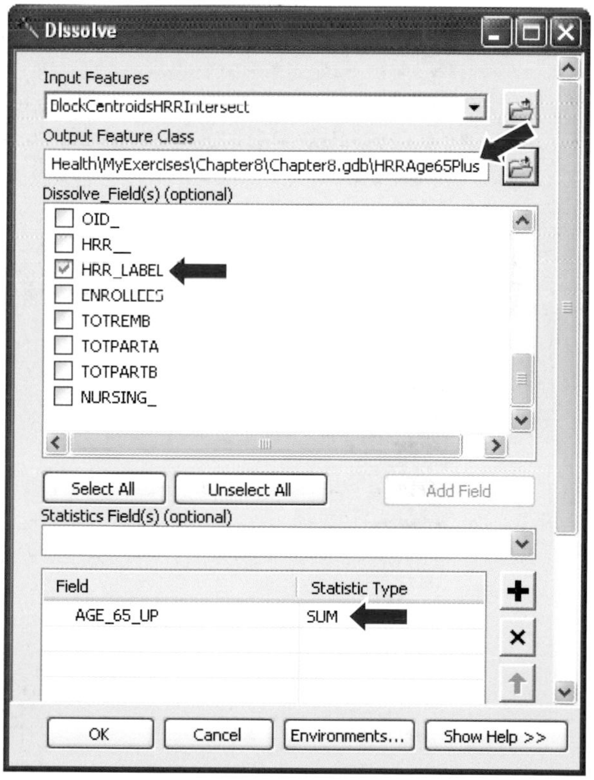

T 8-1

Join the new aggregate data to health referral regions

1 **In the table of contents, right-click HRRAge65Plus and click Open Attribute Table.** The table shows two fields as a result of the Summarize option: HRR_LABEL is the health referral region and SUM_AGE_65_UP is the number of elderly persons in each health referral region. ▶

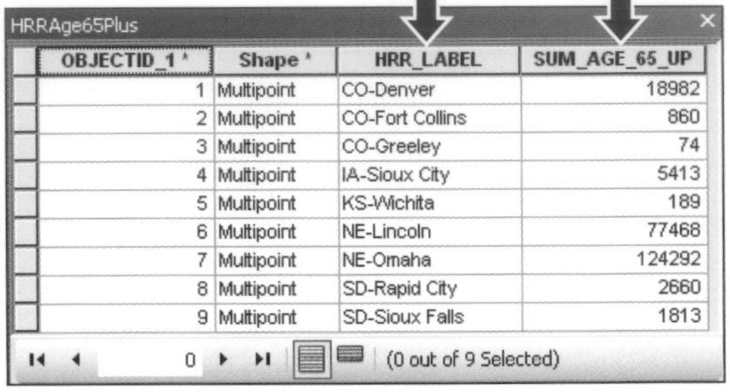

HRRAge65Plus

OBJECTID_1 *	Shape *	HRR_LABEL	SUM_AGE_65_UP
1	Multipoint	CO-Denver	18982
2	Multipoint	CO-Fort Collins	860
3	Multipoint	CO-Greeley	74
4	Multipoint	IA-Sioux City	5413
5	Multipoint	KS-Wichita	189
6	Multipoint	NE-Lincoln	77468
7	Multipoint	NE-Omaha	124292
8	Multipoint	SD-Rapid City	2660
9	Multipoint	SD-Sioux Falls	1813

0 (0 out of 9 Selected)

2 **Close the HRRAge65Plus table.**

3 **If necessary, in the table of contents, click List By Drawing Order and drag Major Cities to the top.**

4 **On the Standard toolbar, click Add Data and add NEHRR from UnitedStates.gdb.** This is a copy of Nebraska health referral regions.

5 **In the table of contents, right-click NEHRR and click Joins and Relates > Join.**

6 **In the Join Data dialog box, match the settings in the figure and click OK.** ▶

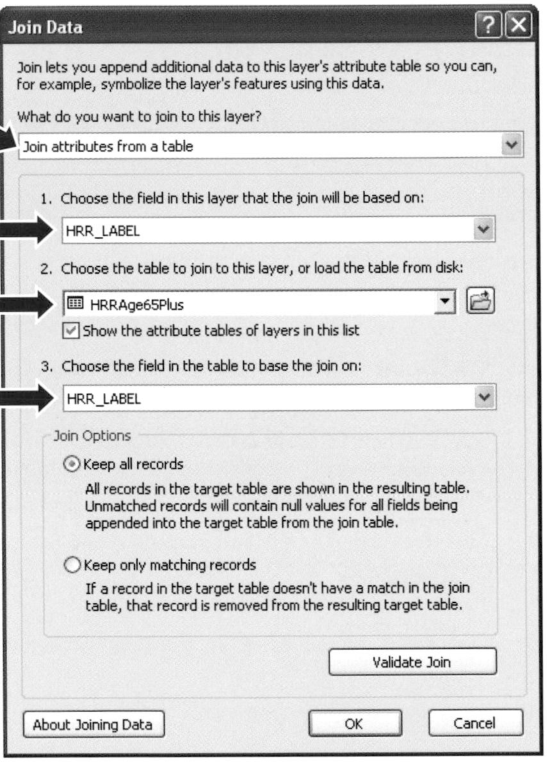

Join Data

Join lets you append additional data to this layer's attribute table so you can, for example, symbolize the layer's features using this data.

What do you want to join to this layer?

Join attributes from a table

1. Choose the field in this layer that the join will be based on:

HRR_LABEL

2. Choose the table to join to this layer, or load the table from disk:

HRRAge65Plus

Show the attribute tables of layers in this list

3. Choose the field in the table to base the join on:

HRR_LABEL

Join Options

Keep all records

All records in the target table are shown in the resulting table. Unmatched records will contain null values for all fields being appended into the target table from the join table.

Keep only matching records

If a record in the target table doesn't have a match in the join table, that record is removed from the resulting target table.

Validate Join

About Joining Data

OK

Cancel

7 **Right-click NEHRR and click Open Attribute Table.** Scroll to the right in the table and see that it now contains the sum of elderly persons.

NEHRR

Shape_Length	Shape_Area	OBJECTID_1 *	HRR_LABEL *	SUM_AGE_65_UP
5773677.095647	477709823642.423	1	CO-Denver	18982
885864.364215	26633592319.2266	2	CO-Fort Collins	860
1367466.001378	7515816647.17835	3	CO-Greeley	74
1353671.875892	45164451270.4334	4	IA-Sioux City	5413
1240664.458992	3457972324.02537	5	KS-Wichita	189
8232345.989202	773153902702.126	6	NE-Lincoln	77468

(0 out of 9 Selected)

8 **Close the table.**

9 **In the table of contents, turn off HRRAge65Plus and rename NEHRR to** Elderly Population by HRR.

Symbolize the elderly population and label enrollees for each region

1 **Right-click Elderly Population by HRR and click Properties and then the Symbology tab.**

2 **On the Symbology tab of the Layer Properties dialog box, match the classifications and settings in the figure and click OK.**

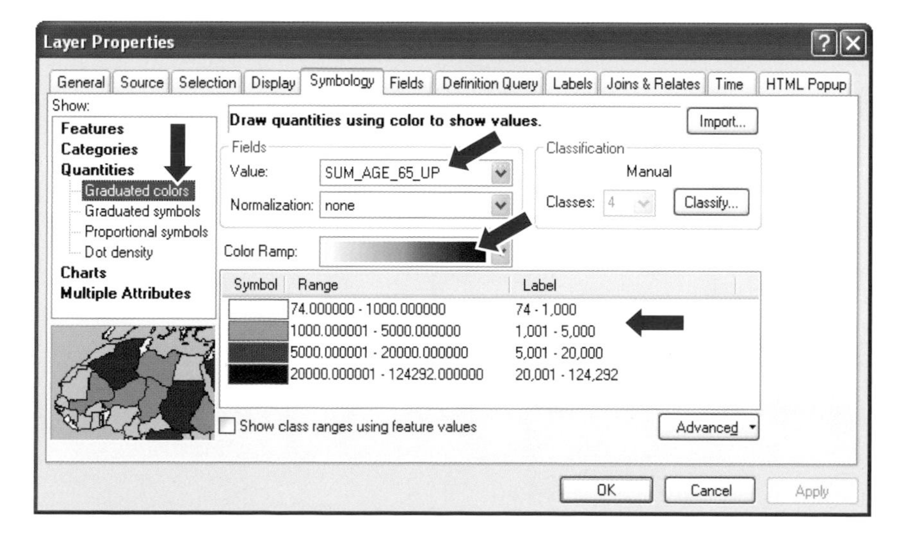

3 Label Elderly Population by HRR using the ENROLLEES field in a Bold font, size 12, and a white halo.

The resulting map shows each health referral region and the number of elderly persons per region. What referral region(s) seems to have a high number of elderly persons compared with a low number of Medicare enrollees?

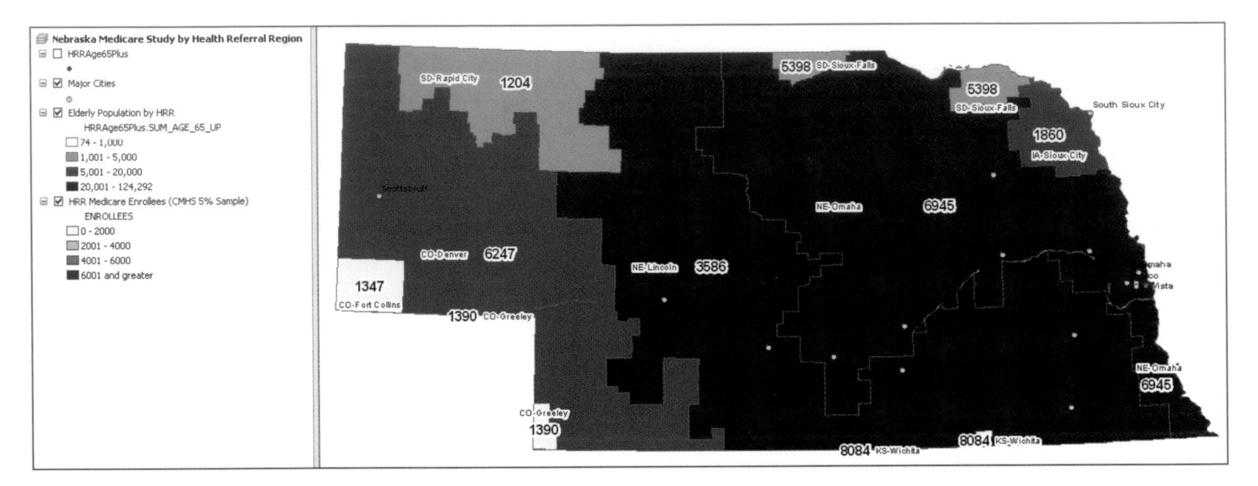

YOUR TURN

Add layers NEHSA (Nebraska Health Service Areas) and NEBlockCentroids from UnitedStates.gdb to your map document and use the Intersect, Dissolve (use HSA_CITY), and Join tools to aggregate the elderly population to HSAs. Add NEHSA again and show the Medicare enrollees as graduated colors. This time show your Health Service Area AGE_65_UP population as graduated symbols. Can you identify service areas that have a high elderly population and a low number of Medicare enrollees?

Save the map document

1 On the File menu, click Save As.

2 Save your map document as Tutorial8-1YourName.mxd **to your Chapter8 folder in MyExercises.** Do not close ArcMap.

Tutorial 8-2

Apportioning poverty data to emergency medical service zones

In this tutorial, you will process spatial data using ArcToolbox instead of the usual ArcMap menu selections. Later, you can automate the procedures by building an ArcToolbox model. Using ArcToolbox, you can implement any series of interactive ArcToolbox steps as a macro or model that can be run as a single step. This saves time and error and having to "reinvent the wheel" for a complex series of steps that you will reuse in a GIS project. Data aggregation and apportionment are ideal candidates for an ArcToolbox model.

A brief description of the layers and tables to be used for input into apportionment follows. Listings of the attributes for each attribute table are included. The layers and data tables were downloaded from the US Census Bureau and EMS Zones is from the City of Pittsburgh Planning Department. The files were renamed to make them more recognizable, extra attributes were deleted, and some attributes were renamed for clarity.

- ***BlkGrpSF3:*** table containing data from the source polygons (block groups) and several SF 3 attributes not available from the Census Bureau at the block level. You will apportion POV65Up, the population age 65 and older living in poverty, from block groups to noncoterminous EMS zones using the block-level SF 1 attribute Age_65_UP as the indicator variable. This assumes that poverty is uniformly distributed over the senior citizen population—clearly an approximation. Notice that you will not need any polygon features of block groups for apportionment. This is because block centroids and polygons are being used for location. Block groups are made up of blocks, and the 15-digit block identifier includes the block group identifier, BlkGrpID, in its first 12 digits. Normally, BlkGrpID is named STFID, but it has been renamed here for clarity.

BlkGrpSF3

OBJECTID_1 *	BlkGrpID	POVUndr18	POV65Up	POP2000
1	420030103001	38	28	657
2	420030103002	0	0	3170
3	420030201001	0	30	938
4	420030201002	0	66	674
5	420030201003	0	0	2752
6	420030201004	6	0	913

0 (0 out of 343 Selected)

- ***BlkGrpSF1:*** table containing block group level data for the SF 1 indicator, AGE_65_UP, and block group identifier, BlkGrpID. Each AGE_65_UP value here is the sum of many blocks from the attribute table of the Blocks layer and is the denominator of a weight used in apportionment.

BlkGrpSF1

OBJECTID *	STATE_FIPS	CNTY_FIPS	STCOFIPS	TRACT	BLKGRP	BlkGrpID *	POP2000	AGE_65_UP	AGE_UNDER_18
1	42	003	42003	010300	1	420030103001	657	139	115
2	42	003	42003	010300	2	420030103002	3170	9	7
3	42	003	42003	020100	1	420030201001	938	61	13
4	42	003	42003	020100	2	420030201002	674	264	8
5	42	003	42003	020100	3	420030201003	2752	35	43
6	42	003	42003	020100	4	420030201004	913	204	27

0 (0 out of 343 Selected)

- ***EMSZones:*** target set of EMS zone polygons for the City of Pittsburgh.

EMSZones

OBJECTID *	Shape *	ZONE	SQ_MILES	Shape_Length	Shape_Area	Shape_Acres
13	Polygon	0	0.34	13611.01561	9462306.480894	217.22
2	Polygon	1	0.28	13584.794931	7809508.968883	179.28
4	Polygon	1	7.88	90183.282091	219819810.743055	5046.3701
12	Polygon	2	6.17	81571.477126	171983868.728634	3948.21
7	Polygon	3	10.52	141509.788648	293180570.649974	6730.5
1	Polygon	4	8.58	80878.610436	239084721.2704	5488.6299
5	Polygon	4	0.23	13264.478689	6425057.318942	147.5
6	Polygon	4	0.08	8997.849247	2124941.630741	48.779999
9	Polygon	5	3.78	48760.820288	105312680.620177	2417.6499
3	Polygon	6	5.59	50944.68849	155769725.754299	3575.98
10	Polygon	7	5.13	55012.134374	143062956.659294	3284.27
14	Polygon	7	3.53	87456.048425	98370939.765898	2258.29
11	Polygon	8	2.25	38634.012245	62701347.035759	1439.42
8	Polygon	9	1.41	38792.512895	39379127.241747	904.02002

0 (0 out of 14 Selected)

In the next figure map, the EMS zones and block group polygons are the ones that were clipped to the city boundary.

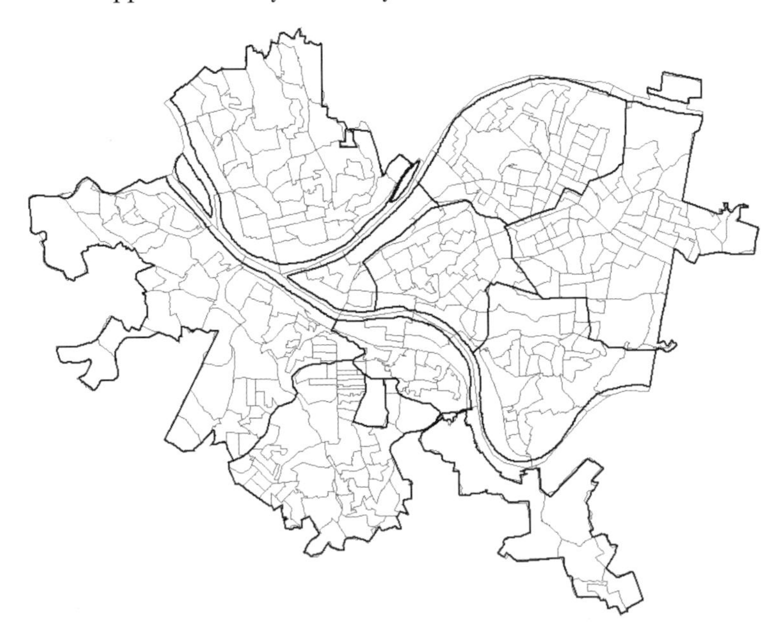

In the next figure map, you can see that the EMS zones and block group polygons were obtained from different sources and digitized independently. Boundaries that in reality are shared do not match and have alignment problems. Also, many block groups, such as the one including the pointer symbol, are split between two EMS zones.

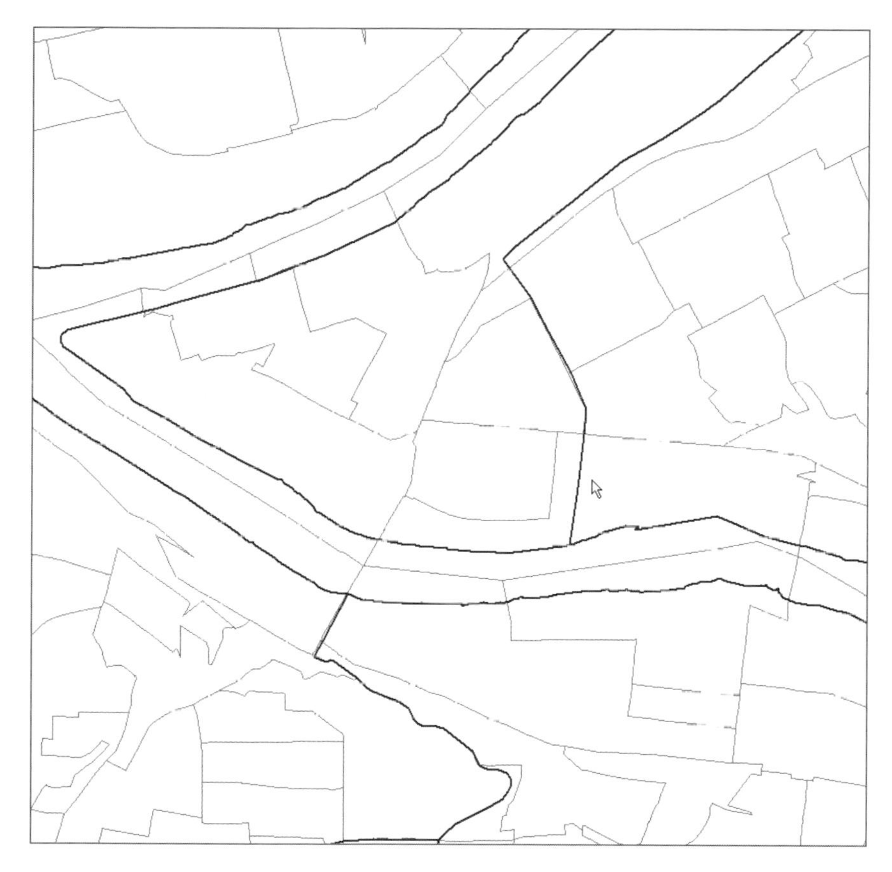

- ***BlockCentroids:*** point features for the centroids of census blocks. BlkID is the block identifier (generally named STFID but renamed here for clarity) and AGE_65_UP is the SF 1 census variable used as the indicator for apportionment.

BlockCentroids

OBJECTID *	BlkID	Shape *	POP2000	AGE_UNDER5	AGE_5_17	AGE_65_UP
1	420030103001000	Point	0	0	0	0
2	420030103001001	Point	0	0	0	0
3	420030103001002	Point	6	0	0	2
4	420030103001003	Point	46	5	4	6
5	420030103001004	Point	33	4	9	6
6	420030103001005	Point	45	5	8	12

1 (0 out of 7467 Selected)

Spatially join EMS zones to block centroids

The first step in the apportionment process is to create a new point feature class that combines the data tables of EMS zones and block centroids through a spatial join.

1 **Start ArcMap and open Tutorial8-2.mxd.**

2 **In the table of contents, click List By Source.** The map opens with all the inputs to apportionment included: three feature classes (BlockCentroids, BlockGroups [polygons not needed], and EMSZones) and two data tables (BlkGrpSF1 and BlkGrpSF3).

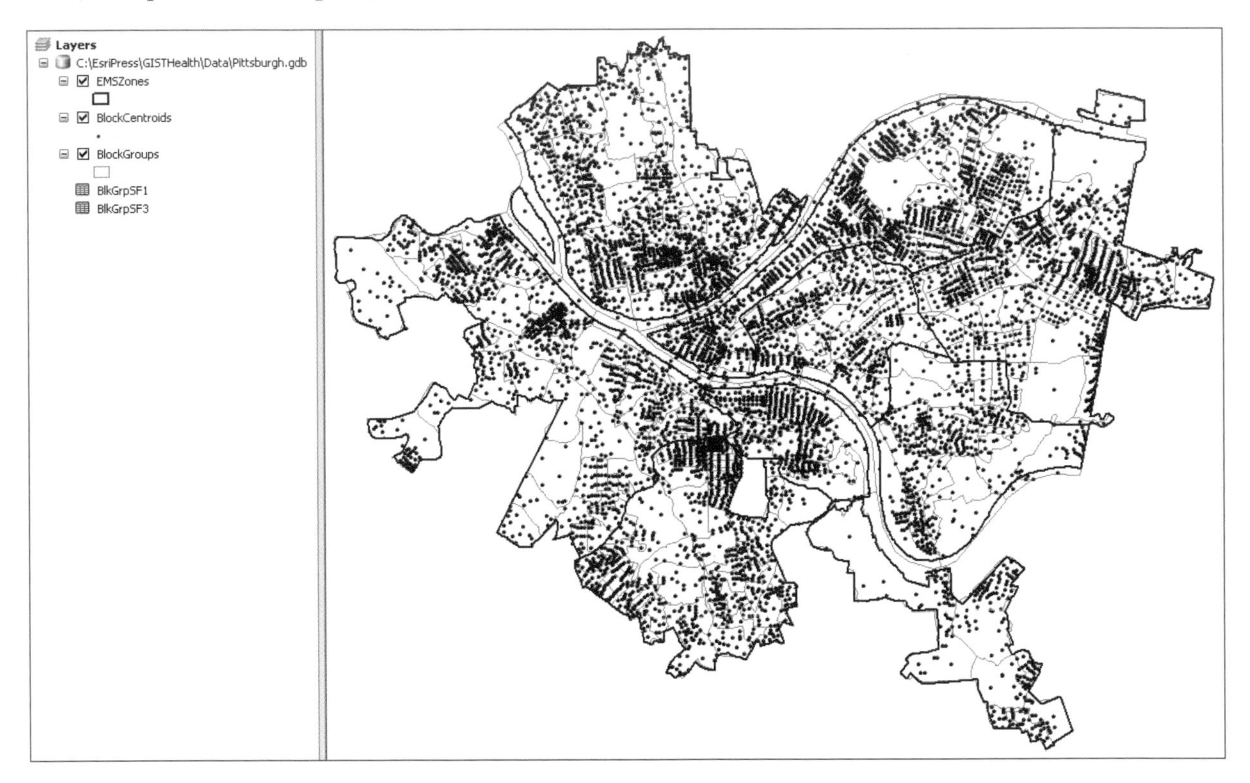

3 **On the Standard toolbar, click ArcToolbox, expand the Analysis toolbox and then the Overlay toolset, and double-click the Intersect tool.**

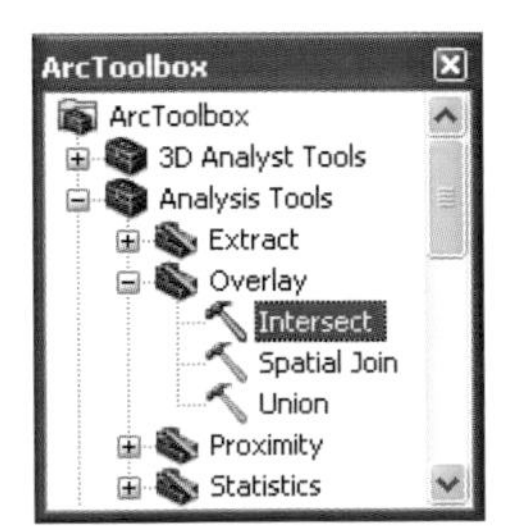

T 8-2

4 **In the Intersect dialog box, match the settings in the figure. Name the output feature class** BlkCentroidsEMS.

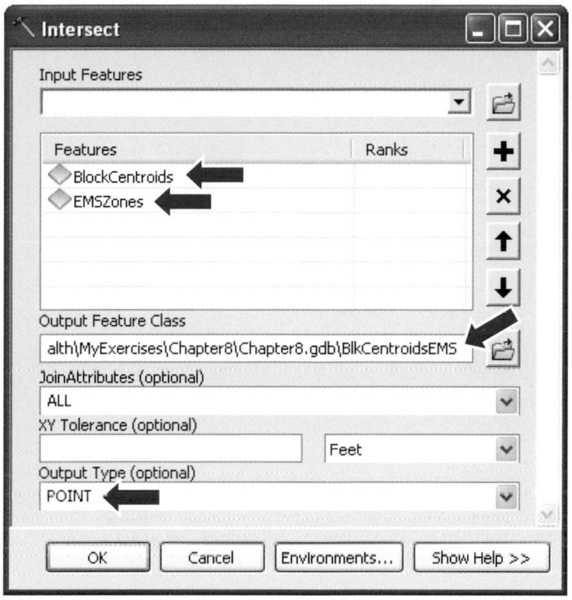

5 **Click OK.**

6 **In the table of contents, right-click BlkCentroidsEMS and click Open Attribute Table.** Notice that the table now has the combined fields of both tables. Key fields are BlkID, POP2000, AGE_UNDER5, AGE_5_17, and AGE_65_UP from the BlockCentroids table and ZONE from the EMSZones table.

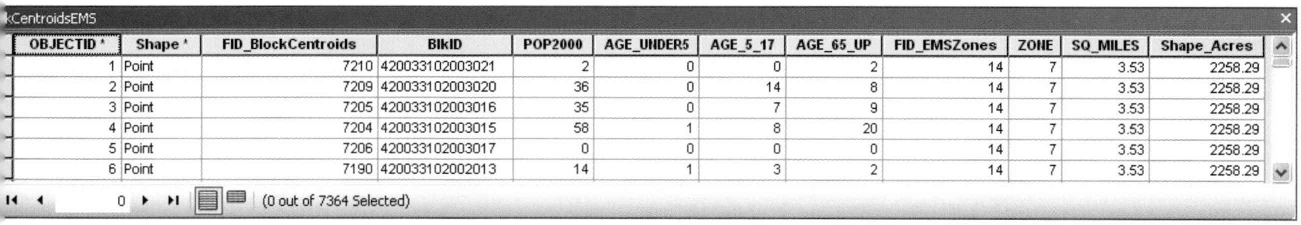

OBJECTID *	Shape *	FID_BlockCentroids	BlkID	POP2000	AGE_UNDER5	AGE_5_17	AGE_65_UP	FID_EMSZones	ZONE	SQ_MILES	Shape_Acres
1	Point	7210	420033102003021	2	0	0	2	14	7	3.53	2258.29
2	Point	7209	420033102003020	36	0	14	8	14	7	3.53	2258.29
3	Point	7205	420033102003016	35	0	7	9	14	7	3.53	2258.29
4	Point	7204	420033102003015	58	1	8	20	14	7	3.53	2258.29
5	Point	7206	420033102003017	0	0	0	0	14	7	3.53	2258.29
6	Point	7190	420033102002013	14	1	3	2	14	7	3.53	2258.29

(0 out of 7364 Selected)

7 **Close the table.**

Use the Mid( ) function to calculate BlkGrpID

The new BlkCentroidsEMS feature class needs the block group ID. This ID is the first 12 characters of the BlkID field so the Mid( ) function is needed to create the block group ID from the BlkID field. You will use the Add and Calculate Field tools in ArcToolbox to perform this function.

1 **In ArcToolbox, expand the Data Management toolbox and then the Fields toolset, and double-click the Add Field tool.**

2 **In the Add Field dialog box, match the settings in the figure and click OK.** ▶

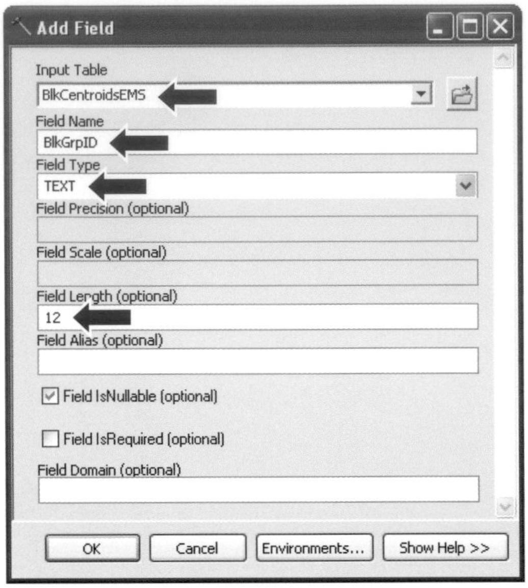

Add Field

Input Table
BlkCentroidsEMS
Field Name
BlkGrpID
Field Type
TEXT
Field Precision (optional)
Field Scale (optional)
Field Length (optional)
12
Field Alias (optional)
Field IsNullable (optional)
Field IsRequired (optional)
Field Domain (optional)
OK Cancel Environments... Show Help >>

3 **In the Fields toolset, double-click the Calculate Field tool.**

4 **In the Calculate Field dialog box, match the Input Table and Field Name settings in the figure, and then click the Field Calculator button to the right of the Expression box.** ▶

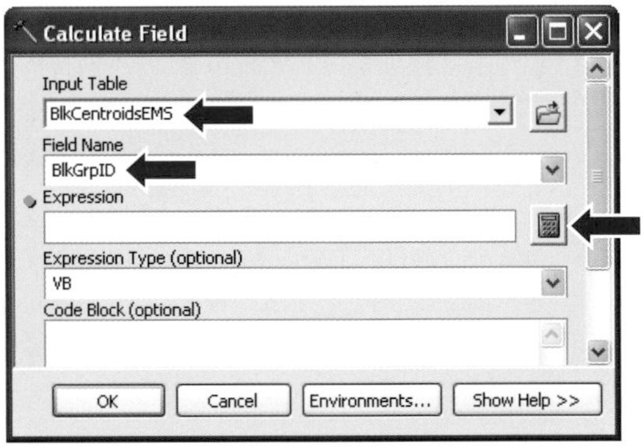

Calculate Field

Input Table
BlkCentroidsEMS
Field Name
BlkGrpID
Expression
Expression Type (optional)
VB
Code Block (optional)
OK Cancel Environments... Show Help >>

5 **Click the expression panel in the lower half of Field Calculator and type the following expression:** Mid([BlkID],1,12). This use of the Mid( ) function extracts the first 12 characters of the text variable BlkID. The first argument of the function is the name of the input text attribute; the second is an integer giving the starting position for extraction; and the third is the number of characters to extract. Alternatively, you can double-click the function and field. ▶

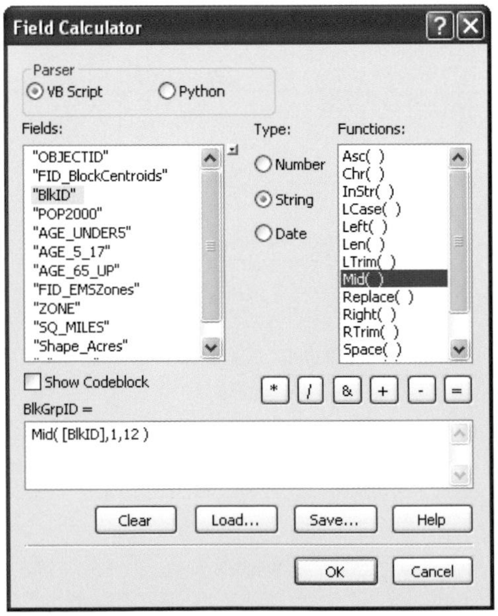

Field Calculator

Parser
VB Script Python
Fields:
"OBJECTID"
"FID_BlockCentroids"
"BlkID"
"POP2000"
"AGE_UNDER5"
"AGE_5_17"
"AGE_65_UP"
"FID_EMSZones"
"ZONE"
"SQ_MILES"
"Shape_Acres"
Type:
Number
String
Date
Functions:
Asc( )
Chr( )
InStr( )
LCase( )
Left( )
Len( )
LTrim( )
Mid( )
Replace( )
Right( )
RTrim( )
Space( )
Show Codeblock
* / & + - =
BlkGrpID =
Mid([BlkID],1,12)
Clear Load... Save... Help
OK Cancel

6 **Click OK in the two open dialog boxes.**

7 **Open the BlkCentroidsEMS attribute table and verify that BlkGrpID is the first 12 digits of BlkID.**

8 **Right-click BlkGrpID and click Sort Ascending.** Notice how all the blocks in the same block group have the same value for BlkGrpID, but they have various ZONE codes.

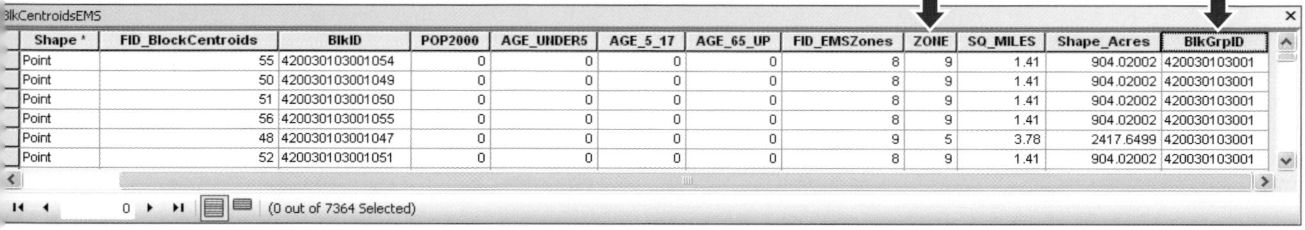

BlkCentroidsEMS

Shape *	FID_BlockCentroids	BlkID	POP2000	AGE_UNDER5	AGE_5_17	AGE_65_UP	FID_EMSZones	ZONE	SQ_MILES	Shape_Acres	BlkGrpID
Point	55	420030103001054	0	0	0	0	8	9	1.41	904.02002	420030103001
Point	50	420030103001049	0	0	0	0	8	9	1.41	904.02002	420030103001
Point	51	420030103001050	0	0	0	0	8	9	1.41	904.02002	420030103001
Point	56	420030103001055	0	0	0	0	8	9	1.41	904.02002	420030103001
Point	48	420030103001047	0	0	0	0	9	5	3.78	2417.6499	420030103001
Point	52	420030103001051	0	0	0	0	8	9	1.41	904.02002	420030103001

0 (0 out of 7364 Selected)

9 **Close the table.**

Create a new Indicator field in BlkCentroidsEMS

In this exercise, you will create a new field in BlkCentroidsEMS called INDICATOR. This field will be populated to include the values of POP_65_UP.

1 **In ArcToolbox, double-click the Add Field tool.**

2 **In the Add Field dialog box, match the settings in the figure and click OK.** ▶

Add Field
Input Table
BlkCentroidsEMS
Field Name
INDICATOR
Field Type
LONG
Field Precision (optional)
Field Scale (optional)
Field Length (optional)
Field Alias (optional)
Field IsNullable (optional)
Field IsRequired (optional)
Field Domain (optional)
OK Cancel Environments... Show Help >>

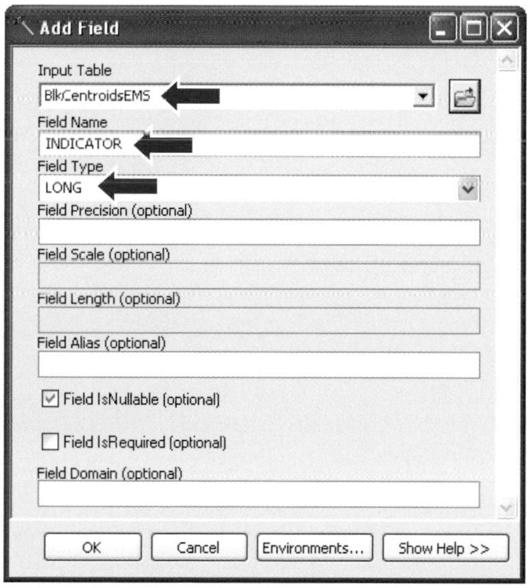

Calculate the new field

Next, you will use the field calculator to populate the INDICATOR field with values from the AGE_65_UP field.

1 **In ArcToolbox, double-click the Calculate Field tool.**

2 **In the Calculate Field dialog box, match the settings in the figure and click OK.** ▶

Calculate Field
Input Table
BlkCentroidsEMS
Field Name
INDICATOR
Expression
[AGE_65_UP]
Expression Type (optional)
VB
Code Block (optional)
OK Cancel Environments... Show Help >>

T 8-2

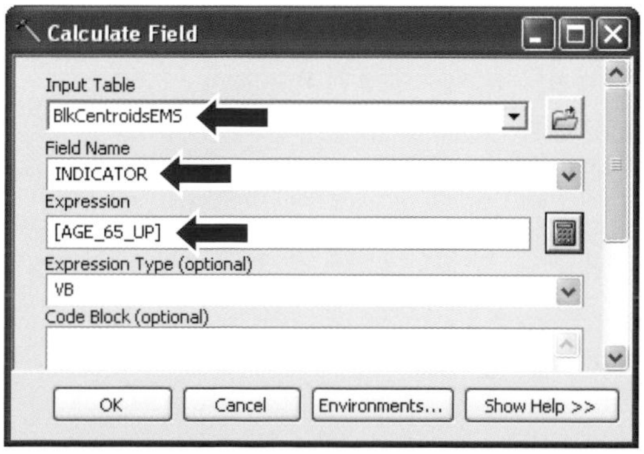

3 Open the BlkCentroidsEMS attribute table and scroll to the right to see the new values for the INDICATOR field. These are the same values as AGE_65_UP.

BlkCentroidsEMS

BlkID	POP2000	AGE_UNDER5	AGE_5_17	AGE_65_UP	FID_EMSZones	ZONE	SQ_MILES	Shape_Acres	BlkGrpID	INDICATOR
420030506001000	54	1	8	19	9	5	3.78	2417.6499	420030506001	19
420030506001008	23	1	0	7	9	5	3.78	2417.6499	420030506001	7
420030506001013	51	3	6	21	9	5	3.78	2417.6499	420030506001	21
420030506001007	19	0	3	1	9	5	3.78	2417.6499	420030506001	1
420030506001006	4	0	0	3	9	5	3.78	2417.6499	420030506001	3
420030506001005	65	3	11	9	9	5	3.78	2417.6499	420030506001	9

0 (0 out of 7364 Selected)

Create another field in BlkCentroidsEMS

Next you will create another field in BlkCentroidsEMS called INT_ID (for Intersection ID) that concatenates BlkGrpID and ZONE.

1 In ArcToolbox, double-click the Add Field tool.

2 In the Add Field dialog box, match the settings in the figure and click OK. ▶

Add Field
Input Table
BlkCentroidsEMS
Field Name
INT_ID
Field Type
TEXT
Field Precision (optional)
Field Scale (optional)
Field Length (optional)
17
Field Alias (optional)
Field IsNullable (optional)
Field IsRequired (optional)
Field Domain (optional)
OK Cancel Environments... Show Help >>

Concatenate fields

1 In ArcToolbox, double-click the Calculate Field tool.

2 In the Calculate Field dialog box, match the settings in the figure, and then click Field Calculator and create the expression shown in the Expression box. Click OK. ▶

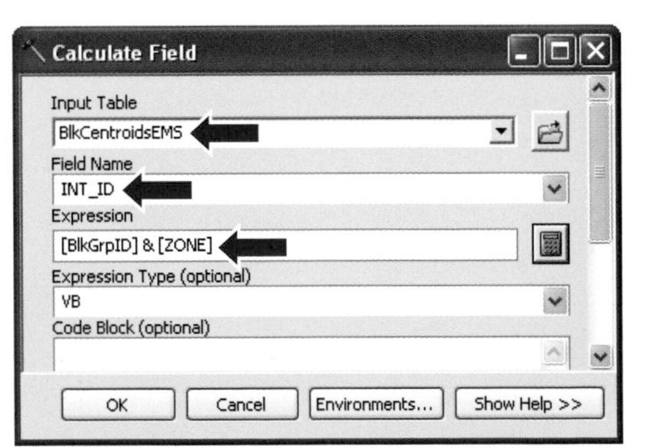

3 Open the BlkCentroidsEMS attribute table and verify that it has the values for the INT_ID field as shown in the figure.

BlkCentroidsEMS

BlkID	POP2000	AGE_UNDER5	AGE_5_17	AGE_65_UP	FID_EMSZones	ZONE	SQ_MILES	Shape_Acres	BlkGrpID	INDICATOR	INT_ID
420030506001000	54	1	8	19	9	5	3.78	2417.6499	420030506001	19	4200305060015
420030506001008	23	1	0	7	9	5	3.78	2417.6499	420030506001	7	4200305060015
420030506001013	51	3	6	21	9	5	3.78	2417.6499	420030506001	21	4200305060015
420030506001007	19	0	3	1	9	5	3.78	2417.6499	420030506001	1	4200305060015
420030506001006	4	0	0	3	9	5	3.78	2417.6499	420030506001	3	4200305060015
420030506001005	65	3	11	9	9	5	3.78	2417.6499	420030506001	9	4200305060015

0 (0 out of 7364 Selected)

Summarize the INDICATOR field by INT_ID using Dissolve

The INDICATOR (AGE_65_UP) field can now be summed by the new INT_ID (BlkGrpID and ZONE) fields. In this exercise, you will aggregate (sum) the data using ArcToolbox tools. The Dissolve tool has the capacity to sum, so that is what you will use. The result will be a new feature class of the aggregated data.

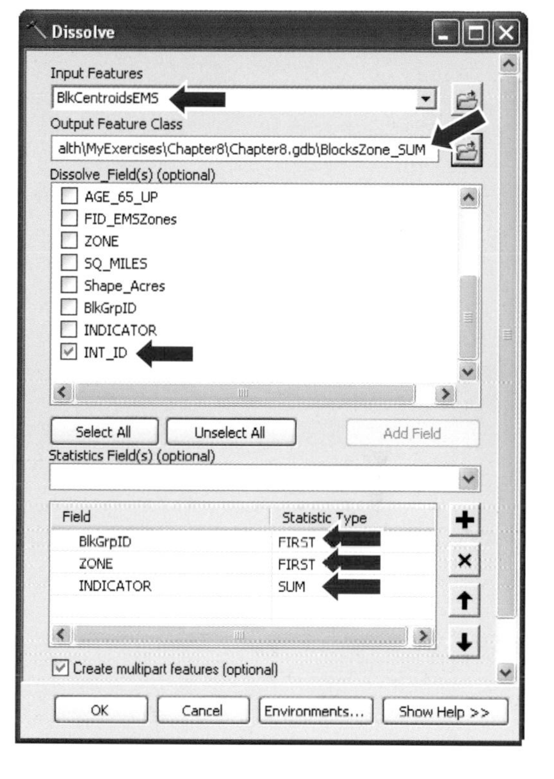

1. **In ArcToolbox, expand the Data Management toolbox and then the Generalization toolset and double-click the Dissolve tool.**

2. **In the Dissolve dialog box, match the settings in the figure. Use the Statistics Field(s) drop-down list to populate the Field column located in the lower portion of the dialog box. Also, be sure to set Statistic Type for each field by clicking the cell just to the right of the field name and choosing one of the statistic types. Name the output feature class** BlocksZone_SUM. The statistic type FIRST is used because these are text fields. This step will simply add these fields to the summary table. ▶

3. **Click OK.**

YOUR TURN

Open the BlocksZone_SUM attribute table and examine the data. You will see that you have created useful data. The SUM_INDICATOR field contains values for the numerator of weights, which was generated from the sum of the AGE_65_UP field for each block group and EMS zone intersected polygon. Close the table.

BlocksZone_SUM

OBJECTID_1 *	Shape *	INT_ID	BlkGrpID	ZONE	SUM_INDICATOR
1	Multipoint	4200301030015	420030103001	5	135
2	Multipoint	4200301030019	420030103001	9	4
3	Multipoint	4200301030029	420030103002	9	9
4	Multipoint	4200302010019	420030201001	9	61
5	Multipoint	4200302010029	420030201002	9	264
6	Multipoint	4200302010039	420030201003	9	35

1 (0 out of 378 Selected)

Add the Denominator field

Next, you will add a field used as the denominator to calculate the weight of block groups within EMS zones.

1. In the Data Management toolbox, expand the Fields toolset and double-click the Add Field tool.

2. In the Add Field dialog box, match the settings in the figure and click OK. ▶

Join BlkGrpSF1 to BlocksZone_SUM

The new DENOMINATOR field is the number of elderly persons over age 65 in each block group. Because this data is not in the BlocksZone_SUM table, you will need to temporarily join it from the BlkGrpSF1 table.

1. In the Data Management toolbox, expand the Joins toolset and double-click the Add Join tool.

2. In the Add Join dialog box, match the settings in the figure and click OK. Ignore the warning message. ▶

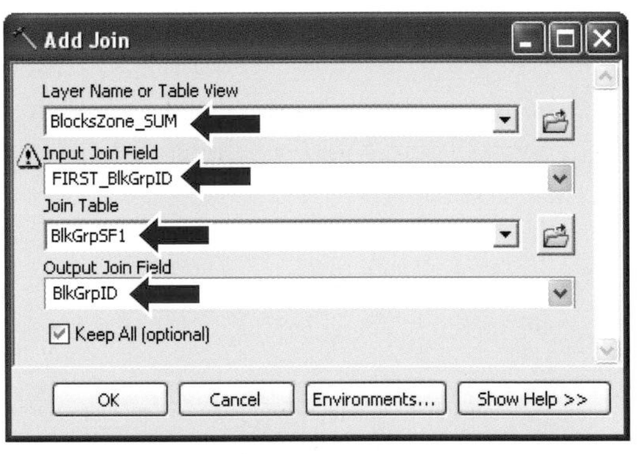

Calculate the DENOMINATOR field

Now that you have the AGE_65_UP field in your Blocks Zone_SUM table, you can calculate the DENOMINATOR field to match these values.

1. In the Fields toolset, double-click the Calculate Field tool.

2. In the Calculate Field dialog box, match the settings in the figure and click OK. ▶

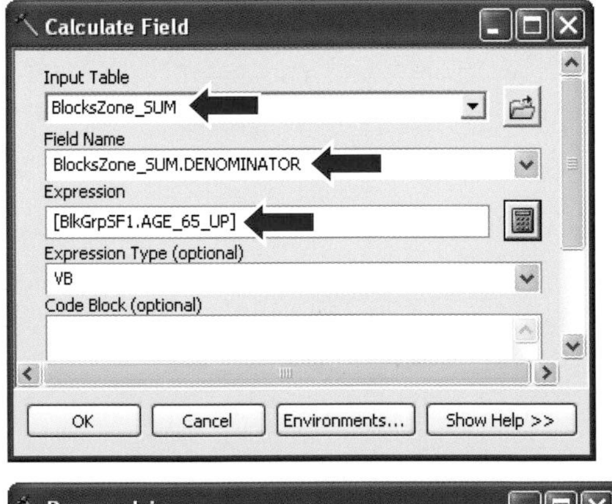

Remove the join from BlocksZone_SUM

1. In the Data Management toolbox, expand the Joins toolset and double-click the Remove Join tool.

2. In the Remove Join dialog box, match the settings in the figure and click OK and Close. ▶

T 8-2

YOUR TURN

Examine the BlocksZone_SUM attribute table and sort ascending by the BlkGrpID field. The apportionment weight for block group 420030201001 is 1 because this block group is entirely inside EMS Zone 9. Block group 420030103001, however, is split between two zones (5 and 9): 135 out of 139 senior citizens (weight = 0.971) are in Zone 5 and the remaining 4 out of 139 (weight = 0.0288) are in Zone 9. You will multiply these weights by the number of senior citizens over age 65 in poverty in the upcoming steps.

BlocksZone_SUM

OBJECTID *	Shape *	INT_ID	BlkGrpID	ZONE	SUM_INDICATOR	DENOMINATOR
1	Multipoint	4200301030015	420030103001	5	135	139
2	Multipoint	4200301030019	420030103001	9	4	139
3	Multipoint	4200301030029	420030103002	9	9	9
4	Multipoint	4200302010019	420030201001	9	61	61
5	Multipoint	4200302010029	420030201002	9	264	264
6	Multipoint	4200302010039	420030201003	9	35	35
7	Multipoint	4200302010049	420030201004	9	204	204

(0 out of 378 Selected)

Calculate the apportionment weights

Next, you will calculate the weight of the elderly population by EMS zone.

1 **In the Data Management Tools toolbox, expand the Fields toolset and double-click the Add Field tool.**

2 **In the Add Field dialog box, match the settings in the figure and click OK.** ▶

Add Field
Input Table: BlocksZone_SUM
Field Name: WEIGHT
Field Type: FLOAT
Field Precision (optional)
Field Scale (optional)
Field Length (optional)
Field Alias (optional)
Field IsNullable (optional)
Field IsRequired (optional)
Field Domain (optional)
OK | Cancel | Environments... | Show Help >>

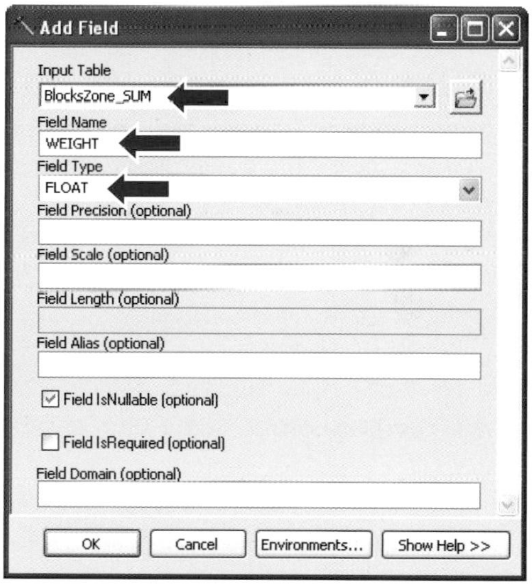

3 **In the Fields toolset, double-click the Calculate Field tool.**

4 **In the Calculate Field dialog box, match the settings in the figure and click OK.** ▶

Calculate Field
Input Table: BlocksZone_SUM
Field Name: WEIGHT
Expression: [SUM_INDICATOR] / [DENOMINATOR]
Expression Type (optional): VB
Code Block (optional)
OK | Cancel | Environments... | Show Help >>

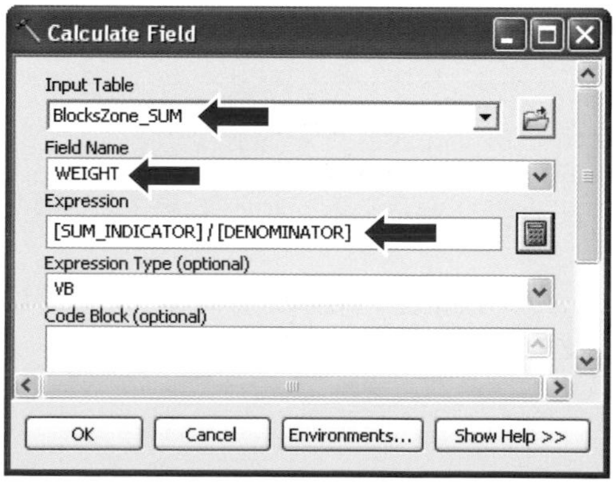

T 8-2

YOUR TURN

Open the attribute table for BlocksZone_SUM and examine the WEIGHT field. A value of 1 means that the block group is entirely within an EMS zone and a fraction means it is split between zones. Close the attribute table.

BlocksZone_SUM

OBJECTID *	Shape *	INT_ID	BlkGrpID	ZONE	SUM_INDICATOR	DENOMINATOR	WEIGHT
1	Multipoint	4200301030015	420030103001	5	135	139	0.971223
2	Multipoint	4200301030019	420030103001	9	4	139	0.028777
3	Multipoint	4200301030029	420030103002	9	9	9	1
4	Multipoint	4200302010019	420030201001	9	61	61	1
5	Multipoint	4200302010029	420030201002	9	264	264	1
6	Multipoint	4200302010039	420030201003	9	35	35	1
7	Multipoint	4200302010049	420030201004	9	204	204	1
8	Multipoint	4200302030015	420030203001	5	5	29	0.172414

0 (0 out of 378 Selected)

Join and calculate poverty data to BlocksZone_SUM

In this exercise, you will calculate the poverty data for the elderly population based on the weighted values you just created. To do so, you will add a new field and temporarily join the poverty data located in the BlkGrpSF3 table.

1 **In the Fields toolset, double-click the Add Field tool.**

2 **In the Add Field dialog box, match the settings in the figure and click OK.** ▶

Add Field
Input Table: BlocksZone_SUM
Field Name: POV_65_PLUS
Field Type: LONG
Field Precision (optional)
Field Scale (optional)
Field Length (optional)
OK | Cancel | Environments... | Show Help >>

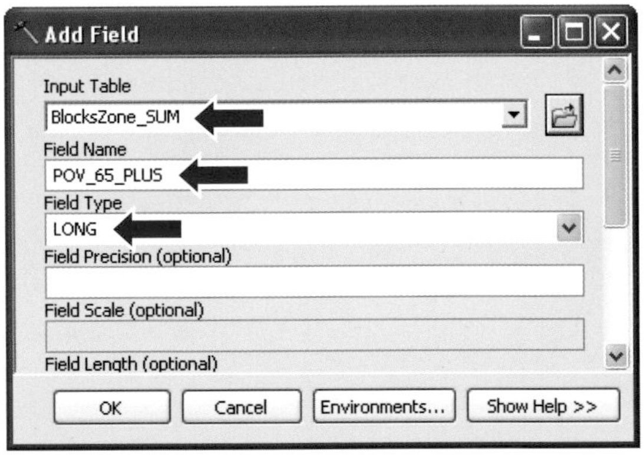

3 **In the Data Management toolbox, expand the Joins toolset and double-click the Add Join tool.**

4 **In the Add Join dialog box, match the settings in the figure and click OK.** Ignore the warning message. ▶

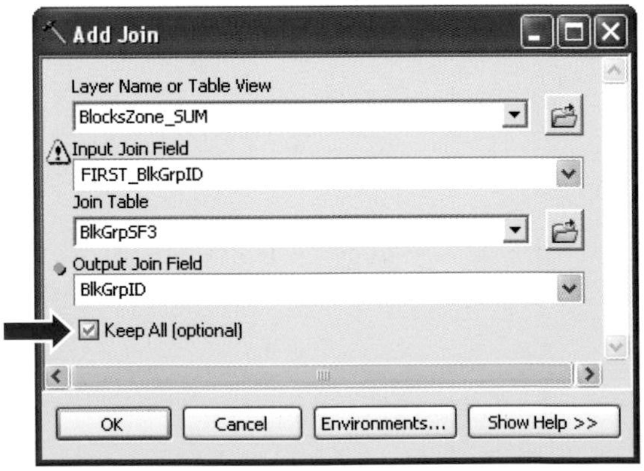

Add Join
Layer Name or Table View: BlocksZone_SUM
Input Join Field: FIRST_BlkGrpID
Join Table: BlkGrpSF3
Output Join Field: BlkGrpID
Keep All (optional)
OK | Cancel | Environments... | Show Help >>

5 **In the Fields toolbox, double-click the Calculate Field tool.**

6 In the Calculate Field dialog box, match the settings in the figure and click OK. ▶

Calculate Field

Input Table: BlocksZone_SUM

Field Name: BlocksZone_SUM.POV_65_PLUS

Expression: [BlocksZone_SUM.WEIGHT] * [BlkGrpSF3.POV65Up]

Expression Type (optional): VB

Code Block (optional)

OK | Cancel | Environments... | Show Help >>

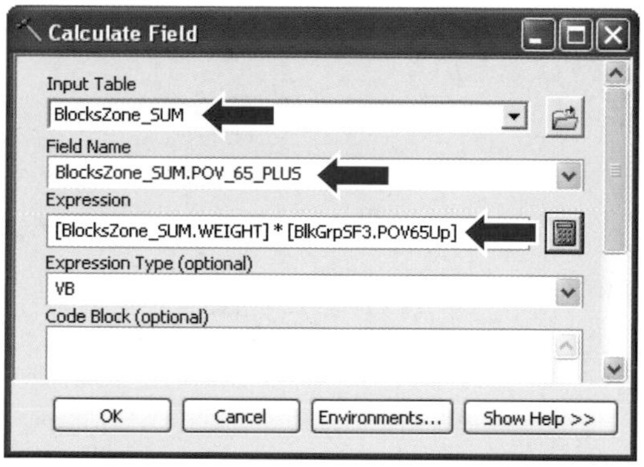

YOUR TURN

Examine the BlocksZone_SUM attribute table and compare it to the one in the figure. See how the weights have split up the SF 3 value for block group 420030103001.

BlocksZone_SUM

OBJECTID *	Shape *	INT_ID	BlkGrpID	ZONE	SUM_INDICATOR	DENOMINATOR	WEIGHT	POV_65_PLUS	POV65Up
1	Multipoint	4200301030015	420030103001	5	135	139	0.971223	27	28
2	Multipoint	4200301030019	420030103001	9	4	139	0.028777	1	28
3	Multipoint	4200301030029	420030103002	9	9	9	1	0	0
4	Multipoint	4200302010019	420030201001	9	61	61	1	30	30
5	Multipoint	4200302010029	420030201002	9	264	264	1	66	66

(2 out of 378 Selected)

Remove the table join from BlocksZone_SUM

You no longer need the BlkGrpSF3 table, so you can remove that join.

1 In the Data Management toolbox, expand the Joins toolset and double-click the Remove Join tool.

2 In the Remove Join dialog box, match the settings in the figure and click OK and Close. ▶

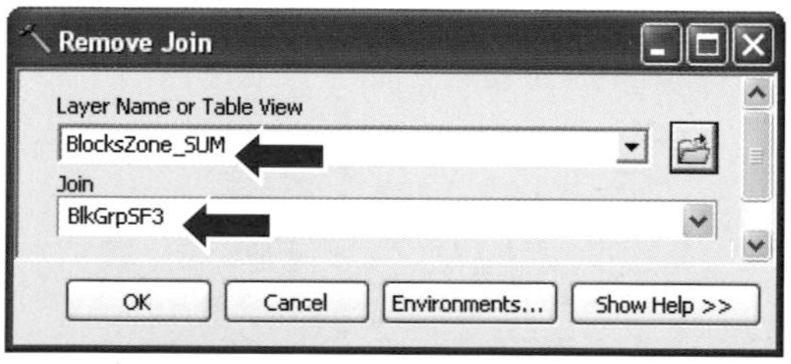

Remove Join

Layer Name or Table View: BlocksZone_SUM

Join: BlkGrpSF3

OK | Cancel | Environments... | Show Help >>

Sum the SF 3 attribute by EMS zone

You can now aggregate the population over age 65 living in poverty to EMS zones.

1 In the Data Management toolbox, expand the Generalization toolset and double-click the Dissolve tool.

2. In the Dissolve dialog box, match the settings in the figure. Name the output feature class POV65_EMS. ▶

3. Click OK.

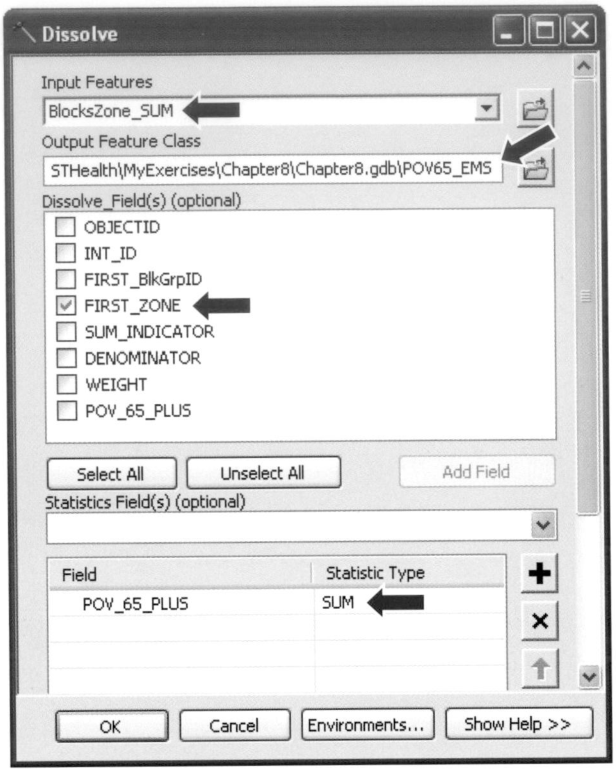

4. In the table of contents, right-click POV65_EMS, open the attribute table, and note the poverty totals for the senior citizen population for each zone. ▶

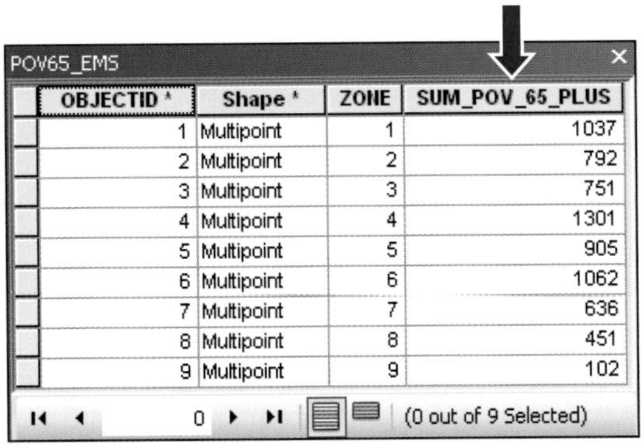

POV65_EMS

OBJECTID *	Shape *	ZONE	SUM_POV_65_PLUS
1	Multipoint	1	1037
2	Multipoint	2	792
3	Multipoint	3	751
4	Multipoint	4	1301
5	Multipoint	5	905
6	Multipoint	6	1062
7	Multipoint	7	636
8	Multipoint	8	451
9	Multipoint	9	102

(0 out of 9 Selected)

5. Close the table.

Join POV65_EMS to EMSZones

You are now ready to join the elderly poverty population to the original EMS zones.

1. In the Joins toolset, double-click Add Join.

2. In the Add Join dialog box, match the settings in the figure and click OK. ▶

3. Open the attribute table for EMSZones to verify that the poverty data was joined.

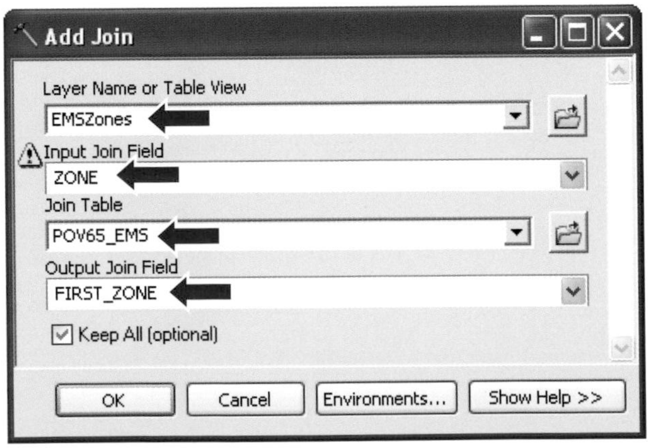

YOUR TURN

Turn off all layers except EMSZones, label the EMS zones using the ZONE field, and create a choropleth map showing the elderly population by EMS zone. What zone has the highest number of senior citizens in poverty?

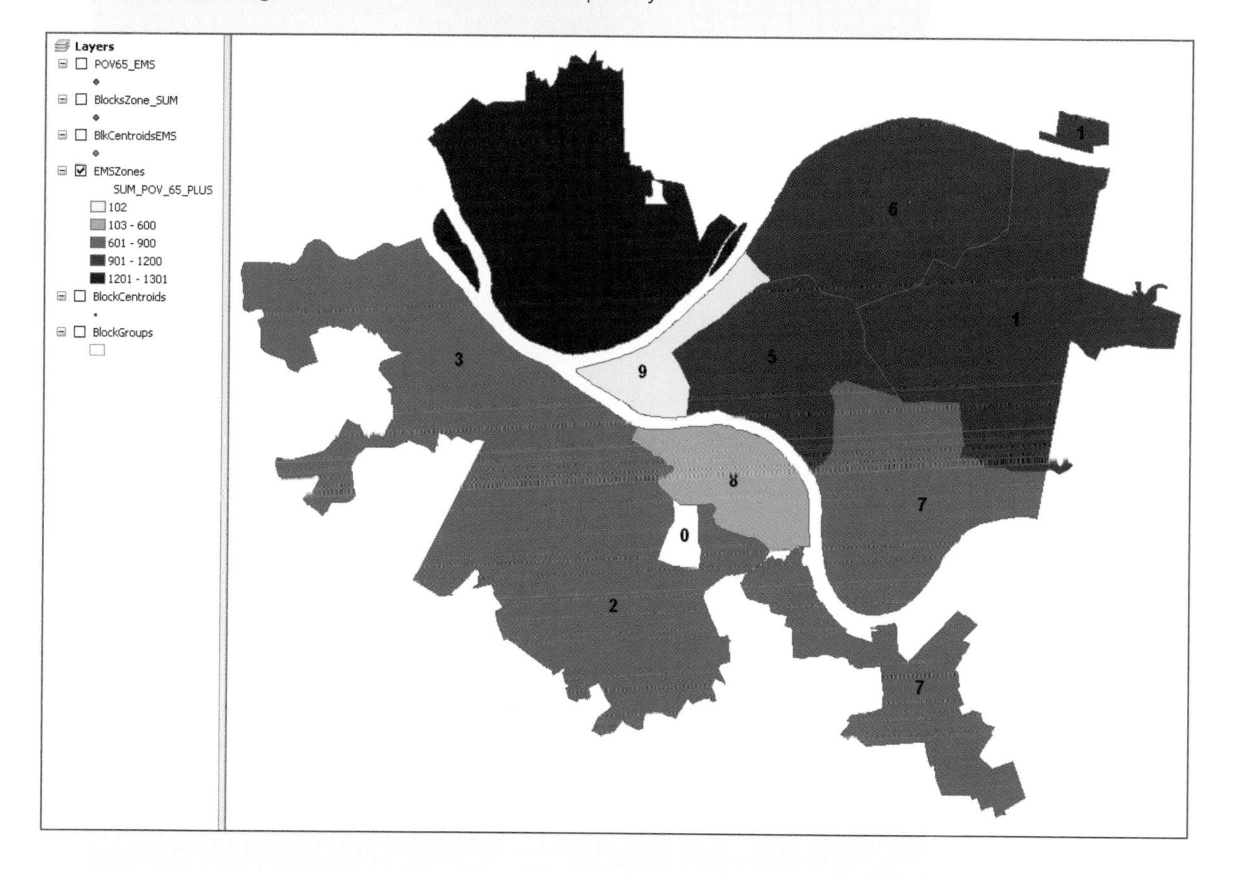

Save the map document

1 **On the File menu, click Save As.**

2 **Save your map document as** Tutorial8-2YourName.mxd **to your Chapter8 folder in MyExercises.** Do not close ArcMap.

Tutorial 8-3
Automating processes using ArcGIS ModelBuilder

Spatial data processing often requires several steps and the use of geoprocessing tools to produce the desired results. ModelBuilder is an ArcGIS application for creating macros—custom programs that document and automate geoprocessing workflows. After you build a model, you can run it once or save it and run it again using different input parameters. In this exercise, you will build a model that contains several steps for aggregating elderly population to health referral regions, similar to the process in tutorial 8-1. However, you will use ArcToolbox functions to automate this process. Before getting started, it is helpful to examine the inputs and outputs of the ArcGIS ModelBuilder application, and then look at the finished model you will build.

Open a map document

1 **In ArcMap, open Tutorial8-3.mxd.** This is a map of Nebraska displaying health referral regions and block centroids.

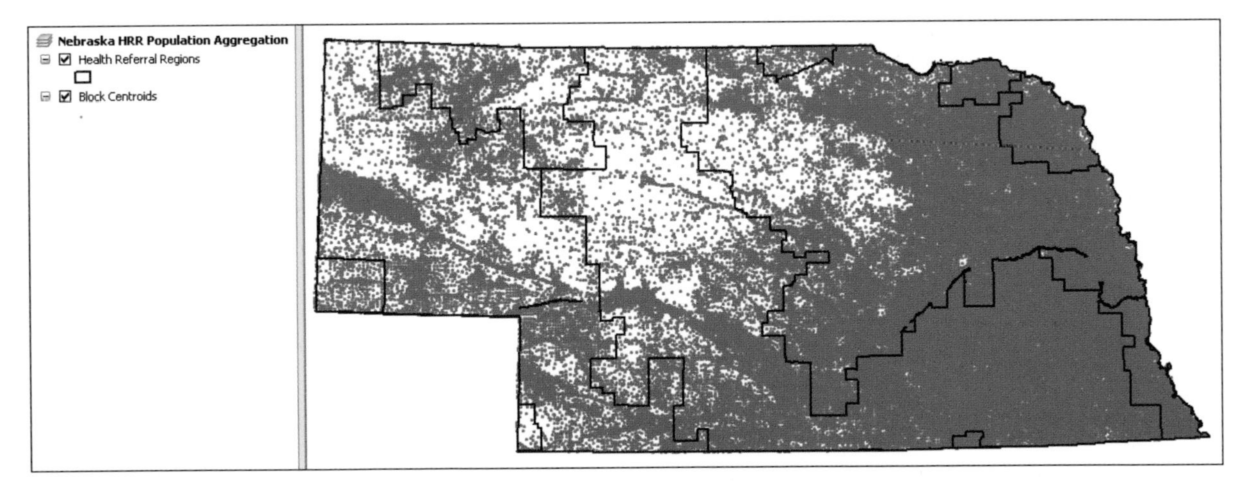

Set geoprocessing options

1 **On the Geoprocessing menu, click Geoprocessing Options.**

2 **If it is not already selected, select the "Overwrite the outputs of geoprocessing operations" check box.** Using this option, you can rerun the model repeatedly without having to delete model outputs first. This saves time when debugging your model and getting it to work properly.

3 **Click OK.**

Create a new model

1 **On the Standard toolbar, click Catalog.**

2 **Browse to your Chapter8 folder in MyExercises, right-click the folder, and click New > Toolbox.**

3 **Rename the toolbox** Chapter8.tbx.

4 **Right-click Chapter8.tbx and click New > Model.** The Model window opens with a blank canvas that you will use to create your model. Note that a toolbox must be created first before a model can be created and saved for later use.

Intersect layers

Now, you will use ArcToolbox to add the Intersect tool. When you pursue model building on your own, you will need to systematically browse through all the tools available to see the types of functionality offered. When you find a tool that you want to learn about, right-click the tool and click Help.

1 **On the Standard toolbar, click ArcToolbox and expand the Analysis toolbox and then the Overlay toolset.**

2 **Drag the Intersect tool into your model.**

3 **Double-click the Intersect process in your model and make selections using the drop-down list in each field as shown in the figure. Name the output feature class** Blocks_X_HRR. ▶

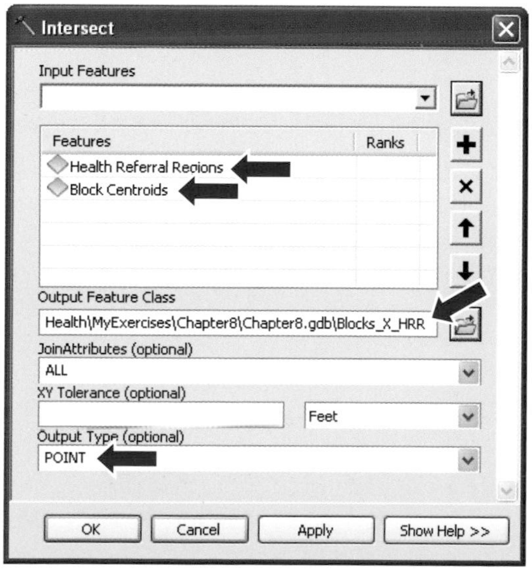

4 **Click OK, and resize and reposition the model elements as shown in the figure by adjusting the size of individual elements and dragging the model elements into place.**

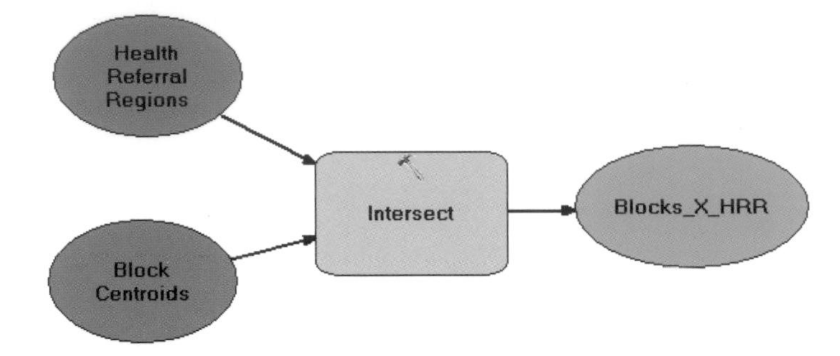

5 **On the Model toolbar, click the Save button.**

Run the partial model

1 **In your model, right-click the Intersect tool, and then click Run.** As the process runs, a report window on the task opens and reports the process status. ▶

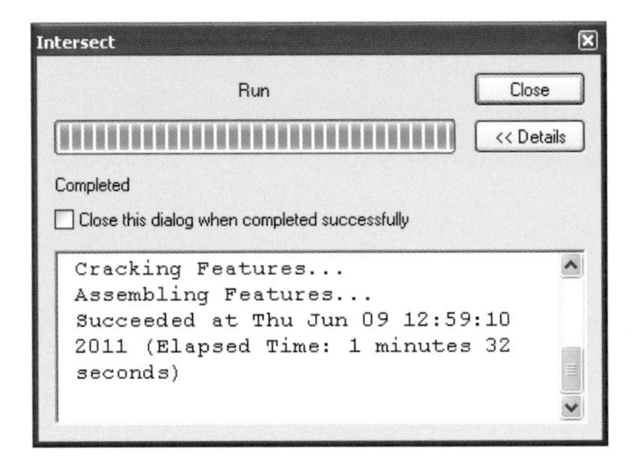

2 **In the Intersect window, click Close.** Drop shadows are added to the model process and its output to indicate that the process has been executed. Note that if you made an error and have to rerun the model, you first have to go to the ModelBuilder Menu bar and click Model > Validate Entire Model, which resets the model.

3 **Right-click the Blocks_X_HRR output of the Intersect process (the green oval), click Add To Display, and save your model.**

4 **In the ArcMap table of contents, open the attribute table for Blocks_X_HRR to verify that the tables were combined.**

5 **Close the table.**

Dissolve blocks

1 **In ArcToolbox, expand the Data Management toolbox and then the Generalization toolset.**

2 Drag the Dissolve tool into your model below the Intersect process.

3 On the ModelBuilder toolbar, click the Connect button, and in the model, click Blocks_X_HRR output from the Intersect process, click the Dissolve process, and in the resulting context menu, click Input Features.

4 On the ModelBuilder toolbar, click the Select button.

5 Double-click the Dissolve process in your model and make selections using the drop-down list in each field as shown in the figure. Name the output feature class HRR_AGE_65_UP. Ignore the warning when clicking AGE_65_UP in the Field column. ▶

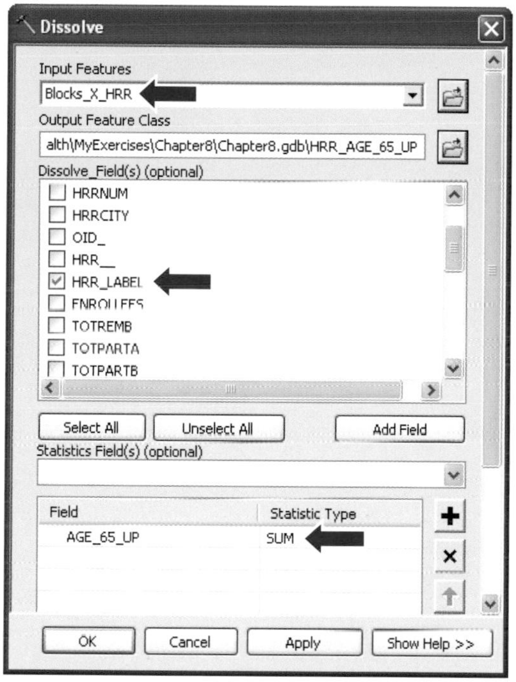

6 Click OK.

7 In your model, right-click the Dissolve process, click Run, and when the model has finished running, close the Dissolve window.

8 Right-click the HRR_AGE_65_UP output of the Dissolve process, click Add To Display, and save your model.

9 In the ArcMap table of contents, open the attribute table for HRR_AGE_65_UP to verify that the field AGE_65_UP was summed, and then close the table.

Join the table

The basic model is almost complete. The last step is to join the dissolved HRR_Age65_UP table to the Nebraska Health Referral Regions polygons.

1 In ArcToolbox, expand the Data Management toolbox and then the Joins toolset.

2 Drag the Add Join tool into your model below the Dissolve process.

3 **On the ModelBuilder toolbar, click the Connect tool, and in the model, click the HRR_AGE_65_UP output from the Dissolve process, click the Add Join process, and in the resulting context menu, click Join Table.**

4 **On the ModelBuilder toolbar, click the Select tool.**

5 **Double-click the Add Join process in your model, make selections using the drop-down list in each remaining field as shown in the figure.** ▶

Add Join
Layer Name or Table View
Health Referral Regions
Input Join Field
HRR_LABEL
Join Table
HRR_AGE_65_UP
Output Join Field
HRR_LABEL
Keep All (optional)
OK Cancel Apply Show Help >>

T 8-3

6 **Specify the Health Referral Regions layer with the recycling arrows. Click OK.** ▶

Health Referral Regions
Block Centroids
HRR_AGE_65_UP
Blocks_X_HRR
Health Referral Regions
Block Centroids

Run and verify the model

The completed model is now ready to run.

1 **On the ModelBuilder Menu bar, click Model > Validate Entire Model.**
This step resets the model. Notice that the drop shadows are removed.

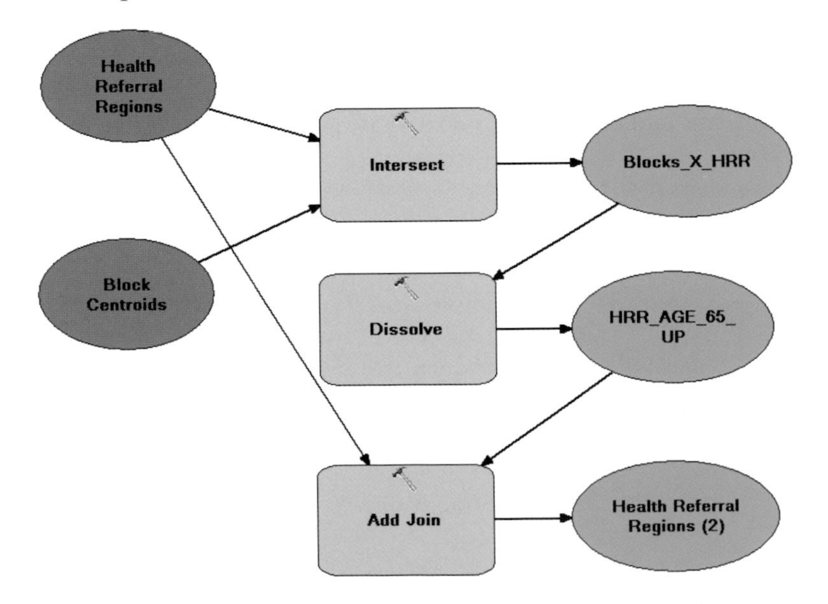

2 Click Model > Run Entire Model.

3 When the model has finished running, click Close.

4 In the ArcMap table of contents, open the attribute table for Health Referral Regions and verify that the SUM_AGE_65_UP field was joined.

Health Referral Regions

Shape *	HRR_BDRY_I	HRRNUM	HRRCITY	OID_	HRR_	HRR_LABEL	ENROLLEES	TOTREMB	TOTPARTA	TOTPARTB	NURSING_	OBJECTID *	Shape_Length	Shape_Area	OBJECTID *	HRR_LABEL	SUM_AGE_65_UP
Polygon	43	103	CO- DENVER	0	103	CO-Denver	6247	6303	3626	2677	484	1	5773677.095647	477709823642.423	1	CO-Denver	18982
Polygon	44	104	CO- FORT COLLINS	1	104	CO-Fort Collins	1347	4929	2630	2296	365	2	885864.364215	26633592319.2266	2	CO-Fort Collins	860
Polygon	46	106	CO- GREELEY	3	106	CO-Greeley	1390	5961	3477	2484	426	3	1367466.001378	7515816647.17835	3	CO-Greeley	74
Polygon	109	196	IA- SIOUX CITY	4	196	IA-Sioux City	1860	4595	2414	2187	293	4	1353671.875892	45164451270.4334	4	IA-Sioux City	5413
Polygon	112	201	KS- WICHITA	6	201	KS-Wichita	8084	5900	3446	2454	365	5	1240664.458992	3457972324.02537	5	KS-Wichita	189
Polygon	171	277	NE- LINCOLN	8	277	NE-Lincoln	3586	5419	3118	2301	436	6	8232345.989202	773153982702.126	6	NE-Lincoln	77468
Polygon	172	278	NE- OMAHA	9	278	NE-Omaha	6945	5480	3190	2291	468	7	9243221.255706	658905376434.787	7	NE-Omaha	124292
Polygon	246	370	SD- RAPID CITY	10	370	SD-Rapid City	1204	5123	2940	2182	464	8	2491862.901154	126495249615.671	8	SD-Rapid City	2660
Polygon	247	371	SD- SIOUX FALLS	11	371	SD-Sioux Falls	5398	4942	2901	2041	470	9	1733307.097666	32617720104.3852	9	SD-Sioux Falls	1813

0 (0 out of 9 Selected)

5 Close the table.

6 On the ModelBuilder toolbar, click Save.

Generalize the model element labels

Your model is capable of being used as a general tool for dissolving any type of polygons. As a first step to generalizing the model, you will change several element labels.

1 In the model, right-click the Health Referral Regions element, click Rename, and type Starting Polygons. Click OK.

2 Similarly, change the labels of the other elements as shown in the figure.

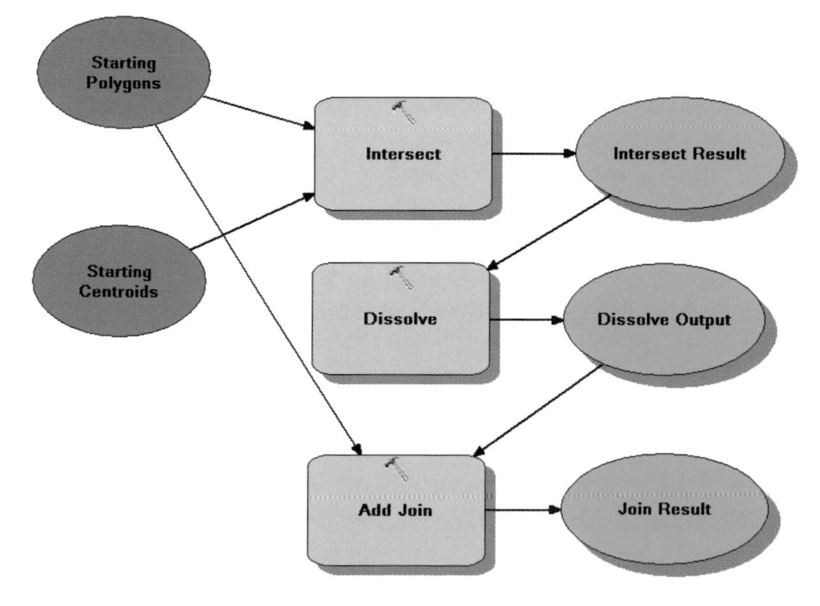

3 On the ModelBuilder toolbar, click Save.

Add model parameters

Your model is currently hardwired with inputs and outputs fixed in processes. Next, you will make several elements into parameters that users can change without needing to modify the model itself. Instead, users will type or make selections in a form that comes up when they open the model, and the model will run using these parameters.

1 **In the model, right-click Starting Polygons and click Model Parameter.** A "P" appears above and to the right of the element, indicating that the user will be asked to browse for an input map layer.

2 **Similarly, make Starting Centroids and Dissolved Output into model parameters.**

Add variables to the model

To be general, the Add Join process needs to get two of its inputs from the user: the Input Join field and the Output Join field. You can make these inputs into parameters, but first you need to create variables to store these parameters in the model.

1 **In the model, right-click the Add Join process and click Variable > From Parameter > Input Join Field.** ArcGIS creates the variable for you.

2 **Click anywhere in the white area of the model to clear selected elements. Move the new variable below and to the left of the Add Join process.**

3 **Make the Input Join field a model parameter by right-clicking it, and then clicking Model Parameter.**

4 **Repeat steps 1–3, except make the variable for the Output Join field of the Add Join process into a model parameter. Move the new element below and to the right of the Add Join process.**

Add labels for documentation

Labels can help document the model. Next, you will add a model title and some notes about the variables to the model.

1 **If necessary, select all model elements and move them to make room at the top for a title label.**

2 Right-click the white area at the top, click Create Label, double-click the resulting label, and type Model to Aggregate Data to Noncoterminous Areas.

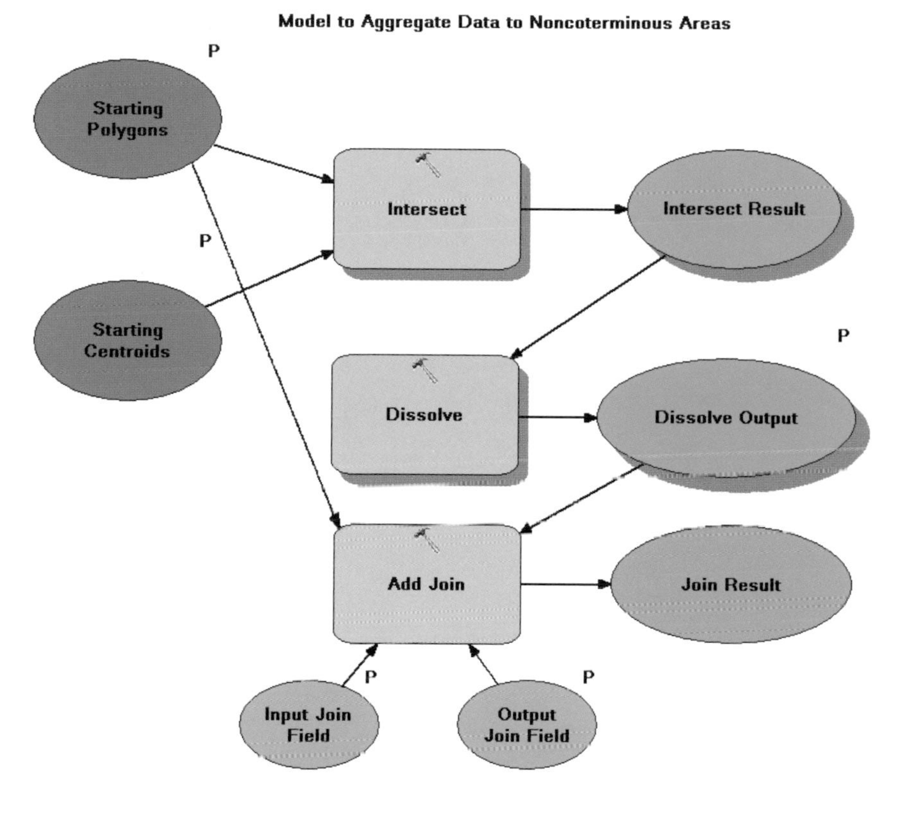

3 On the ModelBuilder toolbar, click Save.

Add model name and description for documentation

You can add Help documentation to model properties in the form that opens when the model is run.

1 On the ModelBuilder Menu bar, click Model > Model Properties.

2 In the Model Properties dialog box, for Name, type AggregrateData **(no spaces) and for Label, type** Aggregate Data for Any Subset of Polygons and Centroids.

3 Select the "Store relative path names (instead of absolute paths)" check box. ▶

4 Click OK.

Model Properties

General | Parameters | Environments | Help | Iteration

Name:
AggregrateData

Label:
Aggregate Data for Any Subset of Polygons and Centroids

Description:

Stylesheet:

☑ Store relative path names (instead of absolute paths)
☑ Always run in foreground

OK | Cancel | Apply

5 On the ModelBuilder toolbar, click Save and close the model window.

Open and run the finished model

The model is stored in Chapter8.tbx and can be opened from there using the Catalog window. Before running the model, however, you must remove all joins from Health Referral Regions. Otherwise, the model will have an error when it attempts to join a table that has already been joined to Health Referral Regions.

1 In the ArcMap table of contents, right-click Health Referral Regions and click Joins and Relates > Remove Join(s) > Remove All Joins.

2 In Catalog, expand Chapter8.tbx, right-click the Aggregate Data for Any Subset of Polygons and Centroids model, click Open, and close the warning at the top of the resulting form.

3 If necessary, change the name of Dissolve Output to HRR_AGE_65_UP **and click Yes to replace the existing file.**

4 Click OK to run the model.

YOUR TURN

In the ArcMap table of contents, remove all layers except Health Referral Regions and Block Centroids, but turn Block Centroids off. Label Health Referral Regions using SUM_AGE_65_UP. The age 65 and up population is the same as that in tutorial 8-1.

Save the map document

1 On the File menu, click Save As.

2 Save your map document as Tutorial8-3YourName.mxd **to your Chapter8 folder in MyExercises.** Close ArcMap.

Summary

A common problem facing GIS analysts is that they obtain aggregate data for one set of polygons but need to transform a different set of polygons. In certain amenable cases, it's easy to make the transformation using simple data aggregation.

In other cases, a good deal of work is needed to achieve an approximate solution. An example is US Census 2000 Summary File 3 (SF 3) data obtained from the Census 2000 long form. This data is available for census block groups and tracts but not for very small census blocks or EMS zones. Thus, SF 3 data needs to be transformed into EMS zones.

In this case, the corresponding approximation is called "apportionment," and this chapter uses a Summary File 1 (SF 1) census variable as an indicator variable. Poverty is assumed to be uniformly spread over the senior citizen population. So, the SF 1 indicator variable for population age 65 and older is used as the indicator for the SF 3 variable population age 65 and older living in poverty. The SF 3 indicator variable is not available for the target polygons, but the SF1 indicator variable is.

You used ArcToolbox to carry out data aggregation. The benefit of using the geoprocessing tools, instead of the usual menu selections in ArcMap, is that they can be built into a macro or model and reused in a single step rather than in a complex series of steps. Automating this process helps you to aggregate data, and tutorial 8-3 helped you to start this process, which is easy to finish on your own.

Assignment 8-1

Map the population in emergency medical service zones

A public-health or emergency medical services director needs to identify the number of people served by emergency medical sites and in EMS zones. Using US Census block centroids and polygons for EMS zones, he can determine the populations served in these areas.

In this assignment, you will use census block centroids for the City of Pittsburgh to determine the total number of people, number of youths, and number of elderly living in EMS zones.

Start with this data

- *\EsriPress\GISTHealth\Data\Pittsburgh.gdb\EMSZones:* polygon features of EMS zones, City of Pittsburgh
- *\EsriPress\GISTHealth\Data\Pittsburgh.gdb\BlockCentroids:* point centroids using US Census 2000 population data, City of Pittsburgh
- *\EsriPress\GISTHealth\DataFiles\Rivers.dxf:* drawing exchange file of rivers, City of Pittsburgh

Create a file geodatabase

Create a file geodatabase called **Assignment8-1YourName.gdb** and save it to your Chapter8 folder in MyAssignments, importing the preceding features into it. Save any new features to your file geodatabase.

Create a model and map that aggregate and compare populations in EMS zones

Create a map document called **Assignment8-1YourName.mxd** and save it to your Chapter8 folder in MyAssignments, using relative paths. Include the preceding layers from your file geodatabase. Import the polygons of the Rivers.dxf file.

In your file geodatabase, create a toolbox called **Assignment8YourName.tbx** and a model called **DataAggregation** that includes three processes (intersect, dissolve, and add join), similar to the model in tutorial 8-3. In the dissolve process, dissolve using the ZONE field and sum all population fields (POP2000, AGE_UNDER5, AGE_15_17, and AGE_65_UP). The result is a sum of population fields, which can be joined to the EMSZones polygon features. Once they are joined, create a new field in EMSZones that adds AGE_UNDER5 and AGE_15_17.

Create a map layout including three data frames that compares the three age populations (total, under age 18, and over age 65) for EMSZones using choropleth maps. In addition, label each zone using all three population figures. Think carefully about your color and classification choices. Rename all data frames and layers appropriately.

Save your map layout as a JPEG image file called **Assignment8-1YourName.jpg** to your Chapter8 folder in MyAssignments.

WHAT TO TURN IN

If your work is to be graded, turn in the following files:

- ***File geodatabase:*** \EsriPress\GISTHealth\MyAssignments\Chapter8\Assignment8-1YourName.gdb
- ***ArcMap document:*** \EsriPress\GISTHealth\MyAssignments\Chapter8\Assignment8-1YourName.mxd
- ***Image file:*** \EsriPress\GISTHealth\MyAssignments\Chapter8\Assignment8-1YourName.jpg

If instructed to do so, instead of individual files, turn in a compressed file, **Assignment8-1YourName.zip**, that includes all the preceding files. Do not include path information in the compressed file.

Assignment 8-2
Map the youth-poverty population in emergency medical service zones

The public health official was impressed with the maps you created in assignment 8-1 and with the output of tutorial 8-2. Your task in this assignment is to now inform the health officials in Pittsburgh how many youths (under age 18) in poverty there are in each EMS zone.

Start with this data

- *\EsriPress\GISTHealth\Data\Pittsburgh.gdb\EMSZones:* polygon features of EMS zones, City of Pittsburgh
- *\EsriPress\GISTHealth\Data\Pittsburgh.gdb\BlockCentroids:* point centroids using US Census 2000 population data, City of Pittsburgh
- *\EsriPress\GISTHealth\DataFiles\Rivers.dxf:* drawing exchange file of rivers, City of Pittsburgh
- *\EsriPress\GISTHealth\Data\Pittsburgh.gdb\BlkGrpSF1:* database of census block groups including youth population in each block group
- *\EsriPress\GISTHealth\Data\Pittsburgh.gdb\BlkGrpSF3:* database of census block groups including youth-poverty population in each block group

Create a file geodatabase

Create a file geodatabase called **Assignment8-2YourName.gdb** and save it to your Chapter8 folder in MyAssignments, importing the preceding features and tables and the polygons of the Rivers.dxf file into it.

Create a map aggregating youth-poverty populations in EMS zones

Create a map document called **Assignment8-2YourName.mxd** and save it to your Chapter8 folder in MyAssignments, using relative paths and adding the layers from your geodatabase.

Use the steps similar to those in tutorial 8-2 to determine the youth-poverty population by EMS zone. Create a choropleth map that is also labeled by a count of youth poverty by EMS zone.

Hints

- *To determine the total youth population, you need to add fields AGE_UNDER5 and AGE_5_17 when calculating the INDICATOR field.*
- *The DENOMINATOR field is AGE_UNDER_18 from the BlkGrpSF1 table.*
- *If you have trouble calculating the WEIGHT field, be sure to select only DENOMINATOR values greater than zero (0). The calculator function cannot divide by zero.*

Create a map layout showing the youth poverty in EMS zones and export the layout as a JPEG image file called **Assignment8-2YourName.jpg** to your Chapter8 folder in MyAssignments.

WHAT TO TURN IN

If your work is to be graded, turn in the following files:

- ***File geodatabase:*** \EsriPress\GISTHealth\MyAssignments\Chapter8\Assignment8-2YourName.gdb
- ***ArcMap document:*** \EsriPress\GISTHealth\MyAssignments\Chapter8\Assignment8-2YourName.mxd
- ***Image file:*** \EsriPress\GISTHealth\MyAssignments\Chapter8\Assignment8-2YourName.jpg

If instructed to do so, instead of individual files, turn in a compressed file, **Assignment8-2YourName.zip**, that includes all the preceding files. Do not include path information in the compressed file.

Chapter 9

Using ArcGIS Spatial Analyst for demand estimation

Objectives

- Process raster-map layers
- Create a hillshade raster layer
- Make a kernel-density map
- Extract raster-value points
- Conduct a raster-based site-suitability study
- Use ArcGIS ModelBuilder to create a risk index

Health-care scenario

Although most heart attacks occur in the home or in the hospital, approximately 20 percent occur in public places. Providing access to automated defibrillators in public places is one innovation that increases the chances of victims surviving heart attacks. One study showed that defibrillators in public places saved twice as many heart attack victims as cardiopulmonary resuscitation (CPR) alone (*Harvard Medical School Family Health Guide* 2004). As a result, health-care policy analysts in Pittsburgh, Pennsylvania, are working on a plan to provide defibrillators in some of Pittsburgh's public places. These analysts would like an estimate of demand or need for this emergency health service. They would also like to understand what factors contribute to heart attacks in public places—for instance, terrain, land use, socioeconomic conditions, and so forth.

A sample of incidents of heart attacks that have taken place in public in Pittsburgh over a five-year period is available for study. The sample was collected using the selection criterion that bystander help could be available, given the point locations of heart attacks. In addition, the policy analysts wish to add the criterion that potential defibrillator sites be located in commercial areas as well as in peak areas of demand.

Solution approach

This study needs a large-scale analysis, down to the block level, to precisely determine where public defibrillators should be located. Given the address data for public-location heart attacks, the corresponding points can be geocoded and mapped. It is then possible to aggregate the points to counts per block and plot choropleth maps as an indicator of demand for defibrillators in public places. Pittsburgh has 7,466 blocks, however. With that many areas, it becomes difficult to use vector graphics. Corresponding choropleth maps, for example, would have areas so small that it becomes impractical to give polygons visible boundaries—there's little room left for color fill. The best treatment for polygons in this case is to plot their centroid points, symbolized by a color ramp to represent magnitudes such as the number of heart attacks. (This differs from a choropleth map that uses polygons.) This sort of point map, however, is difficult to analyze visually and to process analytically.

Hence, a different type of map is needed—one that deals with very small areas or with continuously changing variables that do not work well when depicted as vectors. Raster maps fill this need. They are rectangular arrays of very small, uniform, square cells that are analogous to pixels in an image file (such as a JPEG or GIF file). In addition to recording a value for each cell (such as heart attacks per unit area), raster maps store sufficient data to determine the geographic coordinates of each cell. These coordinates can then be used for plotting and display as background for vector-map layers. Values in the chapter 9 raster map images may vary if you are working with a different version of ArcGIS software.

An additional problem in using choropleth maps to represent demand is that the data for each polygon is a sample and thus carries a degree of sampling error. In other words, the displayed number of heart attacks for each block should be thought of as an underlying mean value for that block, plus random error.

Estimated mean demand is often a more reliable predictor of future demand than raw data because random error gets averaged out—the plus errors tend to cancel out the minus errors. So, it would be better to use a mean surface for heart attacks rather than raw-data maps to predict future demand.

The ArcGIS Spatial Analyst extension has the capacity to create and process raster maps in sophisticated ways. Key to this study is the density-surface estimation capability, which uses data for polygon centroids as input and estimates mean surfaces as output in raster format. In particular, you will use kernel-density estimation to produce a smoothed mean surface for the number of heart attacks per square foot in Pittsburgh. Given this output, it is then possible to make multiple-criteria queries to identify potential locations for public defibrillators.

Raster graphics provide the capability to perform unique GIS analysis, some of which is needed in the current study. One such process is easily combining data from different vector-based geographies. For example, in building a risk index for poverty, you will need to use block and block group map layers as input. Both geographies are easily transformed into the same raster map cells through kernel-density estimation. ArcGIS Spatial Analyst provides raster algebra and an interface to combine multiple raster inputs into a single index. You will use the innovative and well-reasoned approach of so-called "robust" or "improper" linear models (Dawes 1979) to estimate geographic areas of poverty. This kind of model combines two or more independent variables to predict a dependent variable when no dependent-variable data is available. You will build a robust, linear model for poverty, one of the determinants of heart attacks in public places.

The steps to build the robust model are many and complex. So instead of just following along with the steps, you will use ArcGIS ModelBuilder to build a stored macro or model that strings steps together into a single program that can be easily modified, reused, and communicated to others.

Out-of-hospital cardiac-arrest study

Tutorial 9-1
Processing raster-map layers

The map document you will open in this tutorial has map layers that include raster maps from US Geological Survey websites: http://seamless.usgs.gov/website/seamless/viewer.htm for digital elevation (National Elevation Data shaded relief, 1/3 arc second) and http://gisdata.usgs.net/website/MRLC/viewer.php for land use (National Land Cover Data 2001). All raster maps are rectangular in their coordinate systems, but you will use the Pittsburgh boundary as a mask so that cells outside the boundary will have no color and the cells inside will have their assigned colors. In addition, you will use the DEM (digital elevation model) layer to create a hillshade, which has a 3D appearance of topography illuminated by the sun. Placing the hillshade under the land-use layer and giving the land-use layer some transparency makes an attractive and informative map display that provides good background for health data.

Examine raster-map layer properties

1 **Start ArcMap and open Tutorial9-1.mxd.** The vector-map layer called OHCA (out-of-hospital cardiac arrests) is the number of heart attacks over a five-year period per census block that occurred outside of hospitals where bystander help was possible because of location. As expected and by definition, you will see that these heart attacks appear in developed areas. (See facing page.) Next, you will examine properties of the raster layers.

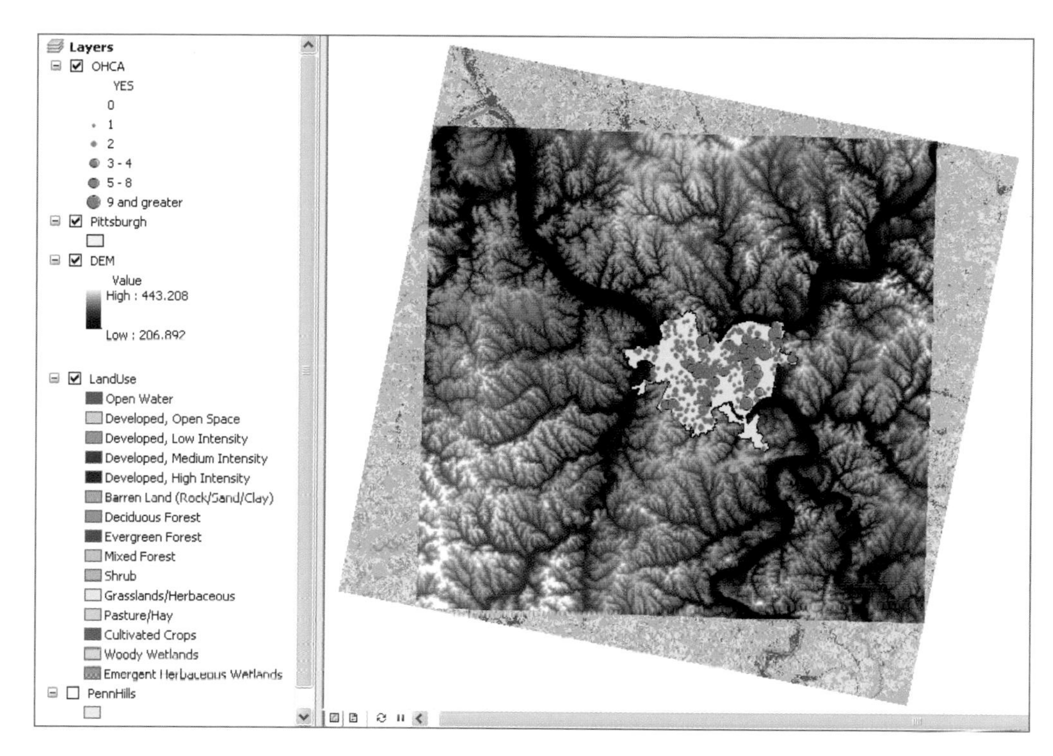

2 In the table of contents, right-click DEM, click Properties, and click the Source tab. All raster maps are rectangular in their coordinate system. This one has 2,106 columns, 1,984 rows, and square cells of 90.70912488 decimal degrees to a side.

3 Scroll down in the Property column until you see the Extent information. Here you can see familiar-looking decimal-degree values for the extent, so this layer is in geographic coordinates. ArcGIS projected the layer to the data frame projection, which is state plane for southern Pennsylvania.

4 Scroll down farther until you see the Statistics information. Each cell or pixel has a single value—elevation in meters—which is stored as a floating point number. The statistics for elevation over the extent include a mean elevation above sea level of 323.7 m and a maximum of 443.2 m.

5 Click OK to close the Layer Properties window.

YOUR TURN

Examine the properties of the land-use layer. Notice that this is a projected layer that uses a projection for the contiguous United States (and the reason why the layer tilts when ArcGIS reprojects it to the local state plane projection). Also notice that the cell size is larger than that of the DEM, 30 m on a side, and that the values are integers corresponding to land-use categories.

Create a file geodatabase

1 **Start ArcCatalog and browse to your Chapter9 folder in MyExercises, right-click Chapter9, and click New > File Geodatabase.**

2 **Rename the geodatabase** Chapter9.gdb.

Set the raster environment

Next, you need to set the environment for using Spatial Analyst tools. Each time you use one of the tools, ArcMap automatically uses the environment settings, which can be a time-saver.

1 **On the Customize menu, click Extensions, select the Spatial Analyst check box, and click Close.** This step loads the Spatial Analyst extension, making its functionality available. Although you won't immediately get a toolbar per se, you will enable links to Spatial Analyst tools. If the extension is not checked here, the Spatial Analyst functions will not be available.

2 **On the Geoprocessing menu, click Environments.**

3 **In the Environment Settings dialog box, click Raster Analysis and type or make selections as shown in the figure. Click OK.** ▶

Extract land use employing a mask

ArcGIS can display a great many raster or image file formats. The land-use layer in your map document is a TIFF file format image downloaded from the USGS site. To process this layer, you must convert it to an Esri format. You can do that by saving it to a file geodatabase. At the same time, you will use the Pittsburgh boundary as a mask to clip the original layer to Pittsburgh's rectangular extent and display only the cells within Pittsburgh's boundary.

1 **On the Standard toolbar, click ArcToolbox.**

2 **In the ArcToolbox window, expand the Spatial Analyst toolbox, then the Extraction toolset, and double-click Extract by Mask.**

3 **In the Extract by Mask dialog box, type or make selections as shown in the figure, naming the output raster** LandUsePgh, **and click OK.** Wait while the extraction is completed. ▶

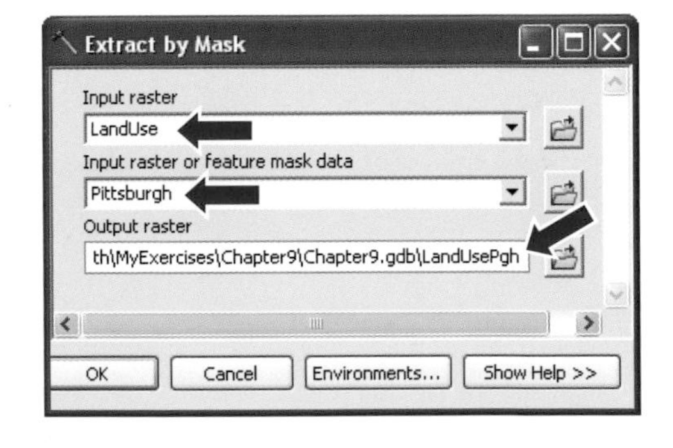

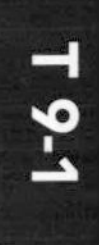

4 In the table of contents, turn off all layers except LandUsePgh.

5 Right-click LandUsePgh and click Zoom To Layer.

ArcMap gave LandUsePgh an arbitrary color ramp (which is unattractive), but next you will add a layer file, created from LandUse, to correctly symbolize the new raster map.

6 Right-click LandUsePgh, click Properties, and click the Symbology tab and then the Import button. Browse through the Data folder to SpatialAnalyst, click LandUse.lyr, click Add, and click OK twice.

The resulting map is informative and attractive; for example, you can see high-density development along Pittsburgh's rivers, and you can see that the clusters of heart attack locations are in developed areas. In the next section, you will give the map a 3D appearance by adding hillshade based on the DEM layer.

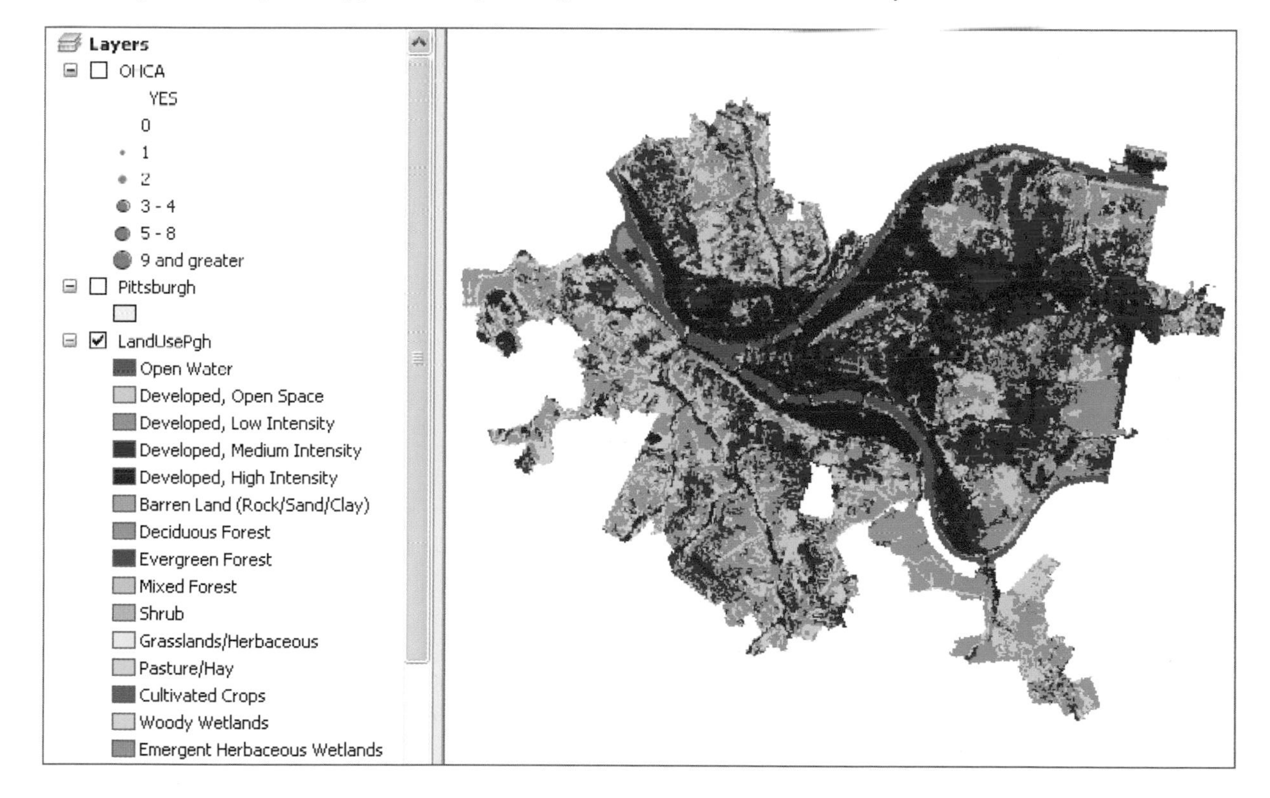

YOUR TURN

Penn Hills is a suburb just outside of Pittsburgh. Extract LandUsePennHills from LandUse using the PennHills layer as a mask. (***Hint:*** *Set PennHills as the mask under Geoprocessing > Environments > Raster Analysis.*) Save as **LandUsePennHills** to Chapter9.gdb in your MyExercises folder. Symbolize the new layer using LandUse.lyr. When finished, turn off all the Penn Hills layers and zoom back to the Pittsburgh layer if necessary. Set the raster mask back to Pittsburgh under Geoprocessing > Environments > Raster Analysis.

Save the map document

1. **On the File menu, click Save As.**

2. **Save your map document as** Tutorial9-1YourName.mxd **to your Chapter9 folder in MyExercises.** Do not close ArcMap.

Tutorial 9-2
Creating a hillshade raster layer

The hillshade function simulates illumination of a surface from an artificial light source representing the sun. Two parameters of this function are the altitude of the light source above the surface horizon in degrees and the angle (azimuth) of the light source relative to true north. The effect of hillshade on a surface, such as elevation above sea level, is striking, providing a 3D appearance relative to light and shadow. You can enhance the display of another raster layer, such as land use, by making it partially transparent and placing hillshade beneath it. That is the objective of this tutorial.

Create hillshade for elevation

In this exercise, you will use the default values of the Hillshade tool for azimuth and altitude. The sun for your map will be in the west (315 degrees) at an elevation of 45 degrees above the horizon.

1 **On the Windows menu, click Search.** Using the Search window to start a Spatial Analyst tool is an alternative to using ArcToolbox.

2 **In the Search text box, type** Hillshade, **press ENTER, and click Hillshade (Spatial Analyst).**

3 **In the Hillshade dialog box, type or make selections as shown in the figure, naming the output raster** HillshadePgh, **and click OK.** Wait while the hillshade layer is created. ▶

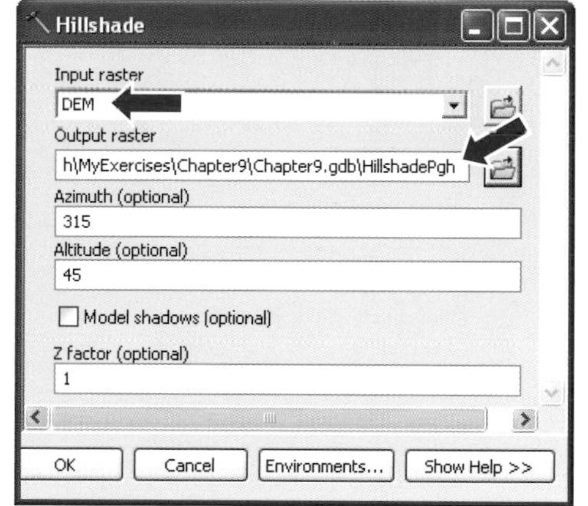

4 **In the table of contents, move HillshadePgh to just below LandUsePgh.**

5 **Right-click HillshadePgh, click Properties, and click the Symbology tab.**

6 **In the Show panel, make sure Stretched is selected, and in the Stretch panel, for Type, click Standard Deviations. Click OK.**

7 **In the table of contents, right-click LandUsePgh, click Properties, and click the Display tab.**

8 In the Transparency box, type 35 **and click OK.**

Now you have the finished product. Heart attack locations are in some developed areas, but not all. Next, you will do additional spatial analysis on population statistics to see if you can determine a major factor affecting the incidence of heart attacks.

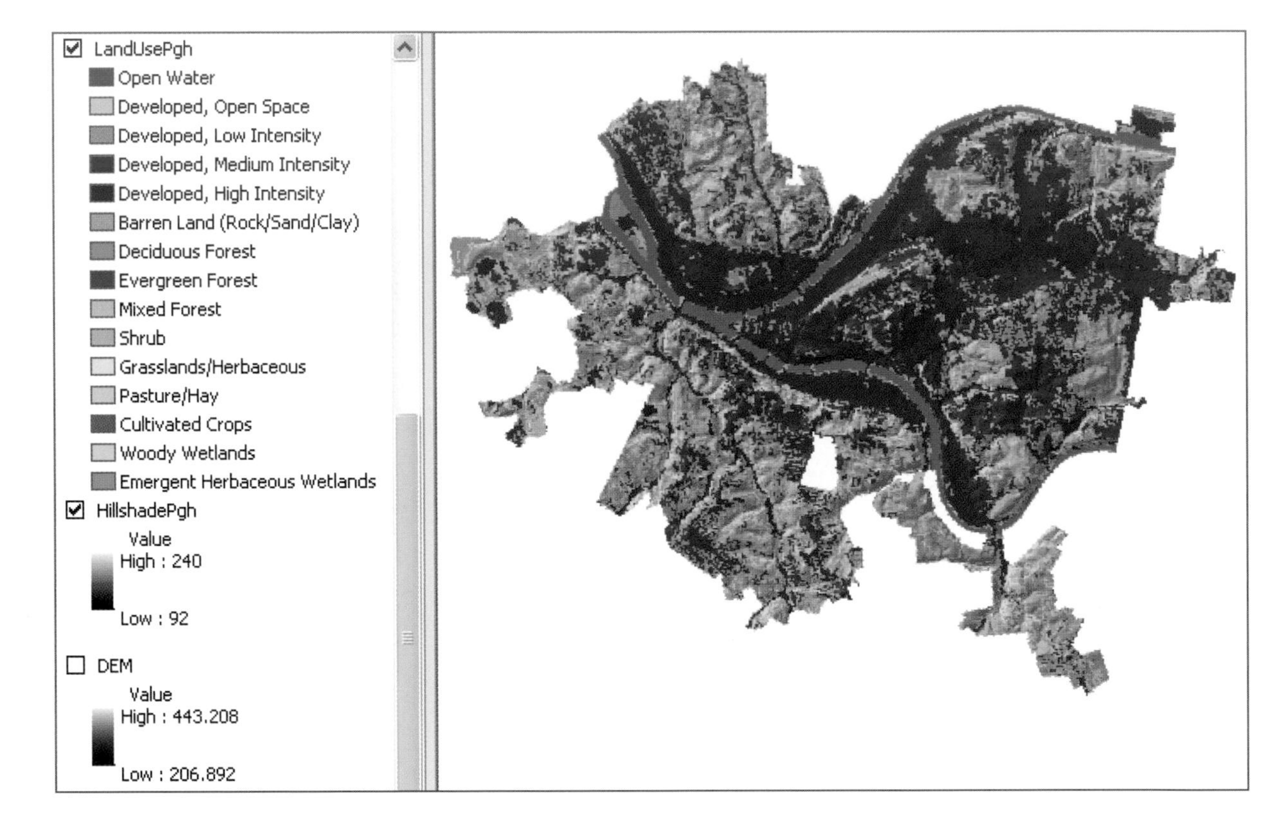

YOUR TURN

Create **HillShadePennHills** and display it under a 35 percent transparent LandUsePennHills.

Save the map document

1 On the File menu, click Save As.

2 Save your map document as Tutorial9-2YourName.mxd **to your Chapter9 folder in MyExercises.** Do not close ArcMap.

Tutorial 9-3
Making a kernel-density map

The incidence of myocardial infarction (heart attacks) outside of hospitals in the United States for people age 35 to 74 is approximately 5.6 per thousand males per year and 4.2 per thousand females per year? (Rosamond et al. 1998). You will use a point feature class of census block centroids in Allegheny County to analyze heart attack incidence as the input to an estimation method called kernel-density smoothing. This method estimates incidence as heart attacks per unit area (density) and has two parameters: cell size and search radius. There is no "science" on how to set these parameters, but the larger the search radius, the smoother the estimated distribution. When smoothing a particular cell, the farther away other points are, the less influence they have. Read ArcGIS for Desktop Help on kernel-density smoothing to learn more about this method.

Assign environment settings and get statistics

The map document you will open in this tutorial shows the observed locations of heart attacks (outside of hospitals and with the potential of bystander assistance) and block centroids symbolized by a color gradient for heart attack incidence, as well as other supporting layers. The attribute table for block centroids has the incidence attribute "Inc." Inc = 0.0042 × [Fem35T74] + 0.0056 × [Male35T74], where Fem35T74 is the population by block of females age 35 to 74 and Male35T74 is the corresponding population for males. The question is whether incidence does a good job of estimating the observed heart attacks in the OHCA point file.

1 **In ArcMap, open Tutorial9-3.mxd.** The map display for estimated incidence using block centroids and point markers is as good as vector graphics allow, but it is difficult to interpret. You will create an alternative representation of incidence by using kernel-density smoothing to estimate the smoothed mean of the spatial distribution.

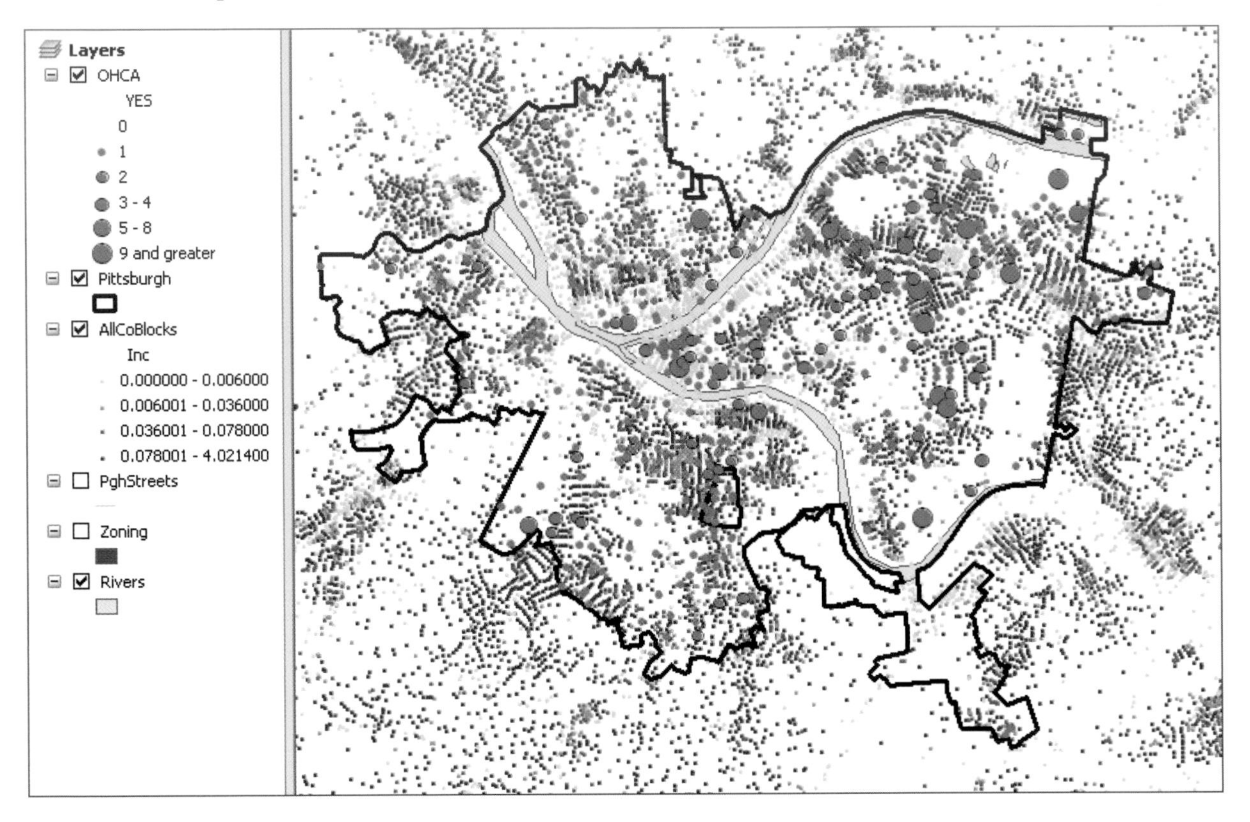

2 On the Geoprocessing menu, click Environments > Raster Analysis, and type or make selections as shown in the figure. ▶

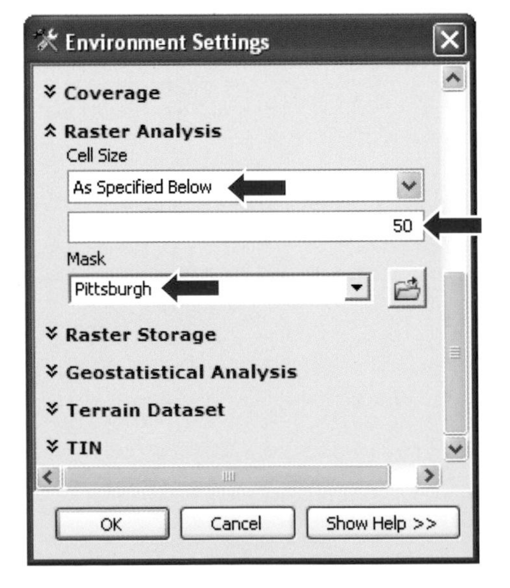

3 **On the Selection menu, click Select By Location, match the settings in the figure, and click OK. ▶**

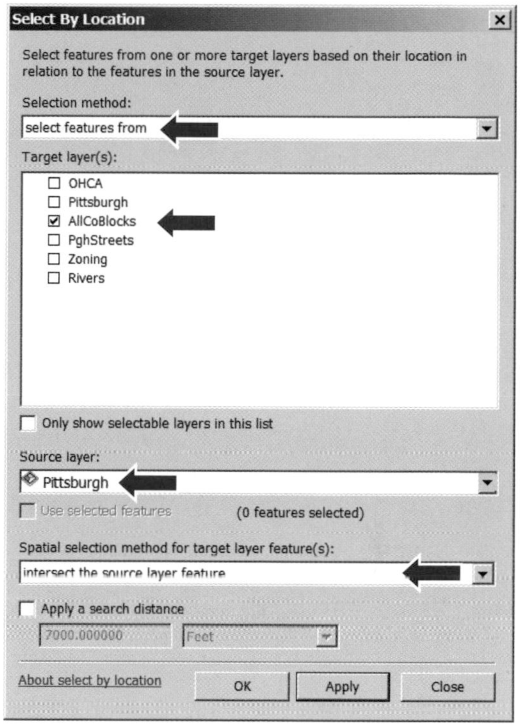

4 **In the table of contents, right-click AllCoBlocks, click Open Attribute Table, right-click the column heading for Inc, and click Statistics.**

Note the sum of Inc, 684 for Pittsburgh, which is the expected annual number of heart attacks in Pittsburgh occurring outside of hospitals. In the following exercise, you will verify that density smoothing preserves this sum in any surface it estimates. Kernel-density smoothing simply spreads the total of incidents around on a smooth surface, preserving the input total number of heart attacks.

5 **Close the Selection Statistics window and the table and clear the selection.**

Select By Location

Select features from one or more target layers based on their location in relation to the features in the source layer.

Selection method:
select features from

Target layer(s):
☐ OHCA
☐ Pittsburgh
☑ AllCoBlocks
☐ PghStreets
☐ Zoning
☐ Rivers

☐ Only show selectable layers in this list

Source layer:
Pittsburgh

☐ Use selected features (0 features selected)

Spatial selection method for target layer feature(s):
intersect the source layer feature

☐ Apply a search distance
7000.000000 Feet

About select by location | OK | Apply | Close

Make a density map for heart attack incidence

The OHCA map layer shows heart attacks per census block in Pittsburgh. Blocks in Pittsburgh average a little less than 300 ft per side in length. Suppose that policy analysts estimate that a defibrillator that's publicly accessible can be made known to residents and retrieved for use as far as 2.5 blocks away from the location. They thus recommend looking at areas that are five blocks by five blocks in size, or 1,500 ft on a side, and locating defibrillators in the center. You will therefore use a 150 ft cell and a 1,500 ft search radius. The 150 ft cell approximates the middle of a street segment, which is the average location of a heart attack.

1 **In the Search text box, type** Kernel density**, press ENTER, and click Kernel Density (Spatial Analyst).**

2 **In the Kernel Density dialog box, type or make selections as shown in the figure. Name the output raster** Kernel1500**. ▶**

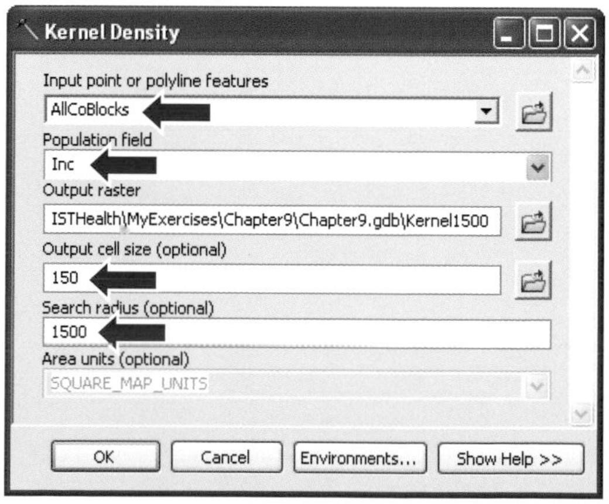

3 **Click OK.**

The resulting surface does not appear useful at this point, but it will after you symbolize it better in the next step.

Kernel Density

Input point or polyline features
AllCoBlocks

Population field
Inc

Output raster
ISTHealth\MyExercises\Chapter9\Chapter9.gdb\Kernel1500

Output cell size (optional)
150

Search radius (optional)
1500

Area units (optional)
SQUARE_MAP_UNITS

OK | Cancel | Environments... | Show Help >>

4 **Right-click Kernel1500, click Properties, click the Symbology tab, and click the Classify button. For Classification Method, click Standard Deviation.**

Standard Deviation is a good option for showing variation in raster grids because it yields a central category and an equal number of categories on either side of the center. That makes dichromatic color scales, such as the one you will use in step 6, more meaningful and easier to interpret. You control the number of categories in the next step by choosing the fraction of standard deviation for creating break points, at every 1, ½, ⅓, ¼, etc., standard deviation.

5 **For Interval Size, click 1/3 Std Dev and click OK.**

6 **Select the color ramp that runs from green to yellow to red and click OK.**

7 **In the table of contents, turn off AllCoBlocks, PghStreets, and Zoning and turn on all other layers.** The estimated incidence matches the clusters of OHCA heart attack data in many, but not all, areas. For example, there is a cluster of heart attacks in Pittsburgh's central business district (the triangle just to the right of where the three rivers join), but the estimated incidence is low there. The problem is that the density map, based on population data, shows expected heart attacks per square foot in reference to where people live, and not necessarily to where they have heart attacks. Many people shop or work in the central business district and have heart attacks there, but few live there.

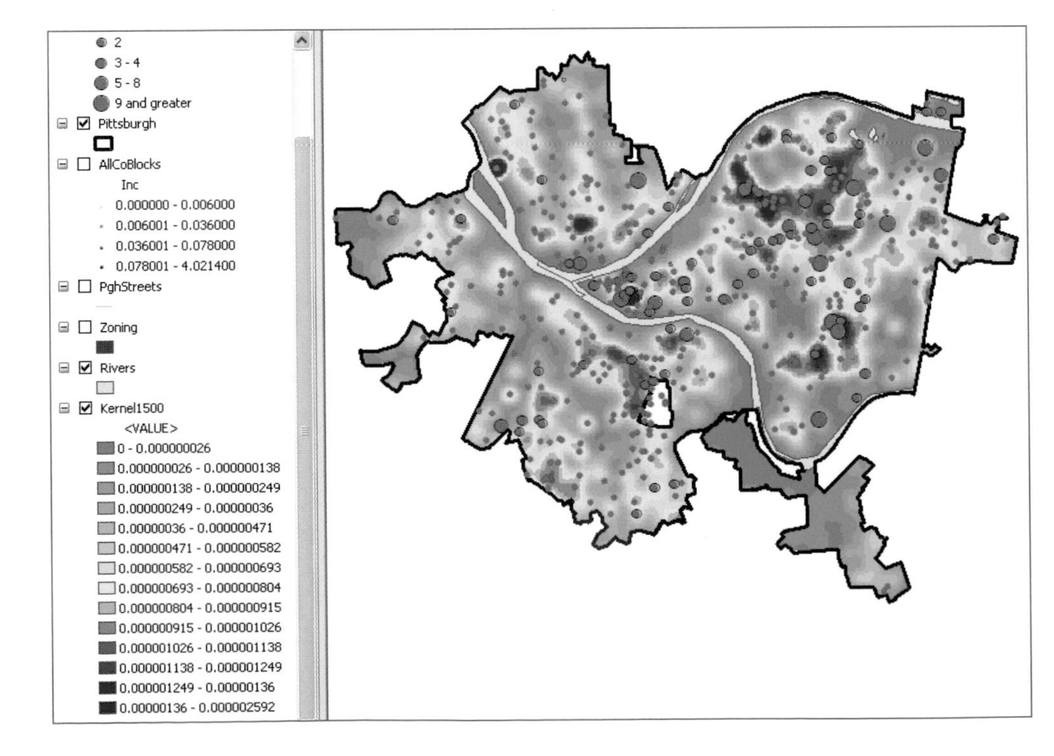

YOUR TURN

Examine the density surface to see if it preserves the total number of heart attacks. The estimated incidence that you found using block centroids was 684. Open the properties of the density surface, click the Symbology tab, and click Classify. There you will find useful statistics: 72,315 cells and a mean of 0.000000415 heart attacks per square foot. Remember that each cell is 150 by 150 ft. Therefore, 150 × 150 × 72,315 × 0.000000415 = 675 heart attacks, which is close to 684. So, what kernel-density smoothing does here is to move around the input number of heart attacks and distribute the incidents smoothly. The kernel-density map is a better estimate of incidence than raw data, because smoothing averages out randomness and provides an estimate of the mean or average surface.

Create a second kernel-density surface for incidence, called **Kernel3000**, keeping all inputs and outputs the same, except use a search radius of 3,000 ft instead of 1,500 ft. Symbolize the output the same as Kernel1500. Keeping Kernel1500 turned on, turn Kernel3000 on and off to see the differences in the two layers. Kernel3000 is more spread out and smoother, but it has the same corresponding number of estimated heart attacks: close to 684.

Save the map document

1. **On the File menu, click Save As.**
2. **Save your map document as** Tutorial9-3YourName.mxd **to your Chapter9 folder in MyExercises.** Do not close ArcMap.

Tutorial 9-4

Extracting raster-value points

Although the estimated densities appear to match the actual heart attack data in OHCA, the match may or may not stand up to closer scrutiny. ArcMap has a tool that extracts point estimates from the raster surface for each point in OHCA. Then you can use the extracted densities multiplied by block areas to estimate the number of heart attacks. If there is a strong correlation between the estimated and actual number of heart attacks, it would be evidence that population by itself is a good predictor of heart attacks.

1 **In the Search text box, type** Extract values to points, **press ENTER, and click Extract Values to Points (Spatial Analyst).**

2 **In the Extract Values to Points dialog box, type or make selections as shown in the figure. Name the output point features** OHCAPredicted.

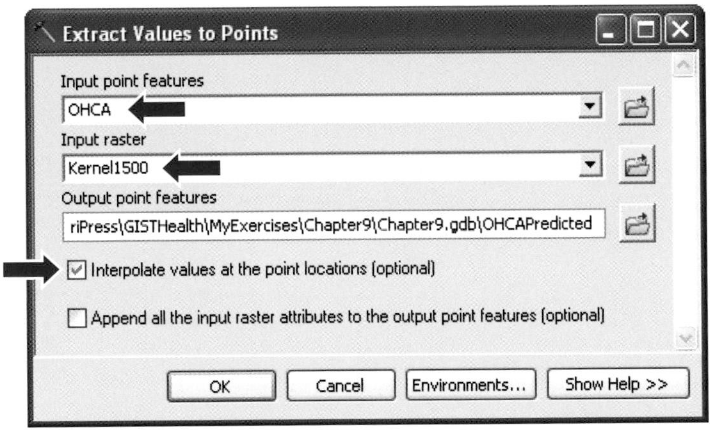

3 **Click OK.** The resulting layer, OHCAPredicted, has an attribute, RASTERVALU, that is an estimate of heart attack density, or heart attacks per square foot, in the vicinity of each block.

Calculate predicted heart attacks

You can expect that the resulting estimate, OHCAPredicted, will be larger than the actual number of heart attacks in OHCA's YES attribute, which is just a subset of all heart attacks (those in which bystander help was possible, given the location).

1 In the table of contents, right-click OHCAPredicted and click Open Attribute Table.

2 Click Table Options > Add Field and add a field called Predicted **using Float for Type.**

3 Right-click the Predicted column heading and click Field Calculator.

4 In the Field Calculator expression panel, create the expression

```
5 * [RASTERVALU] * [Area]
```

and click OK. OHCA data is a five-year sample of heart attacks, and thus the expression includes the multiple 5.

5 Close the attribute table.

A few of the points in OHCA have no raster values near them, so ArcGIS assigns the value -9999 to them to signify missing values. This can be seen in the RASTERVALU field of the OHCAPredicted table. Before looking at a scatterplot of predicted and actual values, you will first select only OHCA points that have positive predicted values.

6 On the Selection menu, click Select By Attributes.

7 For the OHCAPredicted layer, create the expression

```
"Predicted" >= 0
```

and click OK.

8 Right-click OHCAPredicted and click Data > Export Data.

9 Export selected features as OHCAPredicted2 **and save them to Chapter9.gdb.**

10 Click Yes to add the layer to the map.

11 Clear the selected features and turn off the OHCAPredicted layer.

T 9-4

Create a scatterplot of actual vs. predicted heart attacks

Although Pittsburgh has a total of 7,466 blocks, only 1,509 blocks had heart attacks. The scatterplot that you will construct later in this chapter includes data for only these 1,509 blocks but should ideally include the balance of the total blocks, which included actual values of zero (0) but predicted values that were sometimes much larger than zero. Nevertheless, you will be able to get an indication of the correlation between predicted and actual heart attacks. Adding the total balance of blocks would only make the correlation worse, but the correlation is actually already very low, as you will see in this exercise.

1 **On the View menu, click Graphs > Create Graph.**

2 **In the Create Graph Wizard, type or make selections as shown in the figure.**

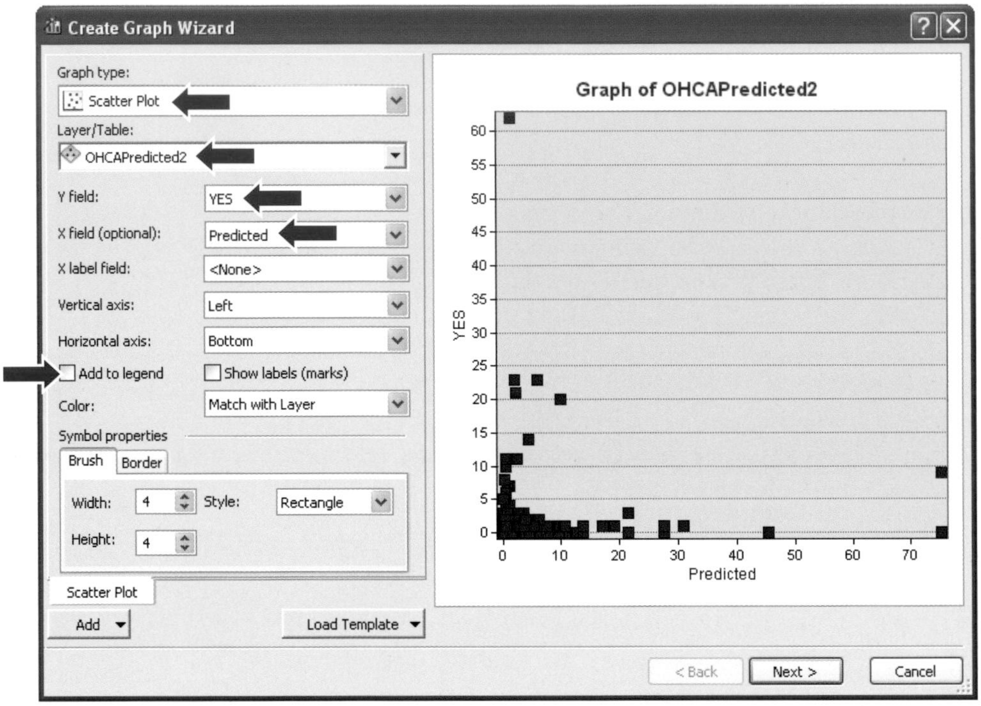

3 **Click Next > Finish.** At the scale of blocks, the predicted values seem to correlate poorly with the actual values. A good correlation would have a graph showing actual (YES attribute) and predicted values scattering around a 45-degree slope line. This scatterplot shows no correlation at all. If you export the corresponding data to a statistical package or Microsoft Excel, you would find that the correlation coefficient between predicted and actual values is only 0.0899, which is very low. Evidently, factors other than where the population resides affect the locations and clustering of heart attacks occurring outside of hospitals.

Save the map document

1 **On the File menu, click Save As.**

2 **Save your map document as** Tutorial9-4YourName.mxd **to your Chapter9 folder in MyExercises.** Do not close ArcMap.

Tutorial 9-5

Conducting a raster-based site-suitability study

The objective of your study is to find locations that have high heart attack rates and that have heart defibrillators accessible to the public. The solution approach includes using kernel-density smoothing on the available heart attack data to remove randomness from the spatial distribution. Kernel-density smoothing provides a more reliable estimate of demand for defibrillators. An assumption is that any location within commercial areas provides needed public accessibility.

Open a map document

A vector-map layer is available for commercial-area boundaries. To conduct a raster-based analysis, you need to convert this map layer into a raster layer. This is the first task you will undertake in this tutorial.

1 **In ArcMap, open Tutorial9-5.mxd.** The map document shows the observed locations of heart attacks (outside of hospitals and with the potential of bystander assistance), a 600 ft buffer of commercially zoned areas in Pittsburgh, and other supporting layers. The 600 ft (or two-block) buffer of commercial areas includes adjacent noncommercial areas that have sufficient access to defibrillators.

2 **On the Geoprocessing menu, click Environments > Raster Analysis and type or make selections as shown in the figure. Click OK.** ▶

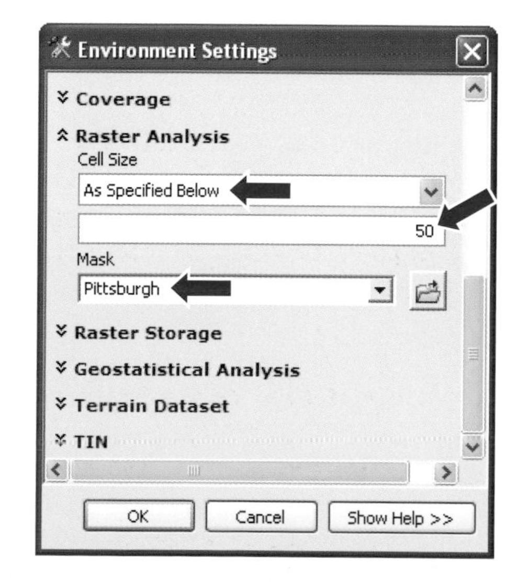

Convert a feature buffer to a raster dataset

The ZoningCommercialBuffer layer has two polygons and corresponding records and a single attribute: Commercial. The Commercial value of 1 corresponds to commercial land use or land within 600 ft of commercial land use. The other value, 0, represents the balance of Pittsburgh and includes all other zoned land uses. You will convert this vector layer to a raster dataset using a conversion tool. First, however, you need to select both records in the vector file to convert them.

1. **In the table of contents, right-click the ZoningCommercialBuffer layer and click Open Attribute table.**

2. **Select both records by clicking the row selector of the first row and dragging the mouse to select both rows. Then close the table.**

3. **In the Search text box, type** Feature to Raster**, press ENTER, and click Feature to Raster (Conversion).**

4. **In the Feature to Raster dialog box, type or make selections as shown in the figure and name the output raster** Commercial**. Click OK.** ▶

Feature to Raster
Input features
ZoningCommercialBuffer
Field
Commercial
Output raster
:\EsriPress\GISTHealth\MyExercises\Chapter9\Chapter9.gdb\Commercial
Output cell size (optional)
50
OK Cancel Environments... Show Help >>

5. **In the table of contents, remove the ZoningCommercialBuffer layer and turn off the OHCA layer.**

6. **Right-click Commercial, click Properties, and click the Symbology tab. In the Show panel, click Unique Values and symbolize the new Commercial area with two colors: white for noncommercial (0) and gray for commercial (1).**

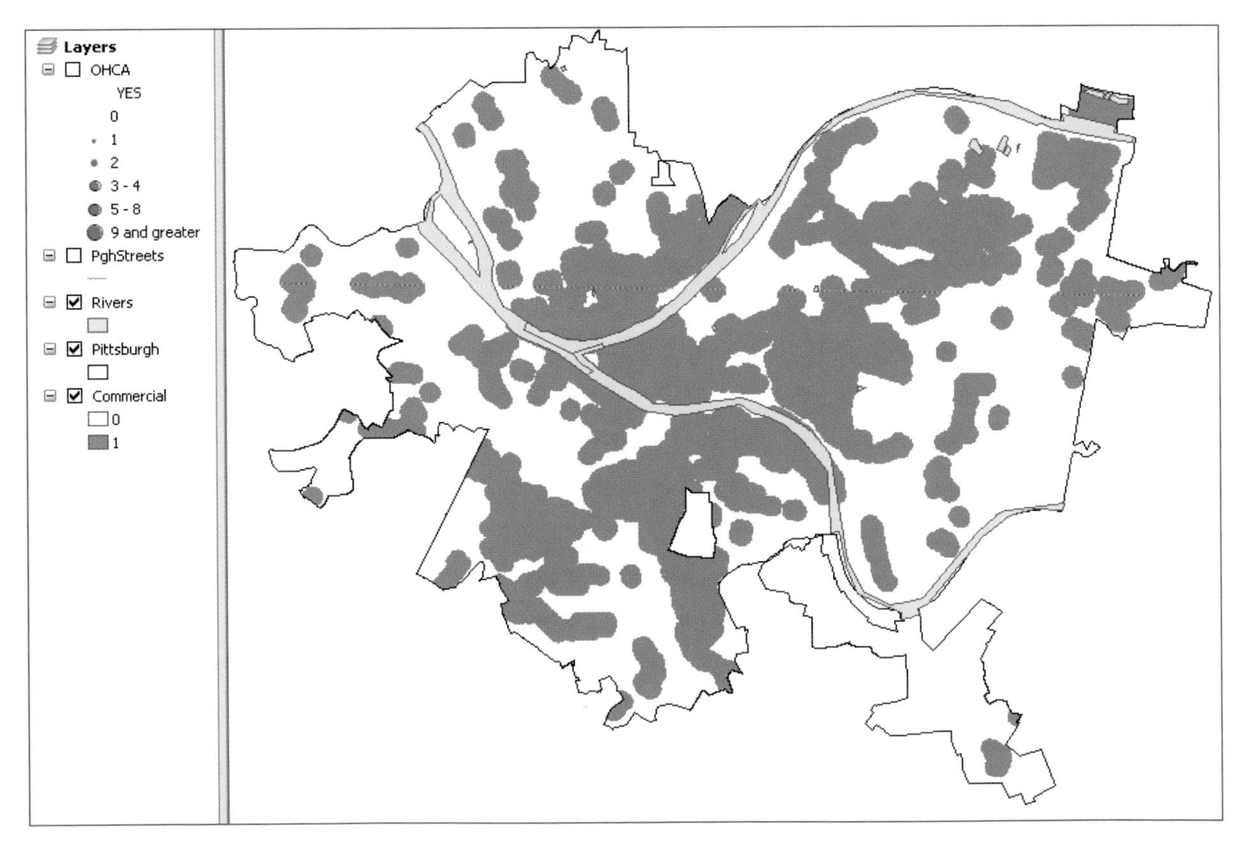

YOUR TURN

Create a kernel-density map based on the YES attribute of the OHCA point layer using 150 ft cells, a search radius of 1,500 ft, and area units of SQUARE_FEET. Call the new raster layer **HeartAttack** and save it to Chapter9.gdb. Symbolize the layer using the standard deviation method and an interval size of 1/3 Std Dev. Use the color ramp that runs from green to yellow to red. Try turning the OHCA layer on and off to see how well the density surface represents heart attacks, and then remove the OHCA layer. The resulting raster map is shown in the figure.

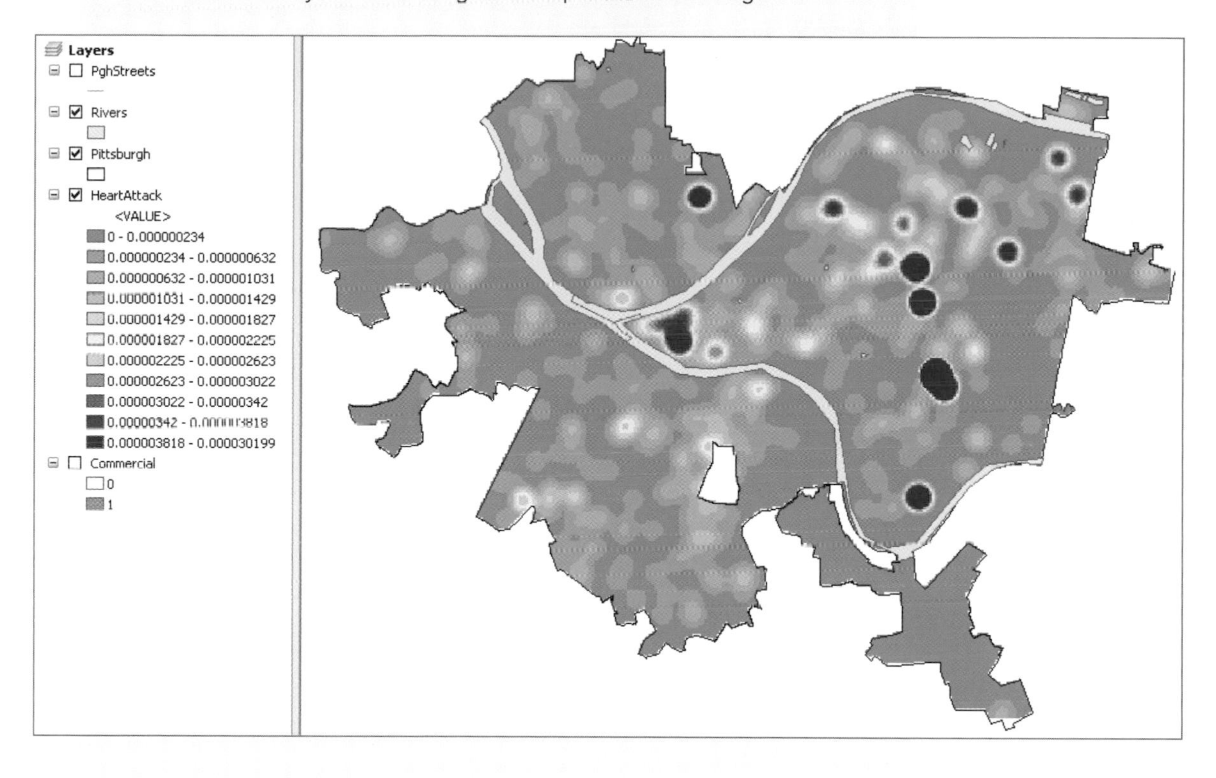

Query a raster dataset using a single criterion and Reclassify

In this exercise, you will first reclassify your kernel-density map, HeartAttack, for areas that have sufficiently high heart attack density to merit a defibrillator. Suppose that policy makers are seeking 25-block areas, roughly five blocks on a side, that would have 10 or more heart attacks every five years in locations where bystander help is possible. A square 25-block area is 5×300 ft = 1,500 ft on a side and $1{,}500 \times 1{,}500$ ft = 2.25×10^6 sq ft of area.

Thus, the heart attack density sought is 10 heart attacks / 2.25×10^6 sq ft = 0.000004444 heart attacks per square foot or higher. Although the density map you just created has a continuous range of values, you will next reclassify values into just two values: 0 for cells that have a density less than 0.000004444 and 1 for cells that have a density greater than or equal to 0.000004444.

1. **In the Search text box, type** Reclassify, **press ENTER, and click Reclassify (Spatial Analyst).**

2. **In the Reclassify dialog box, for Input raster, click HeartAttack and click Classify.**

3. **For Classes, click 2, and for Method, click Manual. In the Break Values panel, type** 0.000004444 **to replace 0.000006 and click OK.** The "Old values" column shows values that have only six decimal places, but Spatial Analyst has all nine decimal places in memory.

4. **For "New values," replace the 1 with** 0 **and the 2 with** 1.

5. **Finish filling in the form by typing or making selections as shown in the figure. Name the output raster** HAttackQ1.

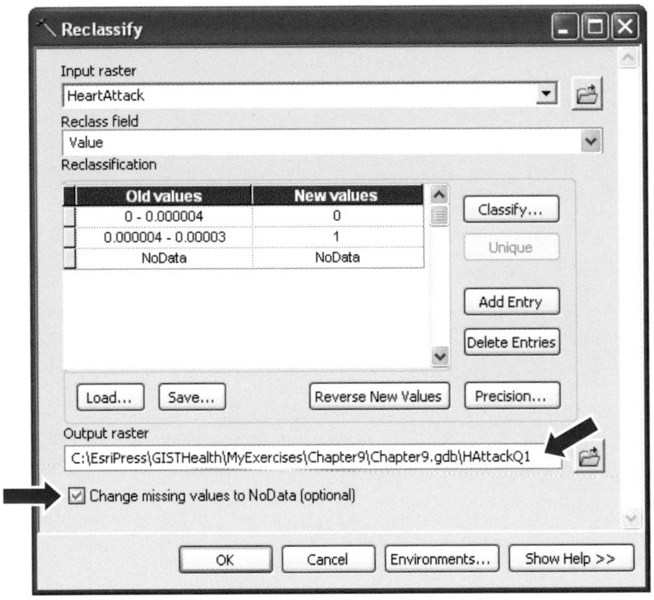

6. **Click OK.**

7. **Symbolize HAttackQ1 so that 0 has no color and 1 is dark blue and make sure that HeartAttack is turned on and below HAttackQ1.** You can see that relatively few peak areas, eight, have sufficiently high heart attack density. (See facing page.) Some of them are likely too small to warrant a defibrillator, but you will not make that determination until you consider all query criteria.

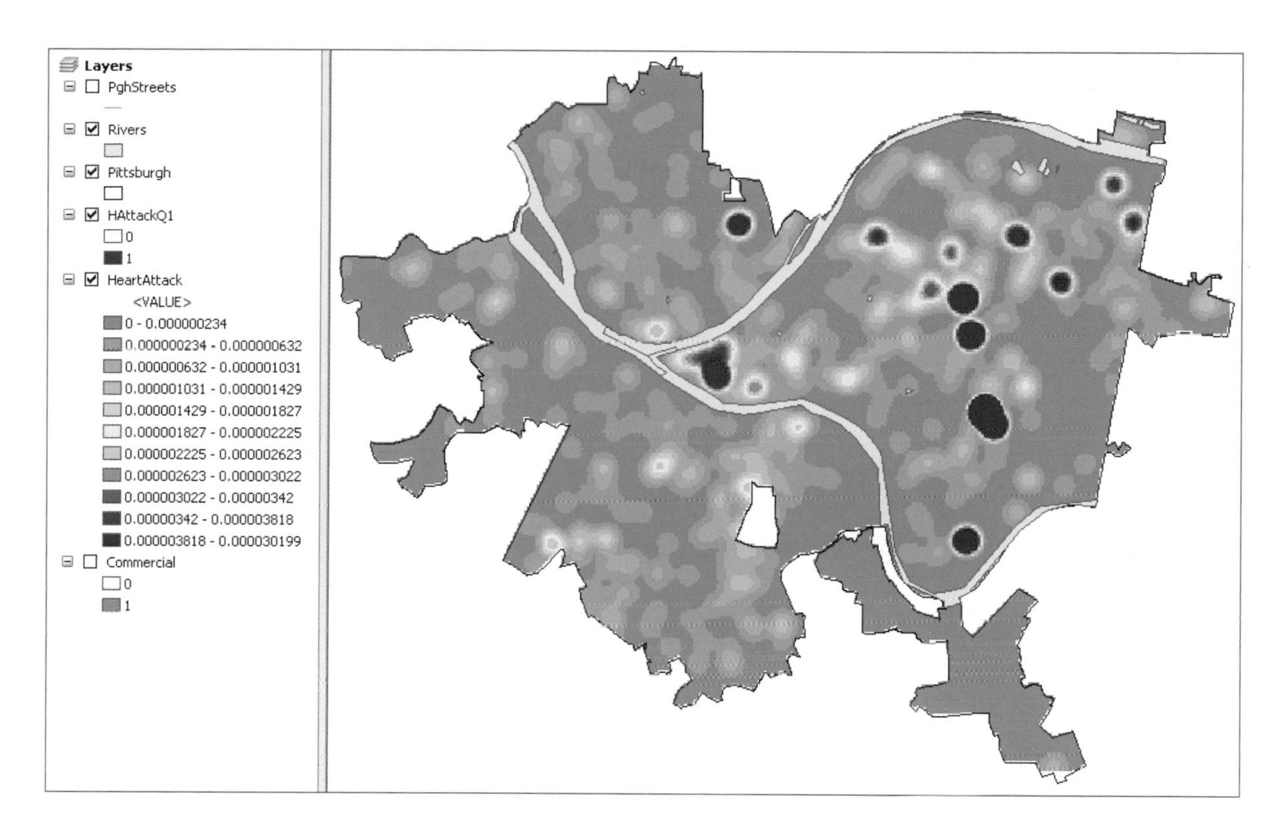

Query a raster dataset using two criteria

Next, you will include a second criterion in the query—locations within the commercial buffer—for suitable defibrillator sites. The Boolean And tool combines two raster datasets by giving all cells the value 0 except where both input cells are 1, in which case the output cell gets the value 1. In this case, the resulting areas defined by cells of value 1 are in both the commercial buffer and the sufficiently high heart attack area of HAttackQ1.

1 **In the Search text box, type** Boolean And**, press ENTER, and click Boolean And (Spatial Analyst).**

2 **In the Boolean And dialog box, type or make selections as shown in the figure and name the output raster** HAttackQ2**. Click OK.**

Boolean And
Input raster or constant value 1
HAttackQ1
Input raster or constant value 2
Commercial
Output raster
C:\EsriPress\GISTHealth\MyExercises\Chapter9\Chapter9.gdb\HAttackQ2
OK Cancel Environments... Show Help >>

3 Resymbolize HAttackQ2 so that 0 has no color and 1 is Tourmaline Green (eighth column, third row of the color chips array) and make sure that HAttackQ1 and HeartAttack are turned on and below HAttackQ2. As you would expect, adding a second criterion using the AND connector has reduced the size of areas that meet the criteria. Three of the formerly promising areas for placement of defibrillators are significantly reduced in size.

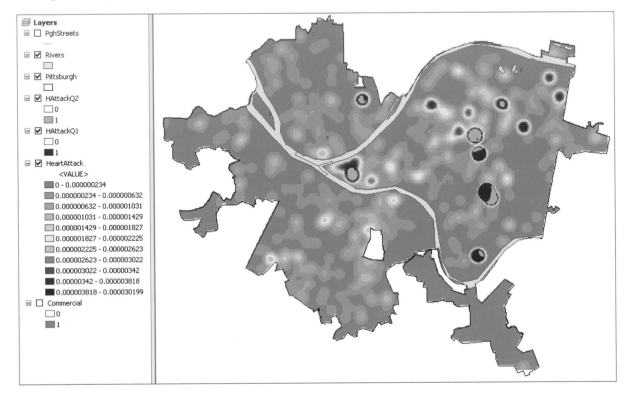

YOUR TURN

Turn on and label the Streets layer using the NAME field. Zoom in on each feasible area to investigate the third criterion—that there be at least 25 blocks, or roughly 2.25 million sq ft, in a square area. Use the Measure tool on the Tools toolbar to measure feasible areas. Which areas remain feasible? Zoom to one of these areas. What would you report back to policy makers?

Save the map document

1 On the File menu, click Save As.

2 Save your map document as Tutorial9-5YourName.mxd **to your Chapter9 folder in MyExercises.** Do not close ArcMap.

Index of poverty risks

Tutorial 9-6
Using ArcGIS ModelBuilder to create a risk index

People who live in poverty often have poor health care, unhealthy diets, and unhealthy habits such as smoking—all factors that contribute to heart attacks. In this tutorial, you will create an index for identifying poverty areas by combining four poverty indicators (O'Hare and Mather 2003): (1) population below the poverty income line, (2) population of female-headed households that have children, (3) population that has less than a high school education, and (4) population of work force males who are unemployed.

Robyn Dawes (1979), a leading researcher on behavioral modeling in the social sciences, provides a simple method for combining these measures into a poverty index. If you have a reasonably good theory that several variables are indicative or predictive of a dependent variable of interest (and whether the dependent variable is observable or not), Dawes makes a good case that all you need to do is to remove scale from each input so that each input has the same weight, and then average the scaled inputs to create a predictive index. A good way to remove scale from a variable is to calculate z-scores, subtracting the mean, and then divide by the standard deviation for each variable.

You can see in the following table that if you simply averaged the four variables, the male unemployed variable arbitrarily gets the highest weight while female-headed households has practically no weight, given the mean of each variable. Z-scores for all four variables, however, have a mean of zero and a standard deviation of 1, so when averaged, they each have equal weight.

Indicator variable	Mean	Standard deviation
Female-headed households with children	1.422	4.431
Less than a high school education	110.060	80.812
Male unemployed	154.500	124.804
Poverty income	126.021	147.188

There are three parts to creating the poverty index. The first part is to calculate the z-score of each of the four indicators. The map layers for the indicators are centroids of blocks for the population of female-headed households with children and centroids of block groups for the other three indicators (which are not available at the more desirable, smaller block level). Thus, to make these layers comparable so that they can be combined into an index, you will transform them into kernel-density maps, using the same 150 ft square grid cells for each. The second part to creating the index then is to create kernel-density maps for all four input variables. The third part is to use an ArcGIS Spatial Analyst tool to add the surfaces, weighted by 0.25, to average them. You will carry out parts 2 and 3 using ArcGIS ModelBuilder to document the work and provide a model for a reusable tool for creating an index.

Set the geoprocessing environment

The map document you will open in this tutorial has inputs for preparing the poverty index: AllCoBlkGrps, which has block group centroids and needed attributes (NoHighSch2 = population with less than a high school education, Male16Unem = males in the work force who are unemployed, and Poverty = population below poverty income) and AllCoBlocks, which has block centroids and the attribute FHHChld = female-headed households with children.

T 9-6

1 **In ArcMap, open Tutorial9-6.mxd.** The map contains block group centroids and block centroids, with each layer displaying one of the four poverty indicators through a color ramp. You can see that it is difficult to represent the spatial patterns effectively using vector graphics, plus it is difficult to integrate the information from just two spatial distributions out of the four needed for the poverty index. The raster poverty index that you will create will do a better job in both regards.

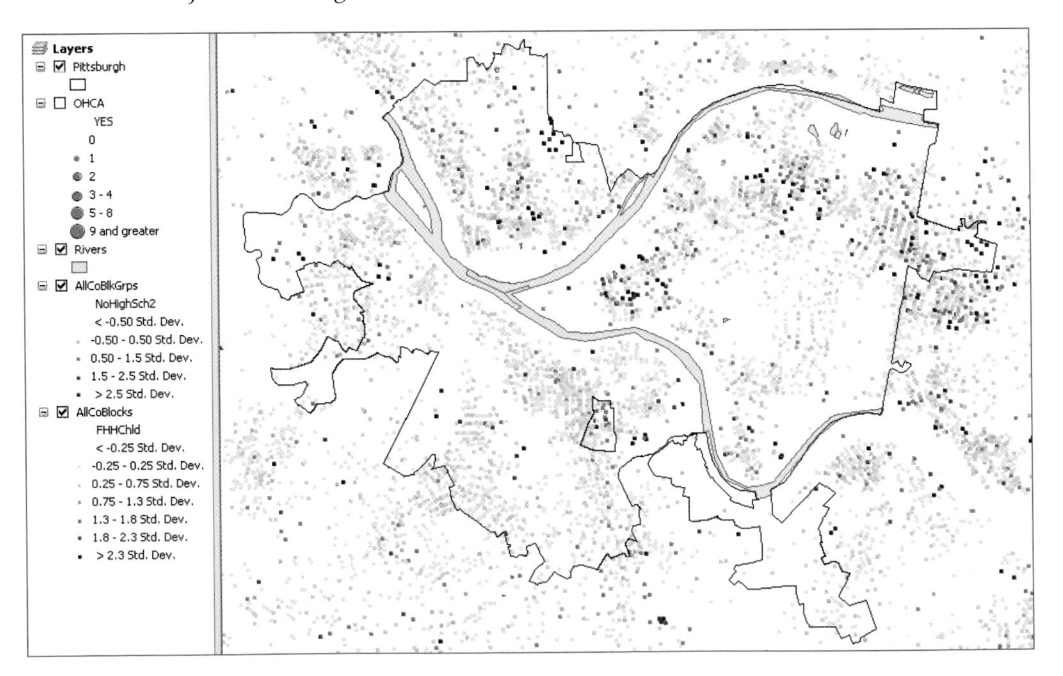

2 **On the Customize menu, click Extensions, select the Spatial Analyst check box if it is not already selected, and click Close.** This step loads the Spatial Analyst extension, so you can use its functionality.

3 **On the Geoprocessing menu, click Geoprocessing Options, and in the Geoprocessing Options dialog box, make selections as shown in the figure. Click OK.**

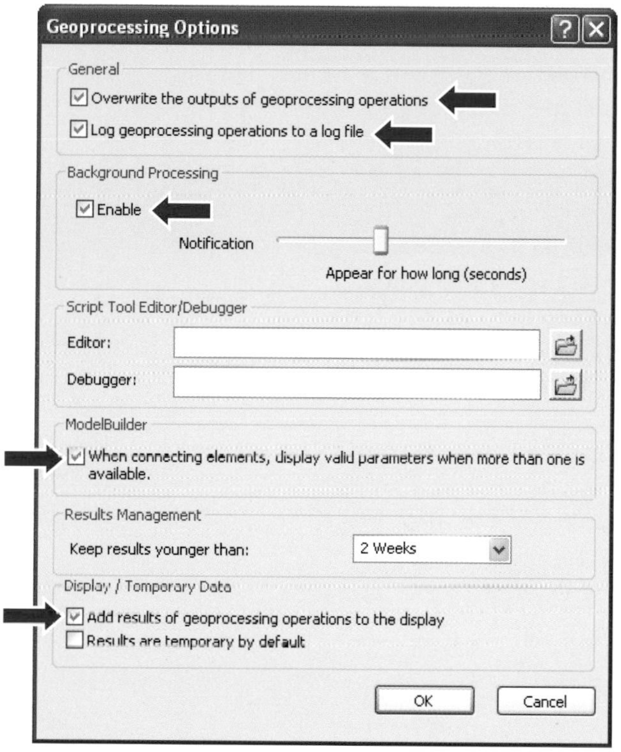

4 **On the Geoprocessing menu, click Environments > Raster Analysis. For Cell Size, click As Specified Below; for Specification, type** 150**; and for Mask, click Pittsburgh. Click OK.**

Standardize the input variables

In this exercise, you will calculate the z-score for one of the input feature classes in an attribute table. To save time, the other three variables already have z-scores ready for use.

1 **In the table of contents, right-click AllCoBlocks and click Open Attribute Table.**

2 **Scroll to the right in the table, right-click FHHChld, and click Statistics.** It is convenient to copy and paste the statistics into Microsoft Notepad, and then later copy and paste them into the field calculator you will be using.

3 In the Statistics of AllCoBlocks window, select all the statistics and press CTRL+C.

4 On your desktop, on the taskbar, click Start, and then click All Programs > Accessories > Notepad.

5 Click inside the Notepad window and press CTRL+V. ▶

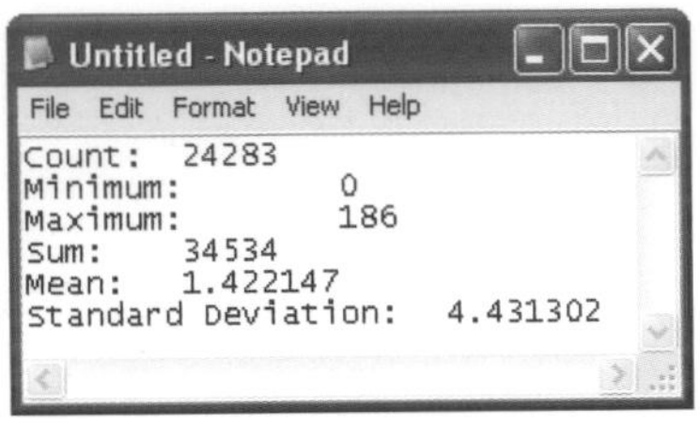

```
Untitled - Notepad
File Edit Format View Help
Count:  24283
Minimum:         0
Maximum:         186
Sum:    34534
Mean:   1.422147
Standard Deviation:   4.431302
```

6 In ArcMap, close the Statistics of AllCoBlocks window, and in the Table window, click Table Options > Add Field. For Name, type ZFHHChld, and for Type, click Float. Click OK.

7 In the table, right-click the column heading for ZFHHChld, click Field Calculator, and create the following expression in the bottom panel of the Field Calculator window by copying and pasting from your Notepad window:

```
( [FHHChld] - 1.422147) / 4.431302
```

8 Click OK. The first six values for the calculated z-scores are shown in the figure. ▶

FHHChld	ZFHHChld
0	-0.320932
0	-0.320932
0	-0.320932
2	0.130403
4	0.581737
1	-0.095265

9 Close the table and Notepad. Do not save the changes.

Create a new toolbox and model

1 On the ArcMap Menu bar, click Windows > Catalog and go to your Chapter9 folder in MyExercises.

2 Right-click Chapter9, click New > Toolbox, and rename the new toolbox UnweightedIndices.tbx.

3 Right-click UnweightedIndices.tbx and click New > Model.

4 On the ModelBuilder Menu bar, click Model > Model Properties.

5 On the General tab, for Name, type PovertyIndex (no spaces allowed), and for Label, type Poverty Index. Click OK and hide the Catalog window.

Create a kernel-density layer for an input

The next task is to create kernel-density layers for the four inputs using the z-scores. After you create model elements for one kernel-density layer, you can easily copy the layer and make adjustments to create the remaining three.

1 **On the ArcMap Menu bar, click Windows > Search.**

2 **In the Search text box, type** Kernel Density, **press ENTER, and drag Kernel Density into the Poverty Index model window.** ▶

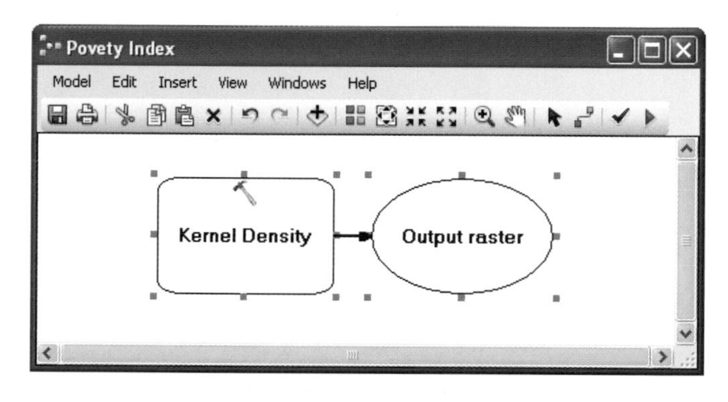

3 **In the model, right-click Kernel Density and click Open.**

4 **In the Kernel Density dialog box, type or make the selections shown in the figure and name the output raster** KDFHHChld. **Click OK.** ▶

5 **Right-click the Kernel Density tool element, click Rename, and change the name to** FHHChld Kernel Density. ▶

6 **Right-click FHHChld Kernel Density and click Run.**

7 **After the model is finished running, click Close.**

8 **Right-click KDFHHChld and click Add To Display.** This layer shows where there is a high concentration of female-headed households that have no children.

9 **Save your model, but do not close it.**

YOUR TURN

Symbolize the new layer using the Classified method, 1/4 standard deviations, and the color ramp that runs from blue to yellow to red. Turn off the point feature layers. The result is as shown in the figure.

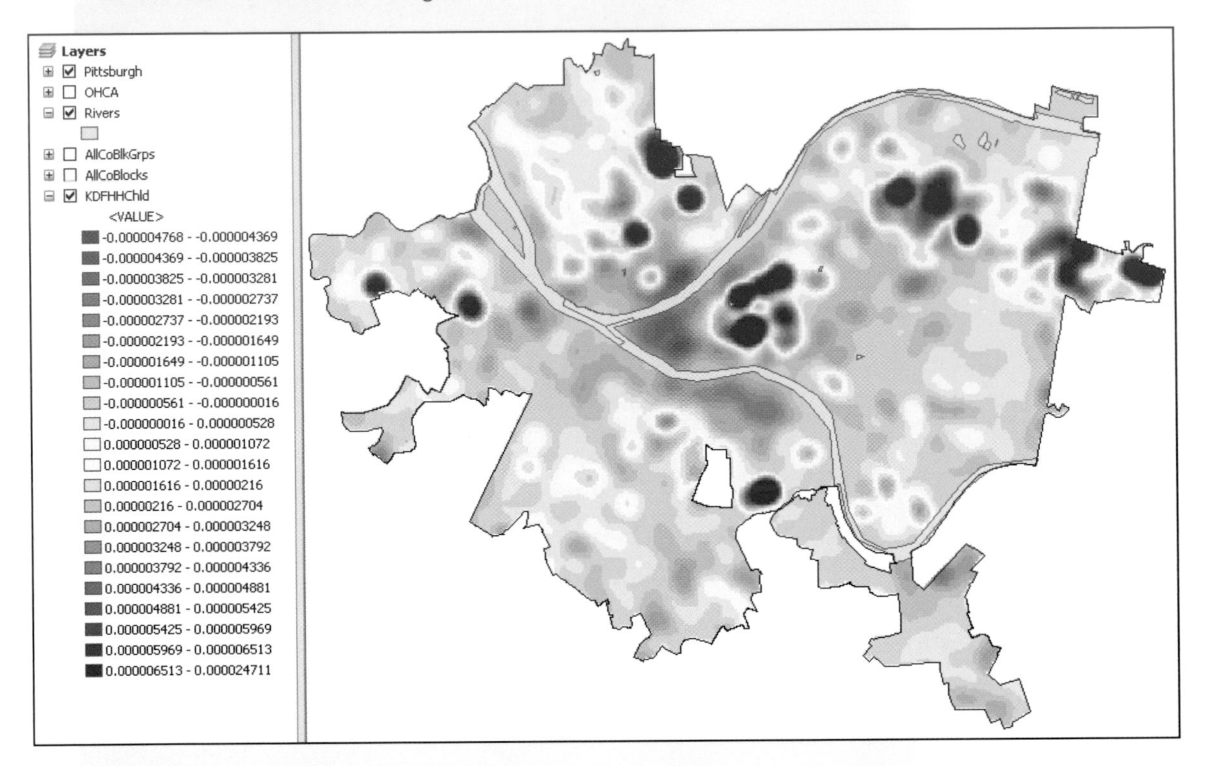

Create a kernel-density layer for a second input

You can reuse the model elements you just built to create other layers. Although blocks work very well for a search radius of 1,500 ft, the remaining three poverty inputs are at the larger block group level and require a larger search radius of 3,000 ft.

1 **In the Model window, right-click FHHChld Kernel Density and click Copy.**

2 **On the ModelBuilder Menu bar, click Edit > Paste.**

3 **In the Model window, right-click the new FHHChld Kernel Density (2) model element and rename it** NoHighSch Kernel Density.

4 **Right-click NoHighSch Kernel Density and click Open.** Ignore the error messages. You will make changes that nullify them.

5 **In the NoHighSch Kernel Density dialog box, type or make selections as shown in the figure and name the output raster** KDNoHighSch. **Click OK.** Note that you will use the input layer AllCoBlkGrps.

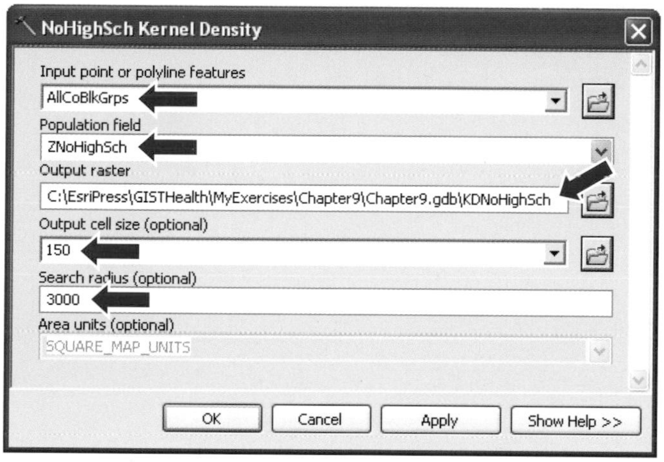

6 **In the Model window, right-click KDFHHChld (2) and rename it** KDNoHighSch.

7 **Right-click NoHighSch Kernel Density and click Run.**

8 **Right-click KDNoHighSch, click Add To Display, and symbolize using 1/4 standard deviation and a color ramp that runs from blue to yellow to red.**

YOUR TURN

Copy and paste the NoHighSch Kernel Density model element into your model twice so you can use the block group attributes ZMaleUnem and ZPoverty to create two new raster layers. See the resulting partial model in the figure for element names that you need to use. Then run each of the two new model elements, add to the display, and resymbolize the resulting map layers. Examine each of the four raster maps. You will see that they have overlapping but different patterns. The index will combine these patterns into a single, overall pattern.

Notice that the model elements for processes acquire drop shadows in the model window after you run them. To reset the model so that you can run it again if needed, on the ModelBuilder Menu bar, click Model > Validate Entire Model. ArcGIS ModelBuilder resets the model and removes the drop shadows. Save your model.

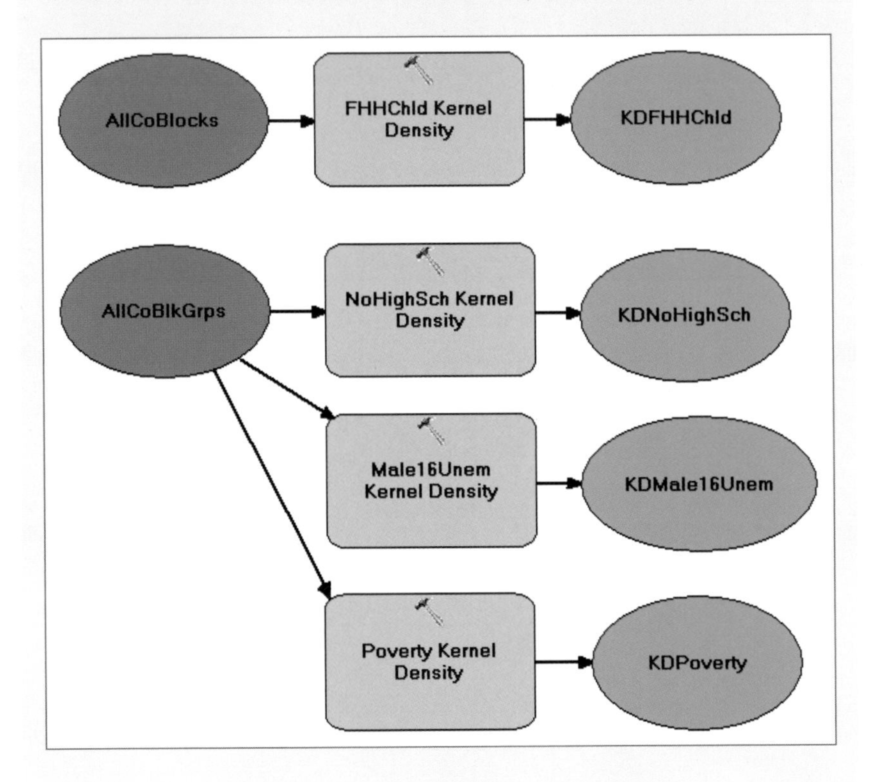

Average multiple kernel-density maps

1 In the Search text box, type Weighted Sum and press ENTER.

2 Drag the Weighted Sum (Spatial Analyst) tool into your model to the right of the kernel-density outputs.

3 **Right-click Weighted Sum, click Open, and in the Weighted Sum dialog box, type or make selections as shown in the figure. Name the output raster** PovertyIndex. If you wish to weight one of the inputs more than the other, simply change the weight value.

Weighted Sum

Input rasters

Raster	Field	Weight
KDFHHChld	VALUE	0.25
KDNoHighSch	VALUE	0.25
KDMale16Unem	VALUE	0.25
KDPoverty	VALUE	0.25

Output raster

C:\EsriPress\GISTHealth\MyExercises\Chapter9\Chapter9.gdb\PovertyIndex

OK Cancel Apply Show Help >>

4 **Click OK and use the model in the figure to complete renaming of the model elements.** You may need to use the Connect tool to complete the model.

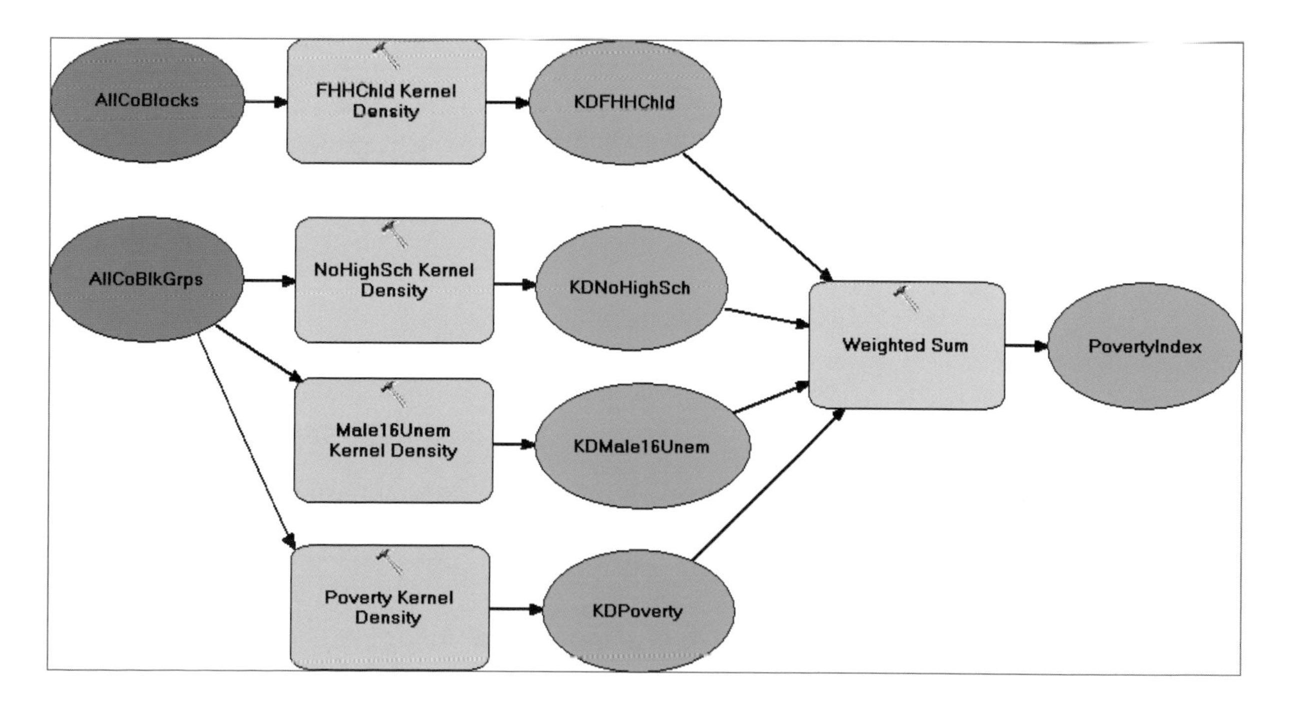

T 9-6

5 Right-click Weighted Sum, click Properties, click the Environments tab, expand Raster Storage, click Raster Statistics > OK. Run the Weighted Sum process and symbolize the results using Stretched in the left panel, standard deviations, and the color ramp that runs from green to yellow to red.

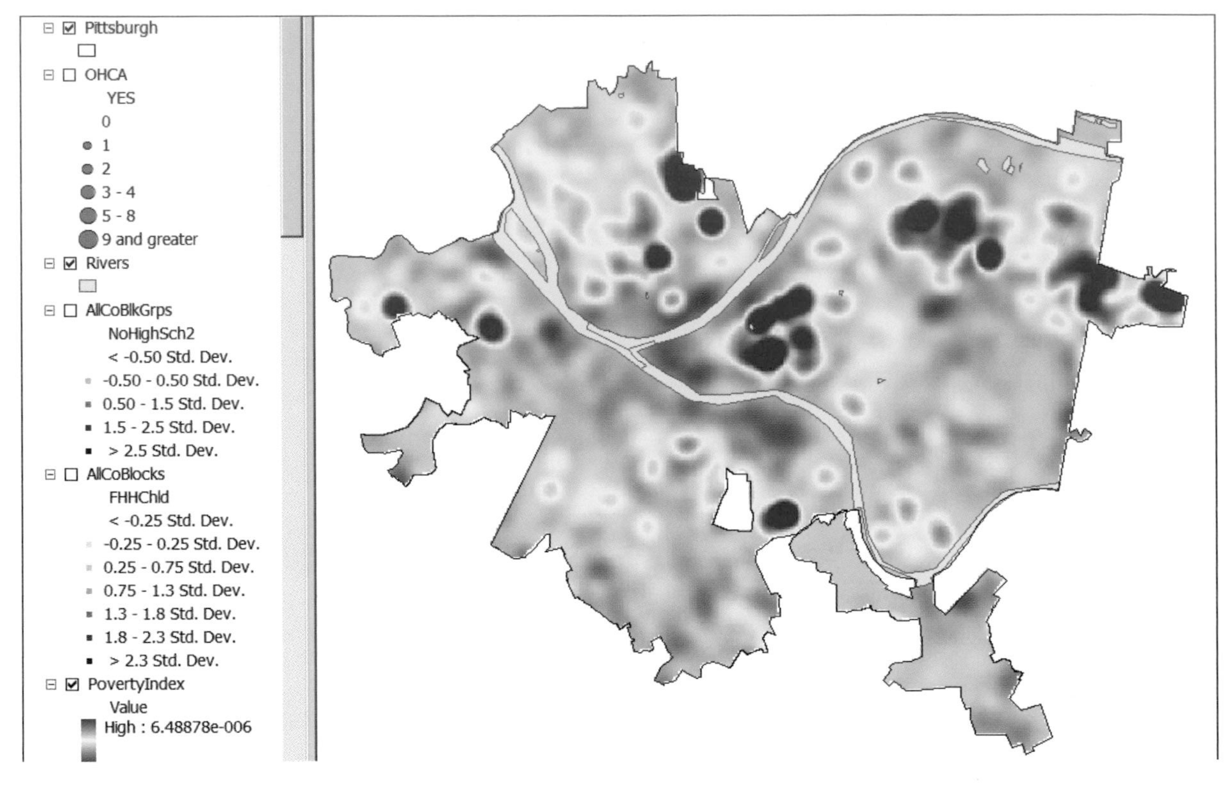

6 Save your model.

Create a poverty contour

Suppose that after consideration, policy analysts want to use the poverty index density of 0.0000009 or higher to define poverty. You will next create a polygon feature class that has the contour line for that "elevation" in the index.

1 In the Search text box, type Contour List **and click the Contour List (Spatial Analyst) tool.**

2 In the Contour List dialog box, type or make selections as shown in the figure and name the output polyline features PovertyContour**.** ▶

Contour List
Input raster
PovertyIndex
Output polyline features
C:\EsriPress\GISTHealth\MyExercises\Chapter9\Chapter9.gdb\PovertyContour
Contour values
0.0000009
OK | Cancel | Environments... | Show Help >>

3 **Click OK and symbolize the PovertyContour layer using an outline width of** 1.15. You now have a set of vector polygons, shown with thick black outlines, that explicitly define poverty areas and can be used for spatial analysis for many policy purposes.

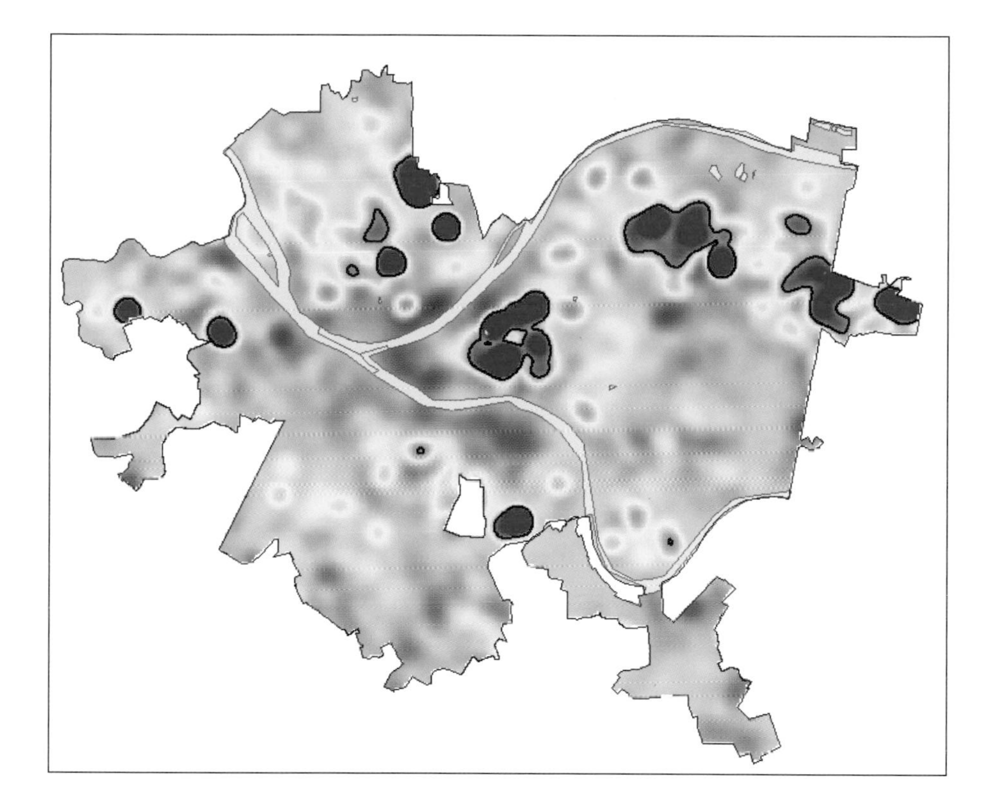

Save the map document

1 **On the File menu, click Save As.**

2 **Save your map document as** Tutorial9-6YourName.mxd **to your Chapter9 folder in MyExercises.** Close ArcMap.

Summary

This study has produced many valuable outputs in support of locating defibrillators in public places in Pittsburgh. You discovered that only a few areas are large enough to meet the criterion for having commercial land uses. You can also show how heart attack incident rates and population determine only a portion of the spatial distribution of heart attacks occurring in public places. Finally, you have constructed a useful index with contour lines defining poverty in Pittsburgh. This is useful for explaining the incidence of heart attacks as well as for many other purposes.

On the technical side, you have become a sophisticated user of raster GIS and the ArcGIS Spatial Analyst extension. You can work with and enhance raster maps for uses such as elevation and land use, using masks to display irregularly shaped study areas and hillshade to provide a realistic three-dimensional appearance. You have a working knowledge of density maps and how to create them using kernel-density smoothing in ArcGIS Spatial Analyst, and you know how to query raster maps for useful information. Finally, you can process raster maps using map algebra to combine them for comparison, and you know how to build impressive macros in ArcGIS ModelBuilder to streamline your work.

Assignment 9-1

Display schools and land use for locating school-based health centers

The first ring of suburbs around urban areas may be candidates for future revitalization as suburban homeowners attempt to downsize their homes or relocate closer to work. In anticipation of this growth in Pittsburgh, suppose that the Allegheny County Health Department plans to create satellite centers in the schools of these suburbs. The centers will provide flu shots, health wellness education programs, lead poisoning prevention programs, and other services. As a starting point for choosing potential schools for these centers, in this assignment, you will prepare a map that shows land use and school locations for the first ring of suburbs.

You will choose the appropriate subset of municipalities in Allegheny County, create a mask for them, and use the mask to display land use with hillshade. Then you will add a layer for schools and display them in the same area.

Start with this data

- *\EsriPress\GISTHealth\Data\SpatialAnalyst\SpatialAnalyst.gdb\Munic:* polygon layer of municipalities in Allegheny County
- *\EsriPress\GISTHealth\Data\SpatialAnalyst\SpatialAnalyst.gdb\CountySchools:* XY data file that has the names of schools and x,y point coordinates in the NAD 1983 Pennsylvania south state plane projection
- *\EsriPress\GISTHealth\Data\SpatialAnalyst\SpatialAnalyst.gdb\Pittsburgh:* boundary polygon for Pittsburgh
- *\EsriPress\GISTHealth\Data\SpatialAnalyst\LandUse\28910720.tif:* land use for Allegheny County
- *\EsriPress\GISTHealth\Data\SpatialAnalyst\SpatialAnalyst.gdb\DEM:* digital elevation model for Allegheny County
- *\EsriPress\GISTHealth\Data\SpatialAnalyst\LandUse.lyr:* layer file for rendering a land-use raster dataset

Preprocess vector layers

Create a file geodatabase called **Assignment9-1YourName.gdb** and save it to your Chapter9 folder in MyAssignments, adding all new layers that you create into it.

Create a map document called **Assignment9-1YourName.mxd** and save it to your Chapter9 folder in MyAssignments, using relative paths. Include each of the preceding layers. Add the municipalities first so your data frame inherits that layer's projection, which is the local 1983 state plane projection. Add county schools as an XY layer. Turn off Pittsburgh to simplify the next step—creating a ring of suburbs.

Define the first ring of suburbs as those in Munic within 1 mi of Pittsburgh but not including Pittsburgh. Start by making Munic the only selectable layer. Then use Selection > Select By Location and select municipalities that are within 1 mi of Pittsburgh. Use the Select Features tool, press SHIFT, and click inside the Pittsburgh polygon in the Munic layer to clear the selection. Finally, right-click Munic and click Data > Export Data to create Suburbs and add it to your map document. Now select schools that intersect suburbs and create SuburbanSchools.

Process raster layers

Using Suburbs as the mask and a cell size of 50, extract a raster from LandUse called **LandUseSub** and import LandUse.lyr for symbolization. Create a hillshade from DEM called **HillshadeSub**. Make LandUseSub transparent, move it above the hillshade, turn off unneeded layers, and display suburban schools using the shaded land-use layer. Housing will be in the red developed areas.

WHAT TO TURN IN

If your work is to be graded, turn in the following files:

- ***File geodatabase:*** \EsriPress\GISTHealth\MyAssignments\Chapter9\Assignment9-1YourName.gdb
- ***ArcMap document:*** \EsriPress\GISTHealth\MyAssignments\Chapter9\Assignment9-1YourName.mxd

If instructed to do so, instead of individual files, turn in a compressed file, **Assignment9-1YourName.zip**, that includes all the preceding files. Do not include path information in the compressed file.

Assignment 9-2

Determine heart attack fatalities outside of hospitals by gender

Females have more fatal heart attacks outside of hospitals than males, perhaps because symptoms of heart attacks in females are less well known than those in males. Heart attacks outside of hospitals are roughly 1.5 per thousand for males age 35 to 74 and 2.3 per thousand for females in the same age range. In this assignment, you will create two density-map layers—one for males and one for females—using these incidence rates for the municipality of Mount Lebanon in Allegheny County. You will do all raster processing using Spatial Analyst tools in a model.

Start with this data

- *\EsriPress\GISTHealth\Data\SpatialAnalyst\SpatialAnalyst.gdb\Munic:* polygon layer for municipalities in Allegheny County
- *\EsriPress\GISTHealth\Data\SpatialAnalyst\SpatialAnalyst.gdb\AllCoBlocks:* point layer for census block centroids in Allegheny County

Preprocess vector layers

Create a file geodatabase called **Assignment9-2YourName.gdb** and save it to your Chapter9 folder in MyAssignments. Include all new layers and other files that you create.

Create a map document called **Assignment9-2YourName.mxd** and save it to your Chapter9 folder in MyAssignments, using relative paths. Include each of the preceding layers.

Select the Mount Lebanon polygon from Munic and export it as **MtLebanon**. Extract the Mount Lebanon blocks from AllCoBlocks and save them as **MtLebBlocks**. Add floating point fields to the attribute table for MtLebBlocks: MMortInc = 0.0015 × [Male35T74] for the annual number of heart attack fatalities for males age 35 to 74 and FMortInc = 0.0023 × [Fem35T74] for females in the same age range.

Process raster layers

Create kernel-density map layers for MMortInc and FMortInc, using MtLebanon as the mask, a cell size of 100, and a search radius of 1,500 sq ft. Give the outputs descriptive names, add them to the map, and apply the same symbology scheme to both. Symbolize the kernel-density map for females first, and then import that symbolization for the male map.

WHAT TO TURN IN

If your work is to be graded, turn in the following files:

- ***File geodatabase:*** \EsriPress\GISTHealth\MyAssigments\Chapter9\Assignment9-2YourName.gdb
- ***ArcMap document:*** \EsriPress\GISTHealth\MyAssigments\Chapter9\Assignment9-2YourName.mxd

If instructed to do so, instead of individual files, turn in a compressed file, **Assignment9-2YourName.zip**, that includes all the preceding files. Do not include path information in the compressed file.

References

Dawes, R. M. 1979. "The Robust Beauty of Improper Linear Models in Decision Making." *American Psychologist* 7, no. 34: 571–82, doi:10.1037//0003-066X.34.7.571.

Harvard Medical School Family Health Guide. "Public defibrillators," last updated May 2004, http://www.health.harvard.edu/fhg/updates/update0504a.shtml. Accessed July 26, 2008.

O'Hare, W., and M. Mather. 2003. "The Growing Number of Kids in Severely Distressed Neighborhoods: Evidence from the 2000 Census." In *Kids Count*, a publication of the Annie E. Casey Foundation and the Population Reference Bureau, revised October 2003, http://www.aecf.org/upload/publicationfiles/da3622h1280.pdf.

Rosamond, W. D., L. E. Chambless, A. R. Folsom, L. S. Cooper, D. E. Conwill, L. Clegg, C. H. Wang, and G. Heiss. 1998. "Trends in Incidence of Myocardial Infarction and in Mortality Due to Coronary Heart Disease, 1987 to 1994." *New England Journal of Medicine* 339, no. 13: 861–67, doi:10.1056/NEJM199809243391301.

Chapter 10

Studying food-borne-disease outbreaks

Objectives

- Assemble basemaps for emergency preparedness
- Geocode events to trace an outbreak source
- Use buffer analysis to identify affected office buildings
- Use buffer analysis to assess vulnerable populations

You will likely want to use GIS in projects for your own organization, for research, or for other purposes. Using GIS will require you to clarify the problem or issue to be studied, identify a solution that employs GIS, determine what data and other resources are available, and design a workflow that progresses from intermediate answers to final presentations for clients and other audiences. For this type of work, you will use many project management and applied research skills beyond employing the functionality available in ArcGIS.

Chapters 1 through 9 have helped you to build your knowledge of GIS functionality and day-to-day workflows by working on parts or phases of GIS projects. In this chapter and the final chapter, you will work on building case studies and doing independent GIS project work. You will not learn any new GIS functionality but how to structure project work and carry out longer sequences of steps that integrate the knowledge and skills learned in the previous chapters. Chapters 10 and 11 each have a health scenario as before, but there are no step-by-step instructions. Instead, guidelines are provided for carrying out GIS project work, and you are asked to follow them while making your own decisions on what steps to take.

Health-care scenario

According to the Centers for Disease Control and Prevention (CDC), food can transmit more than 200 diseases known to be caused by bacteria or viruses. The CDC estimates that approximately 76 million cases of food-borne illness occur in the United States each year, accounting for 325,000 hospitalizations and 5,000 deaths (Mead et al. 1999). In addition to such naturally occurring threats, health organizations, including state and local health departments, are concerned about food-borne illness in connection with emergency preparedness and homeland security—for example, terrorists could taint food with infectious agents in grocery stores and restaurants.

GIS can be used to track and analyze disease outbreaks caused by food-borne agents, the exposure of populations to risk, and the availability of surrounding health services. Using GIS, you can quickly map reported illnesses from food contamination and then model the populations at risk for other outbreaks.

In this case study, you will prepare maps to analyze scenarios of food-borne-disease outbreaks in Allegheny County, Pennsylvania. Members of the Allegheny County Health Department Food Safety Program inspect and regulate every type of food establishment and investigate food contamination and food-borne illnesses.

Case study requirements

The major deliverable for this case study is a computer folder that contains a file geodatabase (Assignment10YourName.gdb), map documents (as follows), a Microsoft PowerPoint presentation (**Assignment10PresentationYourName.pptx**), and a Microsoft Word document project report (**Assignment10ReportYourName.docx**) suitable for the director of the health department.

An outline and guidelines for the project final report follow. Use each category listed, in the order given, as sections in your report. In addition to the report, create a Microsoft PowerPoint presentation that has bullets for the major parts of each section in your report. The PowerPoint presentation should also include output maps and tables.

Problem definition and solution approach

Write a short introduction that includes the definition of the problem, the solution approach, and the scope of the project, including limitations.

- *Clearly state the problem, opportunity, issue, or objective.* The problem is often a gap between the current state and the desired state of a region—for example, too many uninsured persons in a state or too few safe play areas in the poor parts of a city.
- *Provide an approach to the solution.* The approach identifies performance measures for the phenomenon under investigation. For example, the number or percentage of uninsured adults by county may be a performance measure if programs exist or could exist to reduce the number or percentage, and the percentage of children living within five minutes of a park may be a performance measure if there are or could be housing programs designed to

increase this number. The approach also identifies major data sources and, therefore, helps determine the feasibility of the project.

- *Define the scope or limitations of the project.* Most projects do not have all the resources and data needed to accomplish the desired outcome. Thus, it is important to state the scope of the project and any limitations. For example, the scope might include studying the number of uninsured, but not the availability of other options for health care, such as low-cost clinics. A limitation might be that because of the unavailability of certain data, the study includes only county-level data on the uninsured, even though tract-level census data would be helpful.

Data

Describe the data you will use for your project—its sources, table or layer descriptions, and locations within the project's computer files and folders.

- *Describe the inputs to your project and the data sources.* Search for "Internet citations" on the Internet and pick a style for referencing Web sources. Use that style to provide citations for download sites and other data sources.
- *Within your Chapter10 folder in MyAssignments, create a folder, subfolders, and a file structure for the project.* At a minimum, create a project folder and subfolders for data tables (for attribute data), map layers, and documents.

Methodology

Write a formal description of the methodologies used. For example, if you were describing the methodology used in chapter 7, you could say you used ArcGIS and Microsoft Excel software to create the GIS data and produce results, you placed injury data on the map through geocoding, and you did a proximity analysis using buffers.

- *Create an outline of steps for preparing the data.* These steps, and the steps under the next two bullets, should be detailed enough for a GIS user to be able to carry them out. For example, based on chapter 8, you would (1) delete all columns except identifiers, elderly population (age 65 and older), and poverty measures from the SF 3 census data table and (2) create new columns for the percentage of the elderly population that lives in poverty.
- *Create an outline of steps for constructing GIS data.* For example, based on chapter 7, you would (1) geocode an injury table using a TIGER/Line street map layer to produce the Injuries point layer and (2) classify the Injuries point layer by neighborhood using the neighborhood polygon layer and a spatial join, and so forth.
- *Create an outline of steps for spatial analysis.* For example, based on chapter 7, you would (1) create 500 ft, 1,000 ft, and 5,000 ft buffers for the parks layer and (2) use spatial joins of the buffers and Injuries point layer, and so forth.

Results

This section presents and discusses the output maps and tables and also summarizes the results or findings of the case study. Point out to the reader interesting patterns and limitations and refer to each exhibit by number. Place each map and table on the page following its first mention in the text. In a Microsoft Word document and Microsoft PowerPoint presentation, do the following:

- Prepare professional-quality map layouts and statistical tables of results.
- Write short descriptions of the results, referring to figure and table numbers.

Discussion and future work

In this section, you interpret your results and make recommendations and suggestions for future work that could be done to remove limitations or expand the scope of analysis.

Phase 1
Assemble basemaps

Scenario

During an emergency, analysts need to have data readily available so they can respond quickly and take appropriate action. A real-time monitoring system, equipped with a complete and comprehensive set of GIS base layers, needs to be in place and ready for interactive use by a GIS analyst.

In this phase, use the following layers to create a GIS basemap that could be used to analyze food-borne-disease outbreaks. Use street centerlines for the city of Pittsburgh and geocode food sources by street location. This will allow the health department to quickly identify possible sources of food-borne contamination. Copy all tables and layers to your project folders.

Start with this data

- ***\EsriPress\GISTHealth\Data\ACHD.gdb\PghFoodSources:*** a table of food sources from the Allegheny County Health Department
- ***\EsriPress\GISTHealth\Data\Pittsburgh.gdb\Buildings:*** polygon features of Pittsburgh building outlines
- ***\EsriPress\GISTHealth\Data\Pittsburgh.gdb\Neighborhoods:*** polygon features of neighborhood outlines
- ***\EsriPress\GISTHealth\Data\Pittsburgh.gdb\Sidewalks:*** line features of sidewalks
- ***\EsriPress\GISTHealth\Data\Pittsburgh.gdb\StreetsCL:*** line features of street centerlines

Note: *The data is from food inspections but has been modified to protect privacy.* After geocoding, create separate layers for the following four types of food establishments as determined by the supplied query conditions. This will help epidemiologists and emergency planners quickly analyze which types of establishments might be a potential cause of a food-borne-disease outbreak.

The following table describes the various food sources in the PghFoodSources database:

Bakeries	Bakery or Chain Bakery
Restaurants	Adult Food Service Adult Food Service Fee Exempt Chain Restaurant with Liquor Chain Restaurant without Liquor Restaurant without Liquor Restaurant with Liquor
Grocery stores	Supermarket Chain Supermarket
Convenience stores	Chain Retail Convenience Store

Create basemaps

Create a file geodatabase called **Assignment10YourName.gdb** and save it to your Chapter10 folder in MyAssignments. Import the preceding layers into it.

Create a map document called **Phase1_Basemaps.mxd** and geocode the preceding layers and food sources to Pittsburgh streets.

Rematch as many food locations as possible.

Create a map layout of buildings, streets, sidewalks, neighborhoods, and food sources by type as separate layers.

In your final report, keep a log of the steps you took to rematch your addresses. What are some reasons that the food sources did not match? Describe what additional steps may be needed to get all food sources to match. Include the log as an appendix in your final report.

Phase 2
Trace an outbreak source

Scenario

City hospitals report unusually high numbers of the food-borne illness hepatitis A. The home addresses and work addresses of patients who are possibly infected are available as data. Because you already have a basemap for analysis, you can quickly create a map that shows the residences and work locations of the affected patients to determine possible outbreak locations.

Other information that you know about the patients includes the following:

- None of them ate at restaurants that serve alcohol.
- Most patients were very busy and had quick lunches within two or three blocks of where they worked (about a 500 ft buffer).

Start with this data

- ***Map document from phase 1 of this case study***
- ***\EsriPress\GISTHealth\Data\ACHD.gdb\OutbreakResidences:*** database of home locations for patients who have an outbreak of illness
- ***\EsriPress\GISTHealth\Data\ACHD.gdb\OutbreakWorkLocations:*** database of work locations for patients who have an outbreak of illness

Create outbreak source maps

Import the preceding tables, OutbreakResidences and OutbreakWorkLocations, into your file geodatabase. Start with Phase1_Basemaps.mxd and rename the map document **Phase2_OutbreakSources.mxd**.

Geocode outbreak residences and work locations and add the results to the map composition of phase 1.

Create a map layout that shows the results of your analysis.

What observations do you make from the finished map? Using the preceding information, determine what restaurants are possible sources of the outbreak. In your report, name the restaurants that are possible risks.

Phase 3
Identify affected office buildings

Scenario
Given a known infectious source, it is useful for public health officials to determine the buildings in which likely patrons of an establishment work or live. Then those individuals can be informed of the known infection or violation and advised to seek immediate help if they start to display certain symptoms. In the case of a contagious outbreak of a pathogen from a point source, a similar process can be used to identify buildings for quarantine or evacuation. Again, a walking distance measure can identify buildings containing at-risk or potentially infected individuals.

In this scenario, food safety officials have determined that the fictional restaurant Generic Deli is the source of the food contamination.

Start with this data
- *Map documents and layers from phases 1 and 2 of this case study.*

Create a map identifying affected office buildings
Start with Phase2_OutbreakSources.mxd and rename the map document **Phase3_AffectedOfficeBuildings.mxd.**

Create a map that contains a layer of buildings within the Pittsburgh neighborhood where patients work, a quarter-mile buffer around Generic Deli, and buildings whose centroids are completely within this buffer.

Create a map layout that shows the results of your analysis and a description of how you approached the problem.

Phase 4
Assess vulnerable populations

Scenario
Public health officials need to estimate the areas and populations at risk from an identified infectious source—namely, where potential customers of an identified source reside, how many particularly susceptible individuals (in this case, populations age 5 and under, and 65 and over) might be affected, and what the maximum number of potential cases is. This information would be useful for response planning, including communication of incident details, identification of new cases, and ensuring there are sufficient treatment facilities, supplies of antibiotics, and available personnel.

In this scenario, Pittsburgh's rivers flooded. After the floodwater receded, food establishments within the flood zones reopened. Because of power outages in these areas, the health department needs to inspect these establishments to make sure they have properly disposed of affected food supplies and cleaned food preparation areas and equipment. The health department wants to know the elderly (age 65 and over) and very young (age 5 and under) populations within buffers of one-half mile and one mile of these food sources so they can prioritize their inspections.

Start with this data
- ***Geocoded food sources from phase 1 of this case study***
- ***\EsriPress\GISTHealth\Data\Pittsburgh.gdb\BlockCentroids:*** point shapefile of census blocks that includes Summary File 1 (SF 1) population data
- ***\EsriPress\GISTHealth\Data\Pittsburgh.gdb\FemaFlood:*** polygon shapefile of flood zones

Create maps showing vulnerable populations

Import the preceding features into your file geodatabase and create a map document called **Phase4_VulnerablePopulations.mxd.**

Create maps that show the food establishments within the flood zones, polygon buffers of one-half mile and one mile around these establishments, census block centroids within each buffer, and a count of total population, population age 65 and over, and population age 5 and under, within each buffer. For the one-mile buffer, show populations between one-half mile and one mile. Insert these maps of population data results into your final report and presentation.

WHAT TO TURN IN

If your work is to be graded, turn in the following files:

- ***File geodatabase:*** \EsriPress\GISTHealth\MyAssignments\Chapter10\Assignment10YourName.gdb
- ***ArcMap documents:*** \EsriPress\GISTHealth\MyAssignments\Chapter10\Phase1_Basemaps.mxd, Phase2_OutbreakSources.mxd, Phase3_AffectedOfficeBuildings.mxd, and Phase4_VulnerablePopulations.mxd
- ***Microsoft PowerPoint final presentation:*** \EsriPress\GISTHealth\MyAssignments\Chapter10\Assignment10PresentationYourName.pptx
- ***Microsoft Word document final report:*** \EsriPress\GISTHealth\MyAssignments\Chapter10\Assignment10ReportYourName.docx

If instructed to do so, instead of individual files, turn in a compressed file, **Assignment10YourName.zip**, that includes all the preceding files. Do not include path information in the compressed file.

Reference

Mead, P. S., L. Slutsker, D. Vance, I. F. McCaig, J. S. Bresee, C. Shapiro, P. M. Griffin, and R. V. Tauxe. 1999. "Food-Related Illness and Death in the United States." *Emerging Infectious Diseases* 5, no. 5: 607, doi:10.3201/eid0505.990502.

Chapter 11

Forming local chapters of ACHE

Objectives

- Perform market analysis
- Perform territory analysis
- Track chapter status

In this chapter, as in chapter 10, you will work independently on a case study. A health scenario is provided, as before, but there are no step-by-step instructions. Instead, guidelines are provided for carrying out GIS project work and you are asked to follow them while making your own decisions on what steps to take.

Health-care scenario

The American College of Healthcare Executives (ACHE), based in Chicago, is the leading professional association of health-care executives worldwide. ACHE has a 70-year history of serving executives across the health-care industry by providing new educational opportunities, media products and services, professional credentialing, career development services, and networking opportunities.

To respond to the changing needs of the health-care management profession, ACHE developed a plan to form a network of local independent chapters that are closer to where members live, thus providing better access to standard ACHE programs and benefits.

Recently, the ACHE board of governors formalized its plans to evaluate and develop chapters by starting its Partners for Success chapter deployment project. The final chapter network consists of independent, separate corporations bound by an agreement with ACHE. Existing affiliate groups, part of the Healthcare Executive Groups and Women Health Executive Networks (HEG_WHEN), formed initial ACHE chapters, and new chapters are being developed to fill in gaps in coverage.

One of the major steps of the project is to determine where health-care executive chapters should be located to create better regional coverage. In this case study, you will create maps for this purpose. You will use the maps to determine if the desired market areas are unique and nonoverlapping, and if they cover areas of demand. In this case study scenario, you will have the role of GIS analyst working for ACHE.

There will likely be many opportunities in the future to draw on networks to provide health care, and designing territories of responsibility will be an integral part of this work. GIS analysts will need to carry out similar studies in a competitive environment, mapping both their own territories and those of others.

Case study requirements

As in the previous case study in chapter 10, the major deliverable for this case study is a computer folder (MyAssignments\Chapter11\) containing a file geodatabase (**Assignment11YourName.gdb**), map documents (as follows), a Microsoft PowerPoint presentation (**Assignment11PresentationYourName.pptx**), and a Microsoft Word document final project report (**Assignment11lReportYourName.docx**) suitable for the board of governors of ACHE. Create a folder called **Groups** and subfolders called **DatabasesDistricts123** and **GroupsDissolved** that have the appropriate files saved within. Create a folder called **Outputs** and subfolders called **ChapterStatusMaps** and **MarketingMaps** that have the exported images saved within.

Follow the case study requirements already described in chapter 10 for problem definition and solution approach, data, methodology, results, and discussion and future work.

Phase 1
Create market analysis maps

Scenario

In phase 1, you will perform a market analysis based on ACHE membership data by ZIP Code obtained from ACHE affiliate groups. You will conduct a proximity analysis using 25, 50, 75, and 100 mi concentric buffers of affiliate office locations with members by ZIP Code. The resulting maps will allow ACHE chapter leaders to identify overlapping territories. GIS-generated maps can then be made available to leaders of potential new chapters, who can survey uncovered areas to select counties and ZIP Codes to form new territories.

Figure 11.1 is an example of the type of macro you can build to automate the steps to create maps for a market analysis.

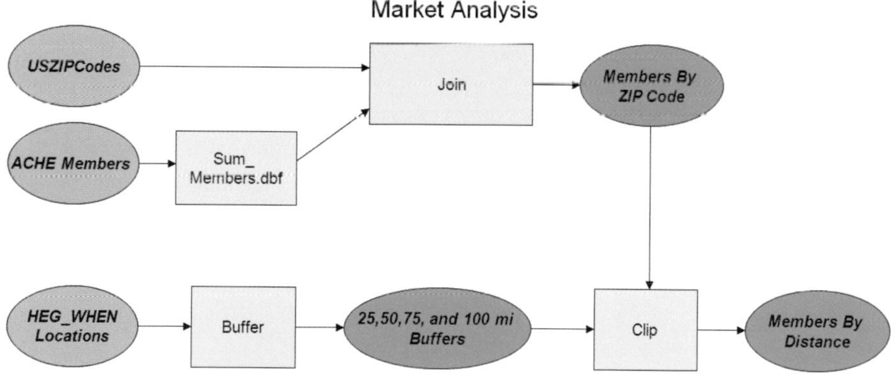

Figure 11.1 Model for building market analysis maps

Start with this data

- ***\EsriPress\GISTHealth\Data\ACHE.gdb\States:*** polygon features of US states including current ACHE districts (field = DISTRICT)
- ***\EsriPress\GISTHealth\Data\ACHE.gdb\ACHEMembers:*** table of current ACHE members by ZIP Code. ***Hint:*** *Summarize the number of ACHE members using the ZIP field, and then join this file to ZIP Code polygons.*
- ***\EsriPress\GISTHealth\Data\ACHE.gdb\HEG_WHEN:*** point features of existing Healthcare Executive Groups and Women Health Executive Networks
- ***\EsriPress\GISTHealth\Data\UnitedStates.gdb\USZipCodes:*** polygon features of ZIP Codes for the United States

Create marketing maps

Import the preceding files into Assignment11YourName.gdb and create a map document called **Phase1_MarketAnalysisMaps.mxd.**

Create a series of maps that include current ACHE districts, a choropleth map of ACHE members by ZIP Code, and multiple buffers of 25, 50, 75, and 100 mi from HEG_WHEN locations.

Phase 2
Create territory analysis maps

Scenario

The ACHE Partners for Success prospectus contains 18 criteria and a number of tools to help leaders of prospective new chapters evaluate their chapter's readiness to become an ACHE chapter. Several of the criteria address territory analysis.

In phase 2 mapping, you will identify overlapping areas. Potential chapter leaders can then make decisions on adding or dropping ZIP Codes or counties from their proposed service areas to eliminate overlaps. The same maps can also be used in negotiations between various adjoining chapters.

Figure 11.2 is an example of the type of macro you can build to automate the steps to create maps for a territory analysis.

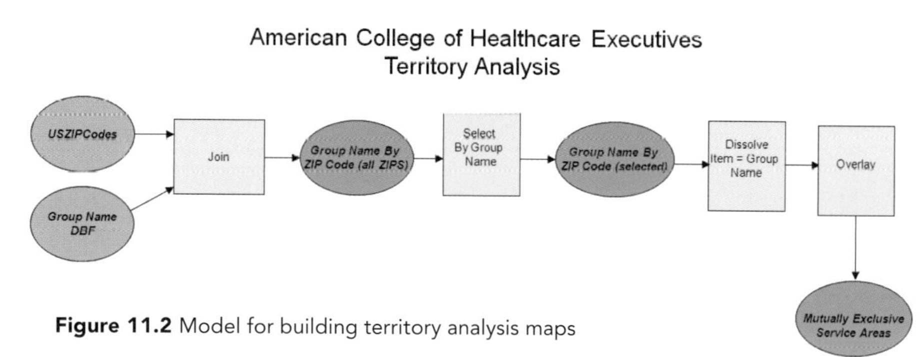

Figure 11.2 Model for building territory analysis maps

Start with this data

- *\EsriPress\GISTHealth\Data\ACHE.gdb\GroupsDistricts1_2_3:* table of ACHE group partners by ZIP Code for districts 1–3
- *\EsriPress\GISTHealth\Data\ACHE.gdb\GroupsDistricts4_5_6:* table of ACHE group partners by ZIP Code for districts 4–6
- *\EsriPress\GISTHealth\Data\UnitedStates.gdb\USZipCodes:* polygon features of ZIP Codes for the United States
- *\EsriPress\GISTHealth\Data\ACHE.gdb\States:* polygon features of US states, including current ACHE districts (field = DISTRICT)
- *ACHE districts:* polygon features created in phase 1 marketing of the case study

Create maps showing territories of overlapping affiliate groups in districts 1, 2, and 3

Import the preceding tables and polygon features into Assignment11YourName.gdb and create a new map document called **Phase2_TerritoryAnalysisMaps.mxd**.

The group-districts database includes affiliate groups that have overlapping ZIP Codes. In order to see the overlap, you need to extract each group to its own database, join the new database of each group to US ZIP Code features, extract just the ZIP Codes for each group, and dissolve based on the group name. Your table of contents should include a separate layer/feature class for each dissolved group territory.

Build a model of the preceding process and include a screen capture of the model in your final presentation and report. ***Hint:*** *If you have trouble repeating the model, remove existing joins on the ZIP Code features before rerunning the model.*

Show each group territory as a transparent polygon or as Hollow fill and an outline to see the groups that overlap.

Create a new feature class of overlapping group territories in New York, Pennsylvania, and Ohio. Show the overlapping areas using a crosshatch fill.

For extra practice, repeat the preceding steps for groups in districts 4, 5, and 6.

These maps will give affiliate group planners and ACHE leaders and staff their first determination of which territories overlap. Affiliate groups that have overlapping territories are required to contact each other to coordinate their boundaries or consider a merger or alliance. When the reshuffling is finished, a new file containing counties and ZIP Codes that make up the realigned territory will be sent to ACHE for remapping.

Territory maps can be reviewed during conference calls, and counties and ZIP Codes can then be added or deleted from a territory.

Phase 3
Track chapter status

Scenario

After potential chapters submit their proposals to be chartered with ACHE, they are given either chartered chapter status or, if not all provisions are met, provisional chapter status.

Chicago ACHE staff use the Chapter Status Tracking System to keep track of an applicant's progress in meeting criteria. The system also tracks unclaimed territory—whole or partial counties not claimed by a chapter. In phase 3 mapping, you will track the status of provisional and chartered ACHE chapters.

Start with this data

- *\EsriPress\GISTHealth\Data\ACHE.gdb\ResolvedPartners:* table of ACHE resolved group partners by ZIP Code
  The ResolvedPartners table contains an item "Status" that has the following values:
  - *PCHP:* Provisional (able to meet 11 of the 18 criteria for chartered status)
  - *CHP:* Chartered (all 18 criteria for becoming an ACHE chapter corporation are met)
- *\EsriPress\GISTHealth\Data\UnitedStates.gdb\USZipCodes:* polygon features of ZIP Codes for the United States

Create chapter status maps

Import the preceding table and polygon features into Assignment11YourName.gdb and create a new map document called **Phase3_TrackingChapterStatus.mxd**.

Create maps showing which chapters are provisional and which are chartered for each ACHE district.

Export your maps as JPEG image files and add them to your final presentation document.

WHAT TO TURN IN

If your work is to be graded, turn in the following files:

- ***File geodatabase:*** \EsriPress\GISTHealth\MyAssignments\Chapter11\Assignment11YourName.gdb
- ***ArcMap documents:*** \EsriPress\GISTHealth\MyAssignments\Chapter11\Phase1_MarketAnalysisMaps.mxd, Phase2_TerritoryAnalysisMaps.mxd, and Phase3_TrackingChapterStatus.mxd
- ***Microsoft PowerPoint final presentation:*** \EsriPress\GISTHealth\MyAssignments\Chapter11\Assignment11PresentationYourName.pptx
- ***Microsoft Word document final report:*** \EsriPress\GISTHealth\MyAssignments\Chapter11\Assignment11ReportYourName.docx
- ***Chapter 11 folders:***
    - \EsriPress\GISTHealth\MyAssignments\Chapter11\Groups\DatabasesDistricts123\
    - \EsriPress\GISTHealth\MyAssignments\Chapter11\Groups\GroupsDissolved\
    - \EsriPress\GISTHealth\MyAssignments\Chapter11\Outputs\ChapterStatusMaps\
    - \EsriPress\GISTHealth\MyAssignments\Chapter11\Outputs\MarketingMaps\

If instructed to do so, instead of individual files, turn in a compressed file, **Assignment11YourName.zip**, that includes all the preceding files. Do not include path information in the compressed file.

Appendix A
Task index

Software tool or concept and tutorial(s) in which it appears

Appendix B
Data source credits

Chapter 1 figure sources include:

Figure 1.1 Lung cancer mortality per 100,000 white males, 2000–2004

- \EsriPress\GISTHealth\Data\UnitedStates.gdb\USMajorCities, from Esri Data & Maps 2004, courtesy of the US Census Bureau.
- \EsriPress\GISTHealth\Data\UnitedStates.gdb\USRivers, from Esri Data & Maps 2004, courtesy of ArcWorld.
- \EsriPress\GISTHealth\Data\UnitedStates.gdb\USLakes, from Esri Data & Maps 2004, courtesy of ArcWorld.
- \EsriPress\GISTHealth\Data\UnitedStates.gdb\USStates, from Esri Data & Maps 2007, courtesy of ArcUSA, US Census Bureau, Esri (Pop2005 field).
- \EsriPress\GISTHealth\Data\UnitedStates.gdb\USCounties, from Esri Data & Maps 2007, courtesy of ArcUSA, US Census Bureau, Esri (Pop2005 field).
- \EsriPress\GISTHealth\Data\NCI.gdb\LungCounty, from The Cancer Mortality Maps website, courtesy of the National Cancer Institute.

Figure 1.2 Locations of serious injuries to child pedestrians in eastern Pittsburgh, Pennsylvania

- \EsriPress\GISTHealth\Data\PedestrianInjuries.gdb\InjuriesJones and InjuriesSmith, courtesy of the Children's Hospital of Pittsburgh.
- Screen captures of http://seamless.usgs.gov, courtesy of the US Geological Survey. All USGS materials, regardless of the media, are entirely in the public domain. There are no user fees, site licenses, or any special agreements, etc., for the public or private use, and/or reuse of any census title. As a tax-funded product, it is all in the public record.
- \EsriPress\GISTHealth\Data\Pittsburgh.gdb\Playgrounds, courtesy of the City of Pittsburgh, Department of City Planning.

Chapter 1 data sources include:

- \EsriPress\GISTHealth\Data\UnitedStates.gdb\USStates, from Esri Data & Maps, 2007, courtesy of ArcUSA, US Census Bureau, Esri (Pop2005 field).
- \EsriPress\GISTHealth\Data\UnitedStates.gdb\USMajorCities, from Esri Data & Maps 2004, courtesy of the US Census Bureau.
- \EsriPress\GISTHealth\Data\UnitedStates.gdb\USRivers, from Esri Data & Maps 2004, courtesy of ArcWorld.
- \EsriPress\GISTHealth\Data\UnitedStates.gdb\USLakes, from Esri Data & Maps 2004, courtesy of ArcWorld.
- \EsriPress\GISTHealth\Data\UnitedStates.gdb\USInterstates, from Esri Data & Maps 2004, courtesy of the US Bureau of Transportation Statistics.
- \EsriPress\GISTHealth\Data\UnitedStates.gdb\USCounties, from Esri Data & Maps 2007, courtesy of ArcUSA, US Census Bureau, Esri (Pop2005 field).
- \EsriPress\GISTHealth\Data\NCI.gdb\LungCounty, from The Cancer Mortality Maps website, courtesy of the National Cancer Institute.
- Screen captures of ArcGIS Online, data courtesy of AND Automotive Navigation Data (Map Data © AND), Tele Atlas North America Inc., US National Park Service, US Geological Survey, and Esri.

Chapter 2 data sources include:

- \EsriPress\GISTHealth\Data\UnitedStates.gdb\USStates, from Esri Data & Maps 2007, courtesy of ArcUSA, US Census Bureau, Esri (Pop2005 field).
- \EsriPress\GISTHealth\Data\UnitedStates.gdb\USMajorCities, from Esri Data & Maps 2004, courtesy of the US Census Bureau.
- \EsriPress\GISTHealth\Data\UnitedStates.gdb\USCounties, from Esri Data & Maps 2007, courtesy of ArcUSA, US Census Bureau, Esri (Pop2005 field).
- \EsriPress\GISTHealth\Data\NCI.gdb\BreState, from The Cancer Mortality Maps website, courtesy of the National Cancer Institute.
- \EsriPress\GISTHealth\Data\NCI.gdb\BreCounty, from The Cancer Mortality Maps website, courtesy of the National Cancer Institute.
- \EsriPress\GISTHealth\Data\NCI.gdb\LungState, from The Cancer Mortality Maps website, courtesy of the National Cancer Institute.
- \EsriPress\GISTHealth\Data\NCI.gdb\LungCounty, from The Cancer Mortality Maps website, courtesy of the National Cancer Institute.

Chapter 3 data sources include:

- \EsriPress\GISTHealth\Data\UnitedStates.gdb\TXCounties, from Esri Data & Maps 2007, courtesy of ArcUSA, US Census Bureau, Esri (Pop2005 field).
- \EsriPress\GISTHealth\Data\UnitedStates.gdb\CACounties, from Esri Data & Maps 2007, courtesy of ArcUSA, US Census Bureau, Esri (Pop2005 field).
- \EsriPress\GISTHealth\Data\UnitedStates.gdb\USCounties, from Esri Data & Maps 2007, courtesy of ArcUSA, US Census Bureau, Esri (Pop2005 field).
- \EsriPress\GISTHealth\Data\UnitedStates.gdb\USMajorCities, from Esri Data & Maps 2004, courtesy of the US Census Bureau.

- \EsriPress\GISTHealth\Data\UnitedStates.gdb\TXTracts, courtesy of US Census Bureau TIGER.
- \EsriPress\GISTHealth\Data\UnitedStates.gdb\HarrisCountyTracts, courtesy of US Census Bureau TIGER.
- \EsriPress\GISTHealth\Data\UnitedStates.gdb\HarrisCountyCities, from Esri Data & Maps 2004, courtesy of the National Atlas of the United States.

Chapter 4 data sources include:

- \EsriPress\GISTHealth\Data\UnitedStates.gdb\USCounties, from Esri Data & Maps 2007, courtesy of ArcUSA, US Census Bureau, Esri (Pop2005 field).
- \EsriPress\GISTHealth\Data\UnitedStates.gdb\USStates, from Esri Data & Maps 2007, courtesy of ArcUSA, US Census Bureau, Esri (Pop2005 field).
- \EsriPress\GISTHealth\Data\UnitedStates.gdb\USLakes, from Esri Data & Maps 2004, courtesy of ArcWorld.
- \EsriPress\GISTHealth\Data\World.gdb\Country, from Esri Data & Maps 2005, courtesy of Esri and the US Census Bureau.
- \EsriPress\GISTHealth\Data\World.gdb\Ocean, from Esri Data & Maps 2005, courtesy of Esri and the US Census Bureau.
- \EsriPress\GISTHealth\Data\NCI.gdb\LungCounty, from The Cancer Mortality Maps website, courtesy of the National Cancer Institute.
- Screen captures of http://hivspatialdata.net/, courtesy of ICF Marco 2011. Measure DHS HIV Spatial Data Repository.
- \EsriPress\GISTHealth\Data\DataFiles\Rivers.dxf, courtesy of US Census Bureau TIGER.
- \EsriPress\GISTHealth\Data\DataFiles\cs42_d00.e00, courtesy of US Census Bureau TIGER.
- \EsriPress\GISTHealth\Data\Pittsburgh.gdb\Neighborhoods, courtesy of the City of Pittsburgh, Department of City Planning.
- \EsriPress\GISTHealth\Data\Pittsburgh.gdb\Sidewalks, courtesy of the City of Pittsburgh, Department of City Planning.
- \EsriPress\GISTHealth\Data\Pittsburgh.gdb\Parks, courtesy of the City of Pittsburgh, Department of City Planning.
- \EsriPress\GISTHealth\Data\Pittsburgh.gdb\Topo25ft, courtesy of the City of Pittsburgh, Department of City Planning.
- \EsriPress\GISTHealth\Data\Pittsburgh.gdb\Buildings, courtesy of the City of Pittsburgh, Department of City Planning.
- \EsriPress\GISTHealth\Data\Pittsburgh.gdb\StreetsCL, courtesy of the City of Pittsburgh, Department of City Planning.
- \EsriPress\GISTHealth\Data\UnitedStates.gdb\PASchools, from Esri Data & Maps 2005, courtesy of the US Geological Survey.
- Screen captures of http://nationalmap.gov/, courtesy of the US Geological Survey. All USGS materials, regardless of the media, are entirely in the public domain. There are no user fees, site licenses, or any special agreements, etc., for the public or private use, and/or reuse of any census title. As a tax-funded product, it is all in the public record.

Chapter 5 data sources include:

- Screen captures of http://www.census.gov, courtesy of the US Census Bureau. All US Census Bureau materials, regardless of the media, are entirely in the public domain. There are no user fees, site licenses, or any special agreements, etc., for the public or private use, and/or reuse of any census title. As a tax-funded product, it is all in the public record.
- Screen captures of http://www.factfinder.census.gov and http://factfinder2.census.gov, courtesy of the US Census Bureau. All US Census Bureau materials, regardless of the media, are entirely in the public domain. There are no user fees, site licenses, or any special agreements, etc., for the public or private use, and/or reuse of any census title. As a tax-funded product, it is all in the public record.
- \EsriPress\GISTHealth\Data\ACHD.gdb\HousingComplaints, courtesy of the Allegheny County Health Department.
- \EsriPress\GISTHealth\Data\ACHD.gdb\Municipalities, courtesy of the US Census Bureau.
- \EsriPress\GISTHealth\Data\ACHD.gdb\Rivers, courtesy of the US Census Bureau.
- \EsriPress\GISTHealth\Data\ACHD.gdb\ElevatedBloodCases_00, courtesy of the Allegheny County Health Department.
- \EsriPress\GISTHealth\Data\ACHD.gdb\ElevatedBloodCases_10, courtesy of the Allegheny County Health Department.
- \EsriPress\GISTHealth\MyExercises\FinishedExercises\Chapter5\dec_00_SF3_H035.zip, courtesy of the US Census Bureau.
- \EsriPress\GISTHealth\MyExercises\FinishedExercises\Chapter5\dec_10_PL_QTPL.zip, courtesy of the US Census Bureau.
- \EsriPress\GISTHealth\MyExercises\FinishedExercises\Chapter5\tl_2010_42003_cousub10.zip, courtesy of the US Census Bureau.
- \EsriPress\GISTHealth\MyExercises\FinishedExercises\Chapter5\tl_2010_42003_tract00.zip, courtesy of the US Census Bureau.
- \EsriPress\GISTHealth\MyExercises\FinishedExercises\Chapter5\tl_2010_42003_tract10.zip, courtesy of the US Census Bureau.

Chapter 6 data sources include:

- \EsriPress\GISTHealth\Data\UnitedStates.gdb\USStates, from Esri Data & Maps 2007, courtesy of ArcUSA, US Census Bureau, Esri (Pop2005 field).
- \EsriPress\GISTHealth\Data\UnitedStates.gdb\USCounties, from Esri Data & Maps 2007, courtesy of ArcUSA, US Census Bureau, Esri (Pop2005 field).
- \EsriPress\GISTHealth\Data\UnitedStates.gdb\PACounties, from Esri Data & Maps 2007, courtesy of ArcUSA, US Census Bureau, Esri (Pop2005 field).
- \EsriPress\GISTHealth\Data\UnitedStates.gdb\PAZIPCodes, from Esri Data & Maps 2007, courtesy of ArcUSA, US Census Bureau, Esri (Pop2005 field).
- \EsriPress\GISTHealth\Data\UnitedStates.gdb\USInterstates, from Esri Data & Maps 2004, courtesy of the US Bureau of Transportation Statistics.
- \EsriPress\GISTHealth\Data\UnitedStates.gdb\PACounties, from Esri Data & Maps 2007, courtesy of ArcUSA, US Census Bureau, Esri (Pop2005 field).

- \EsriPress\GISTHealth\Data\SiteSelection.gdb\Patients, fictitious database.
- \EsriPress\GISTHealth\Data\SiteSelection.gdb\TriStateZipCodes, from Esri Data & Maps 2007, courtesy of Tele Atlas, Esri (Pop2005 field).
- \EsriPress\GISTHealth\Data\SiteSelection.gdb\Streets, courtesy of US Census Bureau TIGER.
- \EsriPress\GISTHealth\Data\SiteSelection.gdb\Hospitals, fictitious database.
- \EsriPress\GISTHealth\Data\SiteSelection.gdb\AlleghenyCountyClinics, courtesy of the US Food and Drug Administration, Department of Health and Human Services.
- \EsriPress\GISTHealth\Data\SiteSelection.gdb\PAClinics, courtesy of the US Food and Drug Administration, Department of Health and Human Services.
- \EsriPress\GISTHealth\Data\SiteSelection.gdb\Tracts, courtesy of US Census Bureau TIGER.

Chapter 7 data sources include:

- \EsriPress\GISTHealth\Data\PedestrianInjuries.gdb\InjuriesJones, courtesy of the Children's Hospital of Pittsburgh.
- \EsriPress\GISTHealth\Data\PedestrianInjuries.gdb\InjuriesSmith, courtesy of the Children's Hospital of Pittsburgh.
- \EsriPress\GISTHealth\Data\PedestrianInjuries.gdb\tgr42003lkA, courtesy of US Census Bureau TIGER.
- \EsriPress\GISTHealth\Data\PedestrianInjuries.gdb\tgr42003ccd00, courtesy of US Census Bureau TIGER.
- \EsriPress\GISTHealth\Data\PedestrianInjuries.gdb\tgr42003wat, courtesy of US Census Bureau TIGER.
- \EsriPress\GISTHealth\Data\PedestrianInjuries.gdb\tgr42003trt00, courtesy of US Census Bureau TIGER.
- \EsriPress\GISTHealth\Data\Pittsburgh.gdb\Parks, courtesy of the City of Pittsburgh, Department of City Planning.
- \EsriPress\GISTHealth\Data\Pittsburgh.gdb\Playgrounds, courtesy of the City of Pittsburgh, Department of City Planning.
- \EsriPress\GISTHealth\Data\Pittsburgh.gdb\Neighborhoods, courtesy of the City of Pittsburgh, Department of City Planning.
- \EsriPress\GISTHealth\Data\Pittsburgh.gdb\ConvenienceStores, courtesy of the Allegheny County Health Department.
- \EsriPress\GISTHealth\Data\Pittsburgh.gdb\BlockCentroids, courtesy of US Census Bureau TIGER.
- \EsriPress\GISTHealth\Data\PedestrianInjuries.gdb\PghCrosswalk, table of census tract numbers and neighborhood names, courtesy of US Census Bureau TIGER.
- \EsriPress\GISTHealth\Data\PedestrianInjuries.gdb\PopPov, table of poverty population and census tract numbers, courtesy of US Census Bureau TIGER.
- \EsriPress\GISTHealth\Data\UnitedStates.gdb\PASchools, from Esri Data & Maps 2005, courtesy of the US Geological Survey.

Chapter 8 figure sources include:

Figure 8.1 County and coterminous census tract boundaries in Pennsylvania

- \EsriPress\GISTHealth\Data\UnitedStates.gdb\PACounties, from Esri Data & Maps 2007, courtesy of ArcUSA, US Census Bureau, Esri (Pop2005 field).

Chapter 8 data sources include:

- \EsriPress\GISTHealth\Data\UnitedStates.gdb\PACounties, from Esri Data & Maps 2007, courtesy of ArcUSA, US Census Bureau, Esri (Pop2005 field).
- \EsriPress\GISTHealth\Data\UnitedStates.gdb\NEBlocks, courtesy of US Census Bureau TIGER.
- \EsriPress\GISTHealth\Data\UnitedStates.gdb\NECities, from Esri Data & Maps 2004, courtesy of the US Census Bureau.
- \EsriPress\GISTHealth\Data\UnitedStates.gdb\NEHRR, from The Dartmouth Atlas of Health Care, courtesy of The Trustees of Dartmouth College.
- \EsriPress\GISTHealth\Data\UnitedStates.gdb\NEHSA, from The Dartmouth Atlas of Health Care, courtesy of The Trustees of Dartmouth College.
- \EsriPress\GISTHealth\Data\Pittsburgh.gdb\EMSZones, courtesy of the City of Pittsburgh, Department of City Planning.
- \EsriPress\GISTHealth\Data\Pittsburgh.gdb\BlkGrpSF1.dbf, courtesy of the US Census Bureau.
- \EsriPress\GISTHealth\Data\Pittsburgh.gdb\BlkGrpSF3.dbf, courtesy of the US Census Bureau.
- \EsriPress\GISTHealth\Data\Pittsburgh.gdb\BlockCentroids, courtesy of US Census Bureau TIGER.
- \EsriPress\GISTHealth\Data\Pittsburgh.gdb\Blocks, courtesy of US Census Bureau TIGER.
- \EsriPress\GISTHealth\Data\Pittsburgh.gdb\BlockGroups, courtesy of US Census Bureau TIGER.

Chapter 9 data sources include:

- \EsriPress\GISTHealth\Data\SpatialAnalyst\SpatialAnalyst.gdb\ZoningCommercialBuffer, courtesy of the City of Pittsburgh, Department of City Planning.
- \EsriPress\GISTHealth\Data\SpatialAnalyst\SpatialAnalyst.gdb\AllCoBlkGrps, courtesy of US Census Bureau TIGER.
- \EsriPress\GISTHealth\Data\SpatialAnalyst\SpatialAnalyst.gdb\AllCoBlks, courtesy of the US Census Bureau.
- \EsriPress\GISTHealth\Data\SpatialAnalyst\SpatialAnalyst.gdb\OHCA, courtesy of the Children's Hospital of Pittsburgh.

- \EsriPress\GISTHealth\Data\SpatialAnalyst\SpatialAnalyst.gdb\PennHills, courtesy of the US Census Bureau.
- \EsriPress\GISTHealth\Data\SpatialAnalyst\SpatialAnalyst.gdb\Pittsburgh, courtesy of the US Census Bureau.
- \EsriPress\GISTHealth\Data\SpatialAnalyst\SpatialAnalyst.gdb\Rivers, courtesy of the US Census Bureau.
- \EsriPress\GISTHealth\Data\Pittsburgh.gdb\StreetsCL, courtesy of the City of Pittsburgh, Department of City Planning.
- \EsriPress\GISTHealth\Data\SpatialAnalyst\SpatialAnalyst.gdb\ZoningCommercialBuffer, courtesy of the City of Pittsburgh, Department of City Planning.
- \EsriPress\GISTHealth\Data\SpatialAnalyst\SpatialAnalyst.gdb\DEM, courtesy of the US Geological Survey.
- \EsriPress\GISTHealth\Data\SpatialAnalyst\SpatialAnalyst.gdb\LandUse, image courtesy of the US Geological Survey.
- \EsriPress\GISTHealth\Data\SpatialAnalyst\SpatialAnalyst.gdb\Munic, courtesy of the US Census Bureau.
- \EsriPress\GISTHealth\Data\SpatialAnalyst\SpatialAnalyst.gdb\CountySchools, from Esri Data & Maps 2007, courtesy of the US Census Bureau.

Chapter 10 data sources include:

- \EsriPress\GISTHealth\Data\Pittsburgh.gdb\Neighborhoods, courtesy of the City of Pittsburgh, Department of City Planning.
- \EsriPress\GISTHealth\Data\Pittsburgh.gdb\StreetsCL, courtesy of the City of Pittsburgh, Department of City Planning.
- \EsriPress\GISTHealth\Data\Pittsburgh.gdb\Sidewalks, courtesy of the City of Pittsburgh, Department of City Planning.
- \EsriPress\GISTHealth\Data\Pittsburgh.gdb\Buildings, courtesy of the City of Pittsburgh, Department of City Planning.
- \EsriPress\GISTHealth\Data\ACHD.gdb\PghFoodSources, courtesy of the Allegheny County Health Department.
- \EsriPress\GISTHealth\Data\ACHD.gdb\OutbreakResidences, fictitious table.
- \EsriPress\GISTHealth\Data\ACHD.gdb\OutbreakWorkLocations, fictitious table.
- \EsriPress\GISTHealth\Data\Pittsburgh.gdb\BlockCentroids, courtesy of US Census Bureau TIGER.
- \EsriPress\GISTHealth\Data\Pittsburgh.gdb\FemaFlood, courtesy of the City of Pittsburgh, Department of City Planning.

Chapter 11 data sources include:

- \EsriPress\GISTHealth\Data\UnitedStates.gdb\USStates, from Esri Data & Maps 2007, courtesy of ArcUSA, US Census, Esri (Pop2005 field).
- \EsriPress\GISTHealth\Data\UnitedStates.gdb\USZipCodes, from Esri Data & Maps 2005, courtesy of TANA/GDT, Esri BIS (Pop2004 field).
- \EsriPress\GISTHealth\Data\ACHE.gdb\ACHEMembers.dbf, courtesy of the American College of Healthcare Executives.
- \EsriPress\GISTHealth\Data\ACHE.gdb\HEG_WHEN, courtesy of the American College of Healthcare Executives.
- \EsriPress\GISTHealth\Data\ACHE.gdb\GroupsDistricts1_2_3.dbf, courtesy of the American College of Healthcare Executives.
- \EsriPress\GISTHealth\Data\ACHE.gdb\GroupsDistricts4_5_6.dbf, courtesy of the American College of Healthcare Executives.
- \EsriPress\GISTHealth\Data\ACHE.gdb\ResolvedPartners.dbf, courtesy of the American College of Healthcare Executives.

Appendix C
Data license agreement

Important: Read carefully before downloading the media.

Environmental Systems Research Institute, Inc. (Esri), is willing to license the data and related materials to you only upon the condition that you accept all of the terms and conditions contained in this license agreement. Please read the terms and conditions carefully before downloading the media. By downloading the media, you are indicating your acceptance of the Esri License Agreement. If you do not agree to the terms and conditions as stated, then Esri is unwilling to license the data and related materials to you.

Esri License Agreement

This is a license agreement, and not an agreement for sale, between you (Licensee) and Environmental Systems Research Institute, Inc. (Esri). This Esri License Agreement (Agreement) gives Licensee certain limited rights to use the data and related materials (Data and Related Materials). All rights not specifically granted in this Agreement are reserved to Esri and its Licensors.

Reservation of Ownership and Grant of License:

Esri and its Licensors retain exclusive rights, title, and ownership to the copy of the Data and Related Materials licensed under this Agreement and, hereby, grant to Licensee a personal, nonexclusive, nontransferable, royalty-free, worldwide license to use the Data and Related Materials based on the terms and conditions of this Agreement. Licensee agrees to use reasonable effort to protect the Data and Related Materials from unauthorized use, reproduction, distribution, or publication.

Proprietary Rights and Copyright:

Licensee acknowledges that the Data and Related Materials are proprietary and confidential property of Esri and its Licensors and are protected by United States copyright laws and applicable international copyright treaties and/or conventions.

Permitted Uses:

Licensee may install the Data and Related Materials onto permanent storage device(s) for Licensee's own internal use.
Licensee may internally use the Data and Related Materials provided by Esri for the stated purpose of GIS training and education.

Uses Not Permitted:

Licensee shall not sell, rent, lease, sublicense, lend, assign, time-share, or transfer, in whole or in part, or provide unlicensed Third Parties access to the Data and Related Materials or portions of the Data and Related Materials, any updates, or Licensee's rights under this Agreement.
Licensee shall not remove or obscure any copyright or trademark notices of Esri or its Licensors.

Term and Termination:

The license granted to Licensee by this Agreement shall commence upon the acceptance of this Agreement and shall continue until such time that Licensee elects in writing to discontinue use of the Data or Related Materials and terminates this Agreement. The Agreement shall automatically terminate without notice if Licensee fails to comply with any provision of this Agreement. Licensee shall then return to Esri the Data and Related Materials. The parties hereby agree that all provisions that operate to protect the rights of Esri and its Licensors shall remain in force should breach occur.

Disclaimer of Warranty:

The Data and Related Materials contained herein are provided "as-is," without warranty of any kind, either express or implied, including, but not limited to, the implied warranties of merchantability, fitness for a particular purpose, or noninfringement. Esri does not warrant that the Data and Related Materials will meet Licensee's needs or expectations, that the use of the Data and Related Materials will be uninterrupted, or that all nonconformities, defects, or errors can or will be corrected. Esri is not inviting reliance on the Data or Related Materials for commercial planning or analysis purposes, and Licensee should always check actual data.

Data Disclaimer:

The Data used herein has been derived from actual spatial or tabular information. In some cases, Esri has manipulated and applied certain assumptions, analyses, and opinions to the Data solely for educational training purposes. Assumptions, analyses, opinions applied, and actual outcomes may vary. Again, Esri is not inviting reliance on this Data, and the Licensee should always verify actual Data and exercise their own professional judgment when interpreting any outcomes.

Limitation of Liability:

Esri shall not be liable for direct, indirect, special, incidental, or consequential damages related to Licensee's use of the Data and Related Materials, even if Esri is advised of the possibility of such damage.

No Implied Waivers:

No failure or delay by Esri or its Licensors in enforcing any right or remedy under this Agreement shall be construed as a waiver of any future or other exercise of such right or remedy by Esri or its Licensors.

Order for Precedence:

Any conflict between the terms of this Agreement and any FAR, DFAR, purchase order, or other terms shall be resolved in favor of the terms expressed in this Agreement, subject to the government's minimum rights unless agreed otherwise.

Export Regulation:

Licensee acknowledges that this Agreement and the performance thereof are subject to compliance with any and all applicable United States laws, regulations, or orders relating to the export of data thereto. Licensee agrees to comply with all laws, regulations, and orders of the United States in regard to any export of such technical data.

Severability:

If any provision(s) of this Agreement shall be held to be invalid, illegal, or unenforceable by a court or other tribunal of competent jurisdiction, the validity, legality, and enforceability of the remaining provisions shall not in any way be affected or impaired thereby.

Governing Law:

This Agreement, entered into in the County of San Bernardino, shall be construed and enforced in accordance with and be governed by the laws of the United States of America and the State of California without reference to conflict of laws principles. The parties hereby consent to the personal jurisdiction of the courts of this county and waive their rights to change venue.

Entire Agreement:

The parties agree that this Agreement constitutes the sole and entire agreement of the parties as to the matter set forth herein and supersedes any previous agreements, understandings, and arrangements between the parties relating hereto.